B. Palmer

P-22

PCC RAD. TECH.
HT D8c
Do Not Remove

Paul F. Laudicina, M.A., R.T. (R)

Professor, Radiological Sciences
Director, Nuclear Medicine Technology
College of DuPage
Glen Ellyn, Illinois

1989

W. B. SAUNDERS COMPANY

Harcourt Brace Jovanovich, Inc.

Philadelphia London Toronto
Montreal Sydney Tokyo

Applied Pathology for Radiographers

W. B. SAUNDERS COMPANY
Harcourt Brace Jovanovich, Inc.

The Curtis Center
Independence Square West
Philadelphia, PA 19106

Library of Congress Cataloging-in-Publication Data

Laudicina, Paul.

Applied pathology for radiographers.

1. Pathology.   I. Title. [DNLM: 1. Pathology. QZ 4 L371a]

RB25.L368   1989   616.07   87–32397

ISBN 0–7216–2143–0

Editor: Margaret Biblis
Developmental Editor: Martha Tanner
Designer: Anne O'Donnell
Production Manager: Carolyn Naylor
Manuscript Editor: Wendy Andresen
Illustration Coordinator: Peg Shaw
Cover Designer: Karen Giacomucci
Indexer: Ellen Murray

Applied Pathology for Radiographers   ISBN 0–7216–2143–0

Last digit is the print number: 9   8   7   6   5   4   3   2   1

Preface

The purpose of this book is to provide the second-year radiography student and the graduate radiographer with a basic working knowledge of pathology as it pertains to diagnostic medical radiography. The text presents those pathological conditions that are most commonly encountered by the staff of the radiology department.

Each chapter begins with an outline. A compilation of related terms follows, listing the disease processes discussed and including terms of special importance in the chapter. The glossary, found at the end of the book, includes all terms listed, as well as their pronunciation and definition. Measurable and reasonable objectives follow the section on related terminology. A general introduction to the chapter comes next, giving the reader an overview of the scope of the chapter. Throughout the text, key words and phrases appear in bold italic type to emphasize their importance.

After the introduction within each chapter, each disease process or condition is presented in a consistent and organized manner. The general information section that is presented first includes important and interesting statistical data. This is then followed by a section on diagnosis. This section is especially significant for the radiographer, since it highlights the various methods of radiological imaging and laboratory tests and procedures that the radiologist uses when making a diagnosis. Each chapter includes examples of normal radiographic studies in addition to those demonstrating specific disease processes. Explanations are provided regarding the advantages and disadvantages of various imaging modalities, the preferred radiographic positions, and most desirable exposure techniques. The treatment section that follows next reflects the latest information regarding the medical and surgical treatment of the disorder. The diseases that are radiographically significant and common are highlighted. It is suggested that the second-year student and graduate radiographer have some previous knowledge of diagnostic imaging, including nuclear medicine, sonography, angiographic special procedures, computed scanning, and magnetic resonance imaging.

Each chapter includes a self-assessment quiz consisting of numerous multiple-choice questions designed to provide readers with an informal method of assessment of what they have learned. An answer key is provided in the back of the text. Finally, each chapter concludes with a set of essay questions, which have the capacity to serve several functions.

These essay questions can be used by students to obtain a more in-depth understanding of the chapter content. The instructor may assign the questions for extra-credit work, term papers, or group projects or may simply use them for discussion to enhance the overall comprehension of the chapter. Readers are encouraged to check their answers and review those portions of the chapter where they have had difficulty. The instructor has the option of using the self-assessment quizzes and study questions in any way that will enhance the reader's knowledge and comprehension.

Although this text is primarily designed for second-year students, the depth and scope can be arranged according to the needs of a particular group. I have found that courses in radiological pathology have been well received by the experienced radiographer working in any clinical environment. I have taught numerous courses, workshops, and seminars in which radiological pathology was the major topic. These courses have been delivered to health professionals working in medical records, occupational therapy, respiratory therapy, and associate-degree nursing, as well as to radiography graduates who desired to update their skills or continue their education.

PAUL F. LAUDICINA

Acknowledgments

Anyone who has taken the time and effort to write a textbook such as this one can understand my wish to give credit where it is due. It is most appropriate to thank individuals who have guided one along the way and who have made significant contributions to one's personal and professional growth. Inspiration, encouragement, and support are necessary ingredients for anyone who wishes to reach a goal or complete a task such as this. For the past 15 years, it has been my goal to write this text. This goal is being realized as a result of the continual love, support, and encouragement that I have received from my entire family, from my professional colleagues, and from students throughout my professional career. They certainly have been a pillar of strength for me.

During my professional career, which has spanned 26 years, many key people provided me with a great deal of guidance, inspiration, and encouragement. I am grateful for the guidance provided me by Stan Wisniewski, R.T. (R), who was my first chief technologist, at the School of Radiologic Technology at Lutheran General Hospital, Park Ridge, Illinois, 1961–1963. I met Margaret Hoing (the first lady of x-ray) when I was a second-year student, in 1962. I also had the opportunity to work with her at a medical center in Park Ridge, Illinois. I was most fortunate in getting to know Margaret Hoing, the radiography pioneer and the person. I spent many hours visiting her and listening to her many recollections of her early life, including her experiences with Ed Jerman, Dr. Coolidge, and other pioneers in radiology.

When I was a fledgling clinical instructor at Resurrection Hospital in Chicago, in 1970, Dr. Alfred Lescher, staff radiologist, aroused my intellectual curiosity about pathology and was instrumental in helping me create a file of teaching films. Dr. Lescher was very gracious in allowing me to observe him reading film and was most patient about answering my many questions regarding pathology. I learned much from him and appreciated the use of his personal texts and references. I would not be a radiography instructor today if it had not been for Mr. Rod Roemer, R.T. (R), and Mr. James Peterson, R.T. (R), of Triton College, River Grove, Illinois, who gave me my first teaching opportunity and to this day are an ever present source of encouragement.

For the past 16 years, I have been a program faculty member and Program Director of the Radiography and Nuclear Medicine programs at College of DuPage in Glen Ellyn, Illinois. These past 16 years have been most rewarding and fulfilling. When it comes to expressing gratitude, I think of my first Academic Dean, Mr. Bill Gooch, who hired me out from my protective clinical environment and really made me feel welcome in a very new and frightening environment. Two individuals who till this day are still providing me with a great deal of support, counsel, and encouragement are Mr. Richard Wood, Executive Dean of Instruction, and Ms. Betsy Cabatit-Segal, the Associate Dean of Health and Public Services. These are people who were always there when I needed them. Mary Parks, R.T., was responsible for getting me involved in my professional society. Without her encouragement and support, I would not have had the motivation to serve my professional society and receive the benefits that I now enjoy. I wish to express my gratitude to Mark Van Dreunen. M.D., Chief of Radiology, Doug Wean, R.T. (R), and the staff of Edward Hines Jr. Veterans' Administration Hospital for their friendship, assistance, and cooperation in acquiring many pathological studies that I could not find anywhere else.

Last, but not least, the real sources of inspiration for this text are the radiography students of College of DuPage. Over the past 16 years, I have had the pleasure of establishing many long-standing relationships. If it were not for the students and their unending encouragement, support, and thirst for knowledge, I would not have had the strength to finish this text. To the aforementioned individuals, I will be forever grateful.

Contents

Applied Pathology for Radiographers

One

General Principles of Pathology

Related Terminology

congestion
degeneration
dysplasia
edema
empyema
endogenous
exogenous
exudate
frequency
hyperplasia
hypertrophy
iatrogenic
idiopathic
incidence
inflammation
in situ
invasion
ischemia
manifestation
metaplasia
metastasis
morbidity
necrosis
neoplasm
nosocomial
organic
pathogenesis
prevalence

Objectives

Upon completion of Chapter 1, the radiographer will be able to

• Describe the difference between structural and functional disease.

• Describe the changes that occur following injury to the cell.

• Explain the significance of degeneration, necrosis, inflammation, and repair.

• List the fundamental tissues and their relationships to disease.

• Describe the terms that relate to growth disturbances that affect the human body.

• List the five leading causes of death and discuss their implications for the general population.

Pathology

The primary definition of pathology is the study of disease. A disease process is any abnormal change that may take place in the body. Disease is also the body's response to some type of injury. Cellular injury usually results in a compromise of cellular function, as well as a possible change in structure. The various pathological processes that cause disease are an important aspect of pathology. The study of these causes is referred to as *etiology.*

The Disease Process

The disease process develops according to the manner of injury. After injury, the sequence of events that takes place ultimately renders the disease apparent. This sequence of events is termed *pathogenesis,* and the observed changes are referred to as *manifestations.* These manifestations are brought to light by patient complaints and by observations made by the attending physician, often during a physical examination. An important part of this examination is taking the patient's history. Two important aspects of the patient's history are symptoms and signs. Changes that are perceived by the patient are termed *symptoms.* These are in the form of complaints offered by the patient, such as headaches, nausea, aches, and pains. Visual abnormal changes in the patient that may be interpreted by the physician or health professional are termed *signs* and include swelling, discoloration, changes in tissue texture, and so on. An examiner may also use senses such as touch and smell to interpret other signs. Abnormal changes may also be interpreted by diagnostic tests and procedures. Tests and procedures mostly involve the clinical laboratory and diagnostic radiology departments. A *test* involves analysis of specimens obtained from the patient, such as blood, urine, and feces. A *procedure* requires additional manipulation of the patient, such as in a biopsy or endoscopic examination of hollow viscera.

Any change of continuity of tissue or loss of function of a part is usually the result of disease or trauma. The term *lesion* is used widely to include many types of cellular changes that take place for a variety of reasons. Lesions are primarily detected by observation by the naked eye or by a microscope. The disease process can be categorized according to whether or not a lesion is present. All disease processes are categorized into one of two groups: structural or functional disease.

Structural Disease

Structural or organic disease involves physical and biochemical changes within the cells. These structural changes are the result of numerous processes, including hereditary disorders, inflammatory diseases, physical injury or trauma, hyperplasias, and neoplasms or tumors. Structural changes in cells are essentially initiated by two types of agents: those that are external, or *exogenous*, and those that are internal, or *endogenous.* Examples of external agents include trauma, chemical injury, and microbial infections.

Trauma may be caused by direct physical injury to tissue from an external blow, exposure to hot or cold temperatures, and radiation.

Chemical injuries are categorized in the same manner as poisoning, as accidental, suicidal, or homicidal. In general, deaths due to unnatural causes automatically become coroners' cases. Inquiry into any unnatural death requires a thorough investigation, including an autopsy or postmortem examination. In many cases, *forensic* pathologists will be called to assist the coroner or medical examiner in determining the exact cause of death.

Microbial injuries are classified by the type of causative organism. Collectively, these external agents are termed infections. Examples of these infections include bacteria, viruses, fungi, rickettsiae, protozoans, and helminths.

Internal or endogenous agents include vascular insufficiency, immunological/autoimmune reactions and diseases, and disturbances that are the result of abnormal metabolism.

The leading internal causative agent is vascular insufficiency. This condition results in tissue necrosis because of anoxia. The myocardial infarct or sudden heart attack is the leading cause of early death in adults and is largely the result of a compromise in the amount of blood received by the heart muscle. Without oxygen, the muscle dies. The deficiency of blood in the muscle is termed *ischemia.* An area of dead or necrotic tissue is termed an *infarct.* Thus, a myocardial infarct is also referred to as *ischemic necrosis*.

Immunological disorders primarily involve the body's ability to fight disease. The body is capable of producing agents to protect itself. These agents are called antibodies. In some cases, the body turns and attacks itself in a process known as *autoimmune disease*. Erratic reactions of the immune system often result in allergic or hypersensitivity reactions. A significant percentage of the population is hypersensitive to certain allergens in food, clothing, and the environment.

Metabolic disorders include the production of enzymes, hormones, and secretory products. These biochemical disorders can be genetically inherited or acquired as secondary effects of certain diseases. These disorders include proteins, carbohydrates, minerals, vitamins, lipids, and fluid.

Hyperplasias and neoplasias are difficult to categorize because their exact cause is unknown and their early behaviors cannot be distinguished. Diseases of which the causes are unknown are referred to as *idiopathic.* Adverse reactions that might take place while under the care of a physician are termed *iatrogenic*. Despite the efforts of hospital personnel, a patient may acquire an infection in the hospital. Those diseases acquired from the hospital environment are referred to as ***nosocomial*** diseases.

Functional Disease

Any disease that presents no lesion is classified as a functional or physiological disease. Various forms of mental illness fall into this category. Neuroses and psychoses are two common forms of mental illness in which no lesion is usually present. However, it is suspected that some chronic neurogenic disorders could bring about a structural change if the condition is allowed to continue without treatment. One such example is an individual whose mental state initiates the stimulation of the acid-secreting digestive glands. This may eventually result in a lesion such as an ulcer of the gastric or duodenal mucosa. If untreated, this excess acid might inflame and erode the mucosa, possibly resulting in hemorrhage. The erosion of tissue represents a structural change. Other examples of functional disease include the functional bowel syndrome or spastic colon and headaches due to tension or psychosomatic causes.

The Effects of Injury

Degeneration and Necrosis

Degeneration is the initial cell response that takes place following injury. The magnitude, duration, and location of the injury determine the level of cell degeneration. Degeneration also refers to sublethal cell injury. Degeneration is the result of injury caused by exogenous and endogenous agents. ***Necrosis*** is the death of cells, most often resulting from acute injury.

Acute Injury

An acute injury has a sudden onset and runs a short, severe course. The best example of acute injury is probably that associated with ***anoxia***, a lack of oxygen, and ***hypoxia***, reduced oxygen. The level of necrosis is dependent on the requirement of the cell for oxygen. When hypoxia is localized to a specific area, it is referred to as ischemia. The area of ischemic necrosis is then referred to as an infarct. Infarcts are most common in the heart and brain. During ischemic necrosis, the cellular proteins coagulate. Coagulation necrosis is the most common form of infarct that is associated with acute injury.

Thrombi and emboli are the two most common causes of infarct. A ***thrombus*** is a mass of coagulated blood or a clot, which usually adheres to the wall of a vessel. Thrombi themselves may contribute to the narrowing of the lumen of a leg vein, causing the patient a great deal of discomfort. If the thrombus dislodges from the wall, it has the ability to travel in the direction of the venous return and enter the right side of the heart and pulmonary artery.

Some thrombi may dissolve, and others will become lodged in the lungs, creating a pulmonary infarct. In actuality, any particulate matter can qualify as an embolus. A thrombus that has the ability to travel through the venous system is a common type of ***embolus***. Emboli are common after severe trauma and fracture of long bones. Fat and marrow frequently become emboli. Air and cancer tissue are other forms of emboli.

In addition to its association with anoxia, acute injury may result from trauma, infection, and hypersensitivity. Fractures, severe sprains, and muscle strains result in vascular damage and a subsequent amount of degeneration and necrosis. Injuries such as fractures are immobilized so that fractured fragments remain in alignment, a minimum amount of blood is lost, and circulation is resumed as soon as possible. The more severe the fracture, the more severe the necrosis.

Infections can be acquired in many ways, but many of the inflammatory reactions are produced by the body's response to the offending organism. Certain individuals are allergic to particulate matter in the environment, including dust, pollens, and air pollution. Others may be allergic to certain types of food, clothing, medications, and so on. Autoimmune diseases such as rheumatoid arthritis may also provoke an inflammatory response.

Liquefaction necrosis is primarily associated with lesions containing pyogenic bacteria and consisting of cellular debris in the form of a foul-smelling purulent discharge. Caseous necrosis presents a cheese-like appearance and is primarily associated with tuberculin bacteria and specific fungi. Enzymatic fat necrosis is associated with the pancreas and involves the leaking of digestive enzymes, producing a lesion similar to that of caseous necrosis. Gangrenous necrosis is a combination of coagulation necrosis and bacteria that are hosted by the necrotic tissue.

Chronic Injury

When discussing chronic injury, the term ***atrophy*** is most often used. Atrophy is a progressive wasting of any part of the body, usually impairing function or even resulting in a complete loss of that function. Cellular wasting results in a decrease in the size of the cell or a decrease in the number of cells.

Senile atrophy occurs as part of the natural aging process. The brain shrinks in size as it ages, and intellectual functions and memory are eventually impaired. Disuse atrophy is most evident in a fractured limb that has been immobilized by a plaster cast for an extended period of time. When two identical extremities are compared, the circumference of the one that was casted is appreciably smaller, and the muscles have diminished ability to contract. Pressure atrophy occurs as a result of steady pressure on tissue. This is common with an expanding tumor or decubitus ulcers (bedsores). Bedridden patients are regularly rotated in bed to avoid pressure sores, which are prone to develop on prominent areas of the body such as the heels, buttocks, and elbows. Endocrine atrophy results from decreased hormone production. This condition is common during and after menopause, when the breasts and uterus may atrophy as a result of the decrease in estrogen and progesterone. Fatty metamorphosis is the deposition of fat within liver cells. This fat is produced by triglycerides and other lipids that are improperly metabolized and is especially common in patients with chronic alcoholism. The flat plate abdomen film or kidney-ureter-bladder workup (KUB) will often demonstrate hepatomegaly. Gross downward displacement of the upper pole of the right kidney and increased height of the right hemidiaphragm may be observed.

Inflammation

Inflammation is the body's response to injury. It serves to localize and isolate toxic substances while destroying the offending organism. Inflammation sets the stage for wound healing and repair by removing the cellular debris from the area. Initially, the capillaries become engorged and dilated with blood. This capillary filling, termed **congestion**, promotes leakage of fluids and protein into the tissues and allows for the infiltration of leukocytes into the area of injury. The leukocytes engulf and digest the bacteria and help remove it from the area, a process called **phagocytosis.**

Acute Inflammation

There are five indications of acute inflammation, referred to as cardinal signs: red skin (congestion or hyperemia), swelling *(edema)*, heat (the temperature of the skin is less than of the blood), pain (swollen tissue presses nerve endings), and loss of function (because of the natural tendency to protect the injured part).

Chronic Inflammation

Unlike acute inflammation, chronic inflammation lasts for long periods of time, possibly weeks, months, years, or even a lifetime. Chronic inflammation is most often associated with sublethal degeneration. Necrosis is uncommon with chronic inflammation. Individuals with conditions such as asthma, allergy, or hay fever may be affected intermittently or during a particular season. However, during a period of years, some conditions may gradually worsen as a result of the aging process, environment, smoking, employment conditions, and so on. For example, emphysema is a chronic progressive disease that ultimately impairs normal breathing. Many types of chronic diseases are primarily environmental. Individuals working in the farming and manufacturing industries will often develop a chronic inflammatory disease of the lungs from the inhalation of particulate matter. This type of inflammation is described as granulomatous, and benign lung lesions called granulomas will be presented. These diseases will be discussed in Chapter 2.

Transudates

Transudate is serum fluid that passes through a membrane or tissue and is due to increased hydrostatic or decreased osmotic pressure in the vascular system. Transudates are quite watery, have a low protein content, and tend to be more generalized than exudates. Fluid filling the lungs during congestive heart failure is the result of decreased osmotic pressure and is termed **pulmonary edema.** Inflammatory reactions involving pleural, pericardial, and peritoneal cavities are associated with serous discharge.

Exudates

Exudates are a cloudy, thick, protein-rich fluid and are associated with the type of injury. Exudates are created by decreased hydrostatic pressure and increased osmotic pressure. Serous exudate is most common in acute inflammations such as minor burns, resulting in the formation of a blister. A fibrinous exudate produces a layer of fibrinogen, which forms a mesh of fibrin and ultimately becomes a scab. Fibrinous exudates are present in second-degree skin burns and pleural effusions. If the exudate contains high levels of protein and blood, it is referred to as a sanguineous discharge or exudate. A purulent exudate is also referred to as suppurative or pyogenic and contains pus. Pus is a thick, viscous, yellowish fluid composed primarily of dead leukocytes, tissue fluid, and remnants of the offending organism.

Inflammatory Lesions

Inflammatory reactions result in the production of a lesion. The lesions vary according to their level of severity. An **abscess** is a localized spherical lesion filled with pus and pyogenic bacteria, usually staphylococci. Abscesses are found in many areas of the body, including the skin (boils, furuncles, and carbuncles), teeth, appendix, bowel, breast, and lung. Pus that fills a space like the pleural cavity is called empyema. **Cellulitis** is a spreading, diffuse infection most commonly involving streptococcal infection of the subcutaneous tissues. The body is unable to confine the infection to a localized area. Cellulitis is characterized by congestion and edema. Ulcers are depressed or excavated lesions on the skin or mucous membrane. They may appear almost anywhere in the body and may involve many types of organs and structures. The stomach and duodenum may be ulcerated by gastric acids. Pressure sores or decubitus ulcers result from wasting away of tissue in debilitated and bedridden patients.

Repair

Repair is defined as the body's attempt to return to normal. There are two primary types of repair, regeneration and fibrous connective tissue repair.

Regeneration is the replacement of dead tissue with new tissue that is identical in structure and function to that of the original tissue. This is the most desirable form of repair. Complex cells such as found in the lung and in renal glomeruli do not regenerate; thus, injury to these structures is usually permanent.

Fibrous connective tissue repair is the second and less preferred method of repair and is also known as scarring or fibrosis. Tissue that has undergone necrosis is replaced with a dense, tough mass of connective tissue, referred to as a scar. The original structure and function of the cell is not restored.

The process of wound repair is classified into two categories: primary union and secondary union. A wound such as a surgical incision has edges that are in close approximation to each other. Only a very small space exists between the two walls of tissue. This space quickly fills in with collagen, which shrinks and draws the wound edges firmly together. The surface of the wound is then covered over with new epithelium. A wound in which tissue has been avulsed or gouged out from the skin surface leaves a gaping depression with the wound edges far apart. Because of the lack of wound approximation, the wound edges are not able to heal by primary union. Secondary union uses the same process but requires more time for the collagen to fill in the wound. Debris must be removed from the wound before healing begins, and the wound will then heal from its base toward the surface. By the time the wound is healed, a significant scar of fibrous connective tissue is covering the skin. The texture of this scar is markedly different from that of adjacent tissue.

Fundamental Tissues

Epithelial Tissue

Epithelial tissue serves as a lining for body spaces, surfaces, and glands. Squamous, transitional, and columnar cells provide the lining for body surfaces. Stratified squamous epithelium is a multilayered tissue containing keratin that provides the lining for the skin, mouth, pharynx, larynx, esophagus, and anus. Transitional epithelium is also multilayered but does not contain keratin. Transitional cells are unique to the urinary tract and include all urinary anatomy from the kidney to the urethra. Columnar epithelial cells are extremely tall and have the unique characteristic of containing mucus-secreting cells. Columnar epithelium specifically lines the nose, trachea, bronchi, stomach, small and large intestine, and many structures of the exocrine system, such as the ducts of the hepatobiliary system and the breast. Because of its similarity to glands, columnar epithelium is frequently referred to as glandular epithelium. Epithelial cells that line specific organs may also be classified by structure. These structures include glands, tubules, or cords. Examples of glandular organs include the pancreas, salivary glands, thyroid, and breasts. The kidney is an example of an organ that essentially contains tubules. Other organs such as the liver, adrenals, and pituitary gland are arranged in sheets with specialized capillaries, called sinusoids, situated between the sheets of cells.

Connective Tissue

The primary purpose of connective tissue is to bind, support, and connect tissues. Connective tissue cells can be distinguished from epithelial cells by their lack of approximation to other cells and by the substances that they produce. These cells include fibroblasts, which are associated with collagen; chondroblasts, with cartilage; osteocytes, with bone; and endothelium, with blood vessels.

Muscle Tissue

Muscle cells are bundles of long, slender cells that can contract or provide movement. They are responsible for locomotion and play an essential role in performing vital body functions. There are three types of muscle cells: voluntary or striated, involuntary or smooth, and cardiac. Some muscles are attached to bones by tendons. Others are attached to other muscles or to skin.

Nerve Tissue

Nerve tissue cells comprise two groups, axons and supporting cells. The brain and spinal cord make up the central nervous system. The supporting cells of the central nervous system include two types of glial cells, referred to as astrocytes and oligodendroglia. Schwann's cells are the supporting cells in peripheral nerves.

Growth Disturbances

A growth disturbance is any type of lesion or tissue mass that is characterized by the proliferation of cells. There is a direct relationship between the proliferative or reproductive capability of the cell and the occurrence of disease. The greater the rate of proliferation, the greater the disease potential. Thus, surface epithelium and endothelial cells, which undergo continuous replacement, have the greatest susceptibility to a growth disturbance. Connective tissue also has a rapid rate of proliferation, but not to the same degree as epithelial and endothelial cells. Skeletal muscle has a limited ability to reproduce itself, and cardiac muscle is not able to replace itself at all. Thus, growth disturbances of muscle tissue occur rarely. In the central nervous system, neurons and oligodendroglia are incapable of proliferation. Lesions involving nervous tissue are considered rare, compared with those of epithelial tissue.

Hyperplasias and Neoplasms

Growth disturbances can be separated into two categories, hyperplasias and neoplasms. **Hyperplasia** is an absolute increase in the number of cells in a tissue and is an exaggerated response to various stimuli. Hyperplasia often recedes when the causative agent is removed. In contrast to hyperplasia, a **neoplasm** continues to grow even after the offending agent is removed. A neoplasm is an abnormal lesion that has excessive growth as its distinguishing feature. There is no beneficial function of a neoplastic lesion. The growth of most tumors is uncontrolled and is uncoordinated with the local environment. Neoplasms consist of two primary components, the **parenchyma,** which includes the tumor cells, and the **supporting** connective tissue, in which the tumor grows and on which the tumor depends for its blood supply. The stealing of blood is characteristic of most neoplasms, and, as a result, anemia is often present in the early history of many neoplasms.

Neoplasias and hyperplasias arise from cells that undergo replacement. Thus, in the early stages of disease, hyperplasia and neoplasia cannot be distinguished from each other and are often confused. The behavior and structure of most tumors in the early stages are almost identical to hyperplasia. Often a tumor is slow growing and nonaggressive; thus, even with periodic evaluation, sudden changes in structure and behavior are not always noted.

Neoplasms or tumors are separated into two groups, those that are benign and those that are malignant. A **benign** tumor is the least serious of the two and seldom is lethal. Benign brain tumors are often fatal because of their location, rather than their growth. In a **malignant** neoplasm or cancer, growth is uncontrolled. The benign tumor remains discrete in an area, but the malignant tumor invades adjacent and surrounding tissues and structures and follows a path through the bloodstream, the lymphatic channels, and the body spaces. This spread of cancer cells to regional and distant body locations is termed **metastasis**. This subject will be discussed further in Chapter 8.

Often occurring with hyperplasia is hypertrophy. **Hypertrophy** is an increase in cell size. This is not to be confused with hyperplasia, which is an increase in cell numbers. Hypertrophy is most often associated with muscle tissue. Hypertrophy of the muscle lining of the pylorus results in a decrease in the lumen of the pyloric canal and causes a life-threatening condition known as pyloric stenosis. As part of the aging process in males, the prostate gland undergoes hypertrophy and often closes off the urethra at the outlet of the bladder. Elderly men may have great discomfort in the lower back region, partly because of the overdistended urinary bladder owing to difficulty in voiding or inability to void. Both pyloric stenosis and prostatic hypertrophy are discussed elsewhere in this text.

Metaplasia

Metaplasia is said to occur as a cell changes from normal to abnormal. Unlike hyperplasia and neoplasia, a cell undergoing metaplasia has not yet acquired any characteristics of a tumor, but the cell is undergoing a change in structure. In most cases, metaplastic lesions are watched carefully and are evaluated more frequently over shorter spans of time. It is not uncommon for metaplasia to be referred to according to the type of originating cell. For example, in the uterine cavity, squamous cells predominate, thus squamous metaplasia may occur in that site. Another example may be cited in the respiratory tract, where columnar epithelium predominates. The columnar epithelium undergoes a change toward that resembling squamous epithelium. This is another example of squamous metaplasia. Metaplasia is often considered to be a premalignant lesion.

Dysplasia

Dysplasia is an abnormal development of tissue. It is characterized by the loss of normal uniformity of the individual cells. It is most important to note that although dysplasia is not considered a neoplasm, it can precede a malignant change. Unlike the presumed causes of cancer (chemicals, the environment, and so on), the cause of dysplasia is unknown.

There are four types of cancer. **Carcinoma** is cancer that has its origin in epithelial tissue. **Sarcoma** is cancer of connective tissue, **leukemia** is cancer of the blood, and **lymphoma** is cancer of the lymphatic system. The majority of words with the suffix *oma* describe tumors. Some exceptions exist, such as hematoma, which is a blood clot. The names, classifications, and types of neoplasms are discussed further in Chapter 8.

The Leading Causes of Death

Organizations such as the U.S. Department of Health and Human Services and the American Cancer Society annually tabulate statistics on human

Table 1–1. Number of Deaths, Death Rates and Percent of Total Deaths for the 10 Leading Causes of Death: United States, 1985

Rank	Cause of Death	No.	Rate	Percent (%)
	All Caused 1985	2,084,000	874.8	100.0
1	Heart disease	775,890	325.0	37.2
2	Cancer	457,670	191.7	22.0
3	Stroke	152,710	64.0	7.3
4	Accidents	92,070	38.6	4.4
5	Chronic obstructive pulmonary disease	66,630	27.9	3.6
6	Pneumonia and influenza	38,620	16.2	1.9
7	Diabetes	28,620	11.2	1.3
8	Suicide	26,770	11.2	1.1
9	Chronic liver disease	23,580	9.9	1.1
10	Atherosclerosis	328,679	13.9	16.1

Adapted from the U.S. Department of Health and Human Services, Monthly Vital Statistics Report, Vol. 34, No. 13, September 19, 1986.

mortality. These statistics describe many factors regarding health in the United States. Information gathered from death certificates and patient health records is submitted to agencies that compile health statistics. When surveys are taken, a population of 100,000 is sampled.

In 1985, an estimated 2,084,000 deaths occurred in the United States, 47,071 more than in 1984 and the largest annual number ever recorded. This is due primarily to the continuing growth of the population and the higher proportion of senior citizens. The death rates for 1984–1985 essentially remained the same (Table 1–1). However, if we look at the *age-adjusted* death rate, which disregards the effects of aging, the death rate declined 0.83%, and that of men by 7.0 years. Whites continue to have greater longevity than blacks (5.6 years). Males continue to have a higher mortality rate than females for the 15 leading causes of death. The black population had higher rates than the white population for 11 of the 15 leading causes of death. The two leading causes that had lower rates for the black population were chronic obstructive pulmonary disease and suicide (Table 1–2).

Mortality rate is the number of persons dying per year divided by a population sample of 100,000. When discussing mortality rate, the greatest emphasis is placed on the leading causes of death. The five leading causes of death account for 75% of deaths in the United States. A total of 2,084,000 persons died of all causes in 1985. The mortality rate was 874.8 per 100,000.

Heart disease is the leading cause of death in the United States and accounts for 4 of every 10 deaths. In 1985, 775,890 people died of one of many major heart diseases, a mortality rate of 410.7 per 100,000. Of that figure, ischemic heart disease accounted for 540,800 deaths, or a mortality rate of 226.5 per 100,000. Heart disease is the leading cause of death

of both sexes and of all ages and all races (Tables 1–3 and 1–4).

Cancer is the second leading cause of death, accounting for one of every six deaths. Cancers of the lung, colon, gastrointestinal tract, breast, female genital organs, and prostate gland account for about 60% of all cancer deaths. In 1985, 457,670 deaths occurred as a result of cancer, establishing a mortality rate of 191.7 per 100,000. Cancer is the leading cause of death of both sexes in persons between the ages of 45 and 64 years. Cancer is the second leading cause of death for both sexes and for all races.

Cerebrosvascular accident or *stroke* is the third leading cause of death. Stroke accounts for 1 of every 10 deaths and results from injury to or death of specific areas of the brain. Like heart disease, stroke results from altered blood flow and subsequent obstruction of cerebral vessels. Atherosclerosis is the primary cause of the altered blood flow. A stroke can occur as a result of rupture of an aneurysm or weakened vessel wall secondary to hypertension as well as atherosclerosis. Death of a portion of the brain is a cerebral infarct. In 1985, stroke accounted for 152,710 deaths, which is a mortality rate of 64 per 100,000. Stroke is most prevalent in persons between the ages of 45 and 64 and in those older than 65 years.

Trauma is the fourth leading cause of death and is responsible for 1 of every 16 deaths. Automobile accidents are most often responsible for traumatic death. In 1985, traumatic death from all causes resulted in 92,070 deaths and a mortality rate of 38.6 per 100,000. Motor vehicle fatalities accounted for 44,930 deaths, a mortality rate of 18.8 per 100,000. Approximately 50% of automobile fatalities occurred

Table 1–2. Ratio of Age-Adjusted Death Rates for the 15 Leading Causes of Death, by Sex and Race: United States, 1984

Rank	Cause of Death	Male-to-Female Ratio	Black-to-White Ratio
1	Heart disease	1.95	1.31
2	Cancer	1.48	1.34
3	Stroke	1.17	1.82
4	Accidents	2.80	1.17
5	Chronic obstructive pulmonary disease	2.37	0.78
6	Pneumonia and influenza	1.84	1.48
7	Diabetes	1.07	2.27
8	Suicide	3.60	0.52
9	Chronic liver disease	2.20	1.70
10	Atherosclerosis	1.30	1.00
11	Nephritis	1.54	2.73
12	Homicide	3.33	5.36
13	Perinatal causes	1.23	2.38
14	Septicemia	1.38	2.78
15	Congenital	1.10	1.00
	All causes	1.75	1.47

Adapted from The U.S. Department of Health and Human Services, Monthly Vital Statistics Report, Vol. 35, No. 6, Supplement (2), September 26, 1986.

Table 1–3. Deaths and Death Rates for the Five Leading Causes of Death in Specified Race-Sex Groups: United States, 1984

Rank	A	B	C	D	E	F	G
1	Heart	Heart	Heart	Heart	Heart	Heart	Heart
2	Cancer	Cancer	Cancer	Cancer	Cancer	Cancer	Cancer
3	Stroke	Accident	Stroke	Accident	Stroke	Accident	Stroke
4	Accident	Stroke	Pneumonia	Stroke	Diabetes	Stroke	Diabetes
5	COPD	COPD	Accident	Homicide	Accident	Homicide	Accident

Adapted from The U.S. Department of Health and Human Services, Monthly Vital Statistics Report, Vol. 35, No. 6, Supplement (2) September 26, 1986.

Abbreviations: A = all 1984; B = white males; C = white females; D = all other males; E = all other females; F = black males; G = black females; COPD = chronic obstructive pulmonary disease.

when the driver was under the influence of alcohol. In 1983, it was estimated that by the end of 1986, traumatic death would overtake stroke as the third leading cause of deaths. Other leading causes of traumatic death include home accidents, work-related accidents, and sports injuries. Fatal accidents are significantly more common among males than among females. In terms of age-adjusted deaths, trauma is the leading cause of death in ages 1 through 44 (Table 1–4).

Chronic obstructive pulmonary disease (COPD) is the fifth leading cause of death, resulting in more than 74,420 deaths and occurring at a rate of 31.2 per 100,000 population. COPD is also the fifth leading cause of death of white males and is most prevalent in the age-group over 65 years.

Standards of Measure

Frequency

Frequency is the rate of occurrence measured over a given period of time. The period of time used to measure this rate is usually 1 year.

Incidence

Incidence is a measure of the number of newly diagnosed cases in a 1-year period. Although incidence usually refers to a period of 1 year, it can be used to measure any unit of time period. However, it is most useful for periods of short duration.

Prevalence

Prevalence refers to the number of individuals with a particular disease at any point in time. Prevalence is best used when attempting to measure the rate of survival for long periods of time, say 5 years. Because of new technology and research, victims of terminal disease may survive between 5 and 10 years following the initial diagnosis. When a population includes a large number of elderly people, the age-adjusted measurement is commonly employed. In addition to a terminal disease, the elderly patient often suffers from diseases of aging. Thus, at the time of death it is difficult to determine the exact cause of death. The age-adjusted survival rate modifies the rate for those who may have died from other causes based on their age.

Acute Illness

An acute illness is one that has a sudden onset and severe symptoms and runs a short course. Upper respiratory tract infections are common examples, as are accidents and heart attacks. Heart attacks are extremely acute, as well as fatal. Heart attack is the leading cause of early death, followed by stroke and cancer. Acute diseases seem to be more common during infancy and childhood.

Table 1–4. Deaths and Death Rates for the Five Leading Causes of Death in Specified Age Groups: United States, 1984

Rank	All Age Groups	1–4	5–14	15–24	25–44	45–65	65+
1	Heart	Accident	Accident	Accident	Accident	Cancer	Heart disease
2	Cancer	Congenital	Cancer	Suicide	Cancer	Heart disease	Cancer
3	Stroke	Cancer	Congenital	Homicide	Heart disease	Stroke	Stroke
4	Accidents	Heart disease	Homicide	Cancer	Suicide	Accident	Chronic obstructive pulmonary disease
5	Chronic obstructive pulmonary disease	Homicide	Heart disease	Heart disease	Homicide	Chronic diseases Liver disease	Pneumonia influenza

Adapted from The U.S. Department of Health and Human Services, Monthly Vital Statistics Report, Vol. 35, No. 6, Supplement (2), September 26, 1986.

Chronic Illness

A chronic illness is one that lasts weeks, months, years, or even a lifetime. Statistically, it has been proved that chronic disease becomes much more common as one ages. When discussing chronic disease, we would be remiss in not mentioning dental caries, which is the leading chronic disease affecting all age-groups, and periodontal disease is the major reason for tooth loss in adults. Fifty percent of the adult population is afflicted with some form of periodontal disease.

The five leading chronic diseases all involve aging and include degenerative arthritis or osteoarthritis, hypertension, hearing impairment, heart disease, and vision impairment. Among those persons seeking medical assistance, upper respiratory tract infections are the leading acute disease and hypertension is the leading chronic disease.

Prognosis

A prognosis is the predicted course of a disease as well as the prospects for recovery. The earlier the detection, the better chance for recovery.

Self-Assessment Quiz

For each of the following questions, select the one best response and circle the letter that precedes it.

1. An abnormal or functional change in the body is termed
   a. disease
   b. diagnosis
   c. etiology
   d. idiopathic

2. The sequence of events that leads from the cause to the structural or functional change is termed
   a. disease
   b. etiology
   c. pathogenesis
   d. syndrome

3. The study of causes is termed
   a. diagnosis
   b. etiology
   c. pathology
   d. pathogenesis

4. A process of assigning a name to a patient's condition is called
   a. disease
   b. diagnosis
   c. etiology
   d. syndrome

5. Symptoms, signs, and laboratory findings all are what aspects of disease?
   a. biochemical
   b. congenital
   c. manifestations
   d. developmental

6. Evidences of disease as perceived by the patient are known as
   a. lesions
   b. injuries
   c. signs
   d. symptoms

7. A written description of symptoms is called
   a. complaints
   b. signs
   c. manifestations
   d. history

8. Physical observations are also referred to as
   a. signs
   b. symptoms
   c. manifestations
   d. history

9. A lesion may correctly be described as
   a. structural change
   b. organic disease
   c. morphological change
   d. all of the above

10. Injuries, inflammations, proliferations, and neoplasms all are forms of
    a. functional disease
    b. structural disease

11. A congenital disease is one that is
    a. acquired through heredity
    b. acquired by sexual contact
    c. present at birth
    d. functional

12. Physical and chemical substances are examples of
    a. internal agents
    b. external agents

13. When a cell has died because of injury, it is said to have undergone
    a. degeneration
    b. necrosis
    c. inflammation
    d. repair

14. Dead cells are capable of recovery.
    a. true
    b. false

15. Which of the following terms describes sublethal injury?
    a. degeneration
    b. inflammation
    c. necrosis
    d. repair

16. Which of the following involves a vascular and cellular reaction?
    a. degeneration
    b. necrosis
    c. inflammation
    d. repair

17. The preferred method of repair is
    a. degeneration
    b. necrosis
    c. connective tissue repair
    d. regeneration

18. An increase in cell population describes
    a. metaplasia
    b. hypertrophy
    c. neoplasia
    d. hyperplasia

19. Which of the following is described as a proliferative reaction to an external stimulus?
    a. degeneration
    b. hyperplasia
    c. hypoplasia
    d. hypertrophy

20. Which type of tumor remains localized and does not spread?
    a. osteoma
    b. fibrosarcoma
    c. osteosarcoma
    d. lymphoma

21. Which type of disease presents no lesion at its onset?
    a. functional
    b. structural

22. Which of the following are examples of physical agents?
    a. fungi
    b. poisons
    c. atherosclerosis
    d. drugs
    e. fungi, poisons, and drugs

23. Altered blood flow, obstructive disease, and hemorrhage are examples of
    a. exogenous agents
    b. endogenous agents

24. Hypersensitivity or allergic reactions are what type of disorders?
    a. exogenous
    b. immunological
    c. metabolic
    d. microbiological

25. Which of the following describes diseases of unknown cause?
    a. idiopathic
    b. etiology
    c. iatrogenic
    d. nosocomial

26. A disease that is acquired while under the care of a physician is described as
    a. idiopathic
    b. etiological
    c. iatrogenic
    d. nosocomial

27. A disease that is acquired by a patient in a hospital is described as
    a. idiopathic
    b. iatrogenic
    c. pathogenic
    d. nosocomial

28. Obstruction of arteries, brain hemorrhage, and atherosclerosis all are common causes of
    a. heart disease
    b. stroke
    c. diabetes
    d. pneumonia

29. A dilatation of an artery is termed
    a. an aneurysm
    b. a thrombus
    c. a clot
    d. an embolus

30. What is the leading cause of secondary death?
    a. chronic obstructive pulmonary disease
    b. ischemia
    c. pneumonia
    d. stroke

31. Survival rate is usually calculated over a period of how many years?
    a. 2
    b. 3
    c. 5
    d. 10

32. As a person ages, the frequency of acute illness
    a. increases
    b. decreases
    c. does not change

33. The leading chronic disease affecting all age-groups is
    a. pneumonia
    b. diabetes
    c. arteriosclerosis
    d. dental caries

34. An analysis performed on a specimen removed from a patient is known as a
    a. test
    b. procedure

35. Which diagnostic imaging modality uses radioisotopes that are injected into the bloodstream?
    a. nuclear medicine
    b. radiography
    c. radiation therapy
    d. ultrasonography

36. The surgical removal of a small specimen is called
    a. a biopsy
    b. a resection
    c. a test
    d. an autopsy

37. Which of the following terms describes the removal of a small lesion, primarily for the purpose of diagnosis?
    a. incisional biopsy
    b. excisional biopsy
    c. resection
    d. autopsy

38. A tissue biopsy taken during surgery to the laboratory for immediate diagnosis describes a frozen section.
    a. true
    b. false

39. The complete removal of a small lesion for the purpose of diagnosis and treatment is known as
    a. an incisional biopsy
    b. an excisional biopsy
    c. a resection
    d. an incisional biopsy and resection

40. A resection is the surgical removal of a
    a. large specimen
    b. small specimen

41. Which segment of the clinical laboratory is often used to determine organ function?
    a. blood chemistry
    b. bacteriology
    c. hematology
    d. blood bank

42. Which segment of the clinical laboratory is often used in the diagnosis of anemia?
    a. blood chemistry
    b. hematology
    c. microbiology
    d. bacteriology

43. Congestion is associated with
    a. degeneration
    b. inflammation
    c. necrosis
    d. repair

44. A serum fluid that passes through a membrane or tissue as a result of increased hydrostatic pressure is known as
    a. congestion
    b. a transudate
    c. inflammation
    d. an exudate

45. Which of the following are types of epithelial tissue?
    a. squamous and oligodendroglia
    b. transitional and astrocytes
    c. transitional, oligodendroglia, and stratified
    d. oligodendroglia, astrocytes, and stratified
    e. squamous, transitional, and columnar

46. Which of the following cells contain keratin?
    a. connective
    b. epithelial
    c. muscle
    d. nerve

47. Which of the following cells contain collagen?
    a. connective
    b. epithelial
    c. muscle
    d. nerve

48. Astrocytes and oligodendroglia are examples of what type of tissue?
    a. connective
    b. epithelial
    c. muscle
    d. nerve

49. Growth disturbances can be categorized as
    a. inflammatory and invasive
    b. metaplasia and hypertrophy
    c. hyperplasia and metaplasia
    d. hyperplasia and neoplasm

50. An increase in cell size is known as
    a. hypertrophy
    b. hyperemia
    c. hyperplasia
    d. metaplasia
    e. dysplasia

51. An increase in cell numbers or population is called
    a. dysplasia
    b. hyperplasia
    c. metaplasia
    d. hypertrophy

52. Pyloric stenosis is an example of
    a. hypertrophy
    b. hyperplasia
    c. neoplasm
    d. atresia

53. The three leading causes of death are
    a. heart disease, stroke, and diabetes
    b. diabetes, accidents, and cancer
    c. heart disease, stroke, and cancer
    d. stroke, diabetes, and accidents

54. Which of the following are types of cancer?
    a. carcinoma
    b. carcinoma and leukemia
    c. lymphoma and sarcoma
    d. all of the above

55. Which form of heart disease is the leading killer of adults?
    a. congenital heart disease
    b. hypertensive heart disease
    c. ischemic heart disease
    d. valvular disease

56. Accidents are the leading cause of death for which age group?
    a. 1 to 4 years
    b. 5 to 14 years
    c. 15 to 24 years
    d. 25 to 44 years
    e. All of the above

57. The number of newly diagnosed cases in a given time period is called the
    a. frequency
    b. incidence
    c. mortality rate
    d. prevalence

58. The number of people with a disease at a given point in time is known as the
    a. frequency
    b. incidence
    c. mortality rate
    d. prevalence

Study Questions

1. What is the sequence of events that take place following injury?

2. Explain the differences between structural and functional disease.

3. What are autoimmune diseases and what is their impact on the body?

4. What are the characteristics of acute inflammation? Chronic inflammation?

5. List the fundamental tissues of the body and the subtypes of specialized tissues.

6. Distinguish between the different types of growth disturbances.

7. Why is the term age-adjusted used when determining mortality rate?

8. Which races are more likely to have the highest mortality rate? Why?

Two

Respiratory System

Related Terminology

air-bronchogram sign
asthma
atelectasis
azygos vein fissure
bronchiectasis
*chronic obstructive pulmonary
    disease*
croup
cystic fibrosis
emphysema
histoplasmosis
hyaline membrane disease
pneumoconioses
pneumonitis
pneumothorax
silhouette sign
tuberculosis

Objectives

Upon completion of Chapter 2, the radiographer will be able to

- *Explain the radiographic significance of the cardiac silhouette and the silhouette sign.*

- *Describe the various radiographic methods for imaging the diseases of the lungs.*

- *Describe the radiographic appearance of each listed disease process involving the lungs.*

- *Identify the mechanisms that are responsible for the onset of lung disease.*

- *List and describe the laboratory tests that are designed to assess pulmonary function.*

- *Describe the current methods of treatment for the listed lung disorders.*

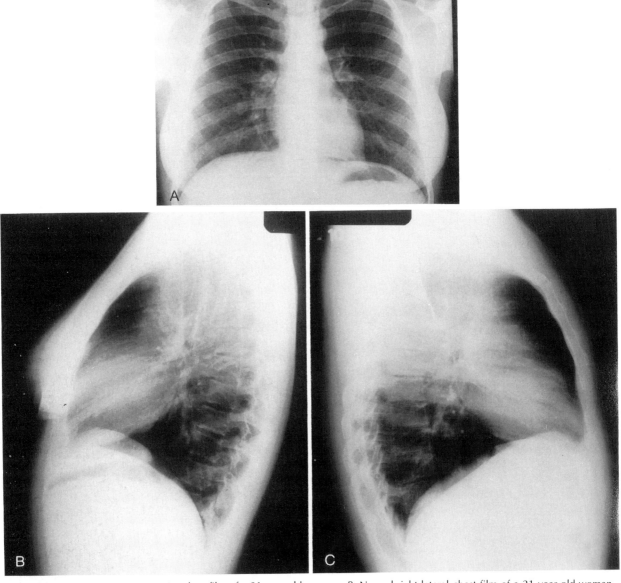

Figure 2–1. *A,* Normal posteroanterior chest film of a 21-year-old woman. *B,* Normal right lateral chest film of a 21-year-old woman. *C,* Normal left lateral chest film of a 34-year-old man.

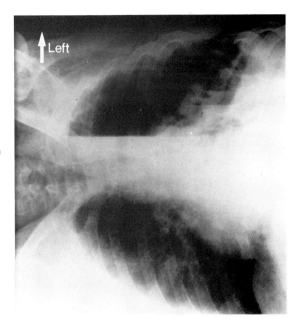

Figure 2–5. Right lateral decubitus chest film for postoperative evaluation of a 51-year-old man.

Radiographs of the chest can be taken with the patient lying in a lateral decubitus position. This can be accomplished by having the patient lie on either side in the lateral recumbent position. The position is named according to the side of the patient that is placed down. Thus, patients who are lying down on their right side are assuming a right lateral decubitus position (Fig. 2–5).

Linear tomography is most useful in visualizing the extent of a lesion within the chest and mediastinum. The tomogram can differentiate a lesion more accurately than a conventional chest radiograph. With the opposite movements of the film and x-ray tube, all anatomy above and below the object plane is blurred. Tomography can accurately discern calcification, cavities, nodules, blood vessels, and, most important, suspected carcinoma (Fig. 2–6).

Bronchography is the radiographic demonstration of the tracheobronchial tree with an oily iodinated contrast agent such as Dionosil. The contrast material reveals an excellent outline of the tracheobronchial structures. Bronchography is used to demonstrate deterioration of the airways caused by long-term inflammatory disease. This is graphically rep-

Figure 2–6. Linear anteroposterior tomogram reveals a bronchogenic neoplasm of the left upper lobe with distal pneumonia. The patient is a woman, age 88.

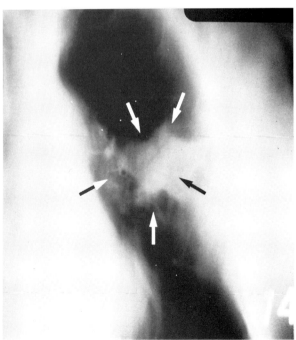

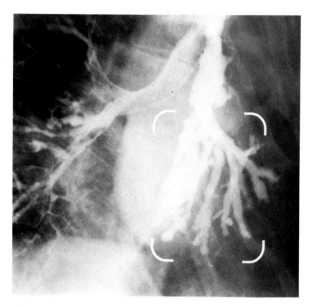

Figure 2–7. Oblique bronchogram study revealing extensive bronchiectasis (brackets) of left lower lung segments.

resented by bronchiectasis, a permanent dilatation of the terminal bronchi in the lower lung segments (Fig. 2–7).

Radionuclide perfusion and ventilation scans are used in conjunction with obstructive disease and pulmonary embolism. To obtain a perfusion scan, a radioactive tracer is injected into the venous system. It then becomes trapped in the pulmonary circulation, where it will provide an image of the distribution of pulmonary blood flow for a scanning camera. A ventilation scan is usually obtained using a radioactive gas such as xenon. The patient is connected to a breathing apparatus, and a bolus of gas is introduced as the patient inhales. The patient then holds his or her breath while an image is made of the initial single-breath distribution of the xenon gas (Fig. 2–8).

In addition to the specific imaging methods, positioning, and techniques, the radiographer should be familiar with normal chest and lung anatomy as seen with the routine projections. The important structures to identify include the diaphragm, the costo-

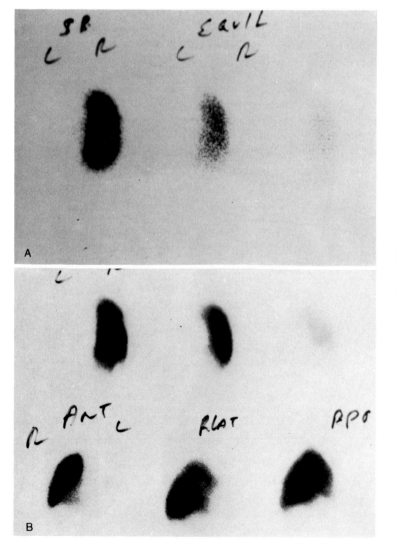

Figure 2–8. *A,* Virtually no ventilation of the left lung but good ventilation of the right lung. *B,* Normal perfusion despite the extent of metastasis and minimal perfusion of the left hilar region.

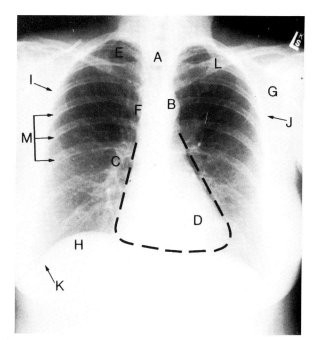

Figure 2–9. Normal posteroanterior chest film. A = trachea; B = aortic arch; C = right pulmonary artery; D = heart; E = right apex; F = hilum; G = left scapula; H = left hemidiaphragm; I = right lung; J = left lung; K = costophrenic angle; L = left clavicle; M = right ribs.

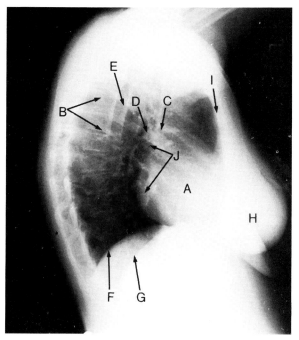

Figure 2–10. Normal left lateral chest film. A = heart; B = dorsal spine; C = right main bronchus; D = left main bronchus; E = trachea; F = left hemidiaphragm; G = right hemidiaphragm; H = breast; I = sternum; J = pulmonary vessels.

phrenic angles, the heart (with emphasis on the right atrium and left ventricle), the right and left hilar regions, the aortic arch, and the superior vena cava. Other areas of importance include the bony structures, such as the anterior ribs, lower cervical and upper three dorsal vertebrae, clavicles, and scapulae (Fig. 2–9). Other landmark visualizations include the trachea, carina, and soft tissues of the axillary and cervical borders. On a lateral view of the chest, the normal anatomy includes the manubrium and body of the sternum, trachea, left bronchus as seen on end, cardiac silhouette, thoracic vertebral bodies, and right and left diaphragmatic domes (Fig. 2–10).

In terms of diagnosis and interpretation of the radiograph, the role of the radiographer is clearly understood; however, one should realize that the radiographer is responsible for producing the product that will be interpreted by the physician. It is the responsibility of the radiographer to take into account all possible variables that may have an effect on the finished radiograph. Obviously, the more knowledge one has, the better he or she can perform a given task. Thus, the more knowledgeable the radiographer, the more functional he or she becomes. With this in mind, it is useful for the radiographer to have an understanding of some of the typical signs of disease on a radiograph of the chest and lungs.

Within the lung interstitium, the intrapulmonary bronchi are not usually visible radiographically because they are aerated and are surrounded by alveolar air. However, whenever a situation exists in which fluids collect within the lung substances, the surrounding parenchyma loses its air as a result of compression. This fluid compression results in the

collapsing of the aerated structures. The areas of fluid consolidation and collapse contrast each other, thus rendering the bronchi visible. This is referred to as the air-bronchogram sign (Fig. 2–11).

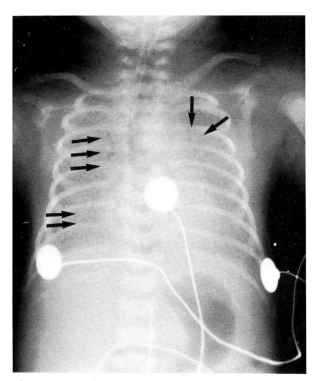

Figure 2–11. Hyaline membrane disease. Arrows indicate the presence of air in the bronchi. This is the air-bronchogram sign and is indicative of alveolar disease. The patient is a 16-month-old boy.

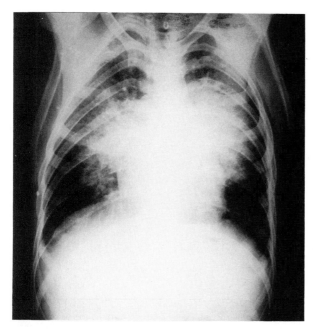

Figure 2–12. Pulmonary edema in a 64-year-old man. Note the obliteration of the right cardiac border. This is referred to as the silhouette sign.

Anatomical structures are recognized on a radiograph because of the many different densities that are present. The outline of the heart is detailed on the radiograph because of the density of the heart itself compared with adjacent structures, especially the air-filled lungs. When different densities are apparent, structures can be differentiated; however, when similar densities occur, such as fluid in contact with the heart, the borders of the heart are obliterated. Loss of the normal radiographic silhouette of a structure is known as the silhouette sign (Fig. 2–12).

Congenital Disorders

Cystic Fibrosis

General Information. Cystic fibrosis is an inherited disease involving dysfunction of the exocrine, or outward-secreting, glands of the body and is the most common cause of childhood pancreatic disease. Cystic fibrosis is not contagious and is not detectable before birth. It is not caused by any maternal illness or action during pregnancy. This disorder is characterized by an accumulation of excessively thick mucus and abnormal secretion of sweat and saliva. In the United States, it is estimated that cystic fibrosis will occur in about 1 in every 2000 births a year, with about 1000 to 2000 new cases being reported annually. It is estimated that the prevalence may be as high as 30,000 cases. It is the most common fatal genetic disease of Caucasian children, but it is also found in significant numbers in blacks and to a lesser degree in Oriental children. Cystic fibrosis affects both sexes and is more common in children of central European ancestry.

Diagnosis. The classic diagnostic feature of cystic fibrosis is the increased *salt* content in sweat. The sweat test is considered to be 99% reliable. The quantitative pilocarpine iontophoresis test (QPIT) is currently the most accurate test used in diagnosing cystic fibrosis.

Radiographically, the chest x-ray reveals collections of thick mucus adhering to the bronchial lining and trapping bacteria, blocking the passage of oxygen. This mucus is very thick, causes infection and obstruction, and is seen as an opaque image on the radiograph. In addition to the bronchial thickening, the x-ray may reveal atelectasis, bronchiectasis, and consolidation in the middle and upper lung fields. When the pancreas is involved, the pancreatic duct blocks the elimination of enzymes from the pancreas to the duodenum. These enzymes are helpful in digesting fats and proteins, which are consequently lost in frequent, bulky, greasy, foul-smelling stools (Fig. 2–13).

Treatment. Because there is no cure for cystic fibrosis, the prognosis is primarily dependent on controlling the effects of the disease. Aerosol inhalation of medications has worked very well for this purpose. These medications include decongestants to shrink swollen membranes, bronchodilators to widen the bronchial passageways, mucolytics to liquefy secretions, and antibiotics to control infections.

In the most severe cases, the patient is bedridden and suffers from pancreatitis and will eventually succumb to pneumonia. Although 50% die by the age of 16, the survival age is increasing as a result of the improved methods of treatment.

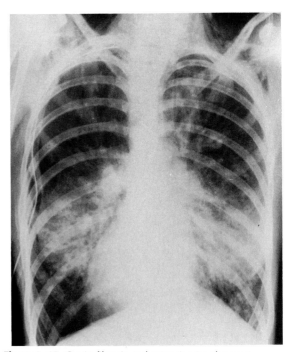

Figure 2–13. Cystic fibrosis and extensive involvement throughout both lungs. Radiolucent appearance indicates thick-walled bronchi that contain mucus secretions and trapped air, indicating endobronchial obstruction. The patient is 14 years old.

Hyaline Membrane Disease

General Information. Hyaline membrane disease is also known as the **respiratory distress syndrome** and is the leading cause of infant mortality. This disease accounts for 40,000 infant deaths annually. It is named for the formation of the hyalin-like membrane lining the distal respiratory passages. Approximately 90% of cases are related to premature birth, and about 50% of the affected infants die within the first 24 hours of life. Sixty percent are born before the 28th week of gestation. A significant number of affected infants are born to diabetic mothers. Hyaline membrane disease is more common in cesarean births.

Hyaline membrane disease is due to a loss or absence of surfactant within the lung. Surfactant is a chemical detergent that is secreted by the epithelium of the alveoli and decreases the surface tension of the fluids lining the alveoli and bronchioles. When the surface tension is kept low, air can pass through the fluid and into the alveoli. If the surface tension is not decreased by adequate supplies of surfactant, the alveoli collapse. This results in widespread atelectasis and inadequate ventilation, with the blood rerouting through the collapsed tissues, resulting in hypoxia and acidosis of the blood. Those newborns who survive the first 72 hours usually recover quickly.

Diagnosis. The chest radiograph is the most significant means of imaging hyaline membrane disease. Present are widespread minute pulmonary **granular** opacities and an **air-bronchogram sign.** The bronchi are seen because they are surrounded by **nonaerated** alveoli. In the more severe cases, the opacities are most prominent. In less severe cases, the air in the bronchi is most obvious (Fig. 2–14).

Treatment. Treatment of this disorder requires vigorous respiratory support with warm humidified oxygen under conditions of positive pressure. Sodium bicarbonate is administered to overcome acidosis. At one time, the danger of infant blindness due to the increased concentration of oxygen was a consideration. Retrolental fibroplasia often occurred in premature infants receiving this treatment. More recently, improved methods of oxygen administration have practically eliminated this complication.

Sudden Infant Death Syndrome

General Information. Sudden infant death syndrome (SIDS), also known as crib death, occurs quite unexpectedly. The infant in most cases is healthy and shows no signs of distress. Studies indicate that SIDS most often occurs between the ages of 3 weeks and 4 months and accounts for about 10,000 infant deaths annually. It is second only to accidents as a major cause of death in children younger than 15 years. SIDS has been found to occur most often in the winter months, to infants born of mothers who are of low socioeconomic status and who are younger than 20. There is also a higher incidence in male and non-Caucasian infants.

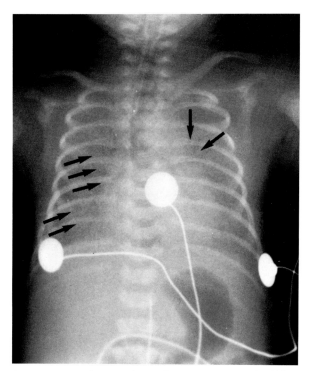

Figure 2–14. Hyaline membrane disease in a 16-month-old boy. The visible streaks of air represent the air-bronchogram sign. There is a diffuse granular appearance with an increase in the reticular network of the lung fields.

Diagnosis. Infants who die of SIDS are usually underweight, and there is some suggestion that this condition is more probable in infants who were born prematurely. Postmortem examinations have been inconclusive thus far, although there is some evidence of abnormal control of lung ventilation, atrophic adrenal glands, and petechiae over the surfaces of the visceral pleura. Families who have a history of prematurity, hyaline membrane disease, seizure disorders, and SIDS have a higher risk of being afflicted a second time. As in hyaline membrane disease, an air-bronchogram sign is present in both frontal and lateral projections.

Treatment. In most cases of SIDS, the infants are found dead in their cribs. When they are found in respiratory distress, emergency resuscitation must be initiated. However, in more cases than not, this syndrome results in the death of the infant. The psychological effects on the family after infant death are significant, because parents feel that they must shoulder the blame and responsibility for the infant's death. Intensive counseling is often necessary. National foundations for SIDS families have been established.

Azygos Vein Fissure

General Information. The azygos vein passes up from the lumbar region to the right side of the fourth thoracic vertebra, where it arches over the right lung. Azygos vein fissure occurs during intrauterine

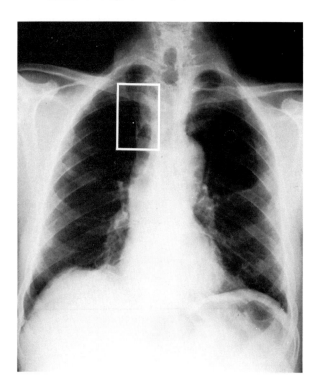

Figure 2–15. Azygos vein and fissure as a curvilinear line in the right apical (rectangle) region. The patient is a 65-year-old man.

development when the vein migrates from the chest wall to lie within the mediastinum. In most cases, this variant is of no clinical significance but could be confused with pneumonia because it is associated with a fluid mass. Azygos vein fissure is present in about 1% of the population.

Diagnosis. Because fluid collects within this fissure, the azygos vein is usually seen at the medial aspect of the fissure. This may be observed on a routine PA projection of the chest (Fig. 2–15).

Treatment. Treatment is not usually required for this normal variant. The differential diagnosis must rule out other disease processes. This condition is rarely significant and is often reported by the radiologist as an incidental finding.

Acute Disorders

Croup

General Information. Croup is a condition characterized by laryngitis with laryngeal spasm. This inflammatory disorder may result in obstruction of the upper airway. It is usually due to a virus, is most common in the winter and affects mostly males from the age of 3 months to 3 years. Fifteen percent of patients having croup also have a documented family history of croup.

Diagnosis. The key sign of this disorder is a *bark-like* cough produced by inflammation, edema, and spasm. Throat cultures are taken to rule out bacterial infection, diphtheria, and foreign body obstruction.

Soft tissue AP projections of the anterior neck area may show *spasm* and *constriction* of air in the airway. During inspiration, there is a croaking sound referred to as stridor. The attacks are usually present at night (Fig. 2–16).

Treatment. When respiratory difficulty arises, the child may be admitted to a hospital. A tent with cool humidity and particulate mist will help liquefy the secretions and reduce spasm.

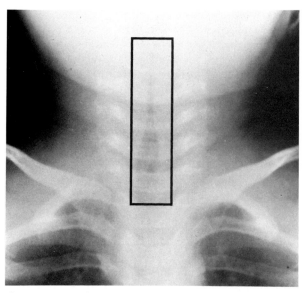

Figure 2–16. Tracheobronchitis or croup in a 2-year-old boy. Soft tissue view of the neck reveals a narrowing of the subglottic region and distension of the hypopharynx (rectangle).

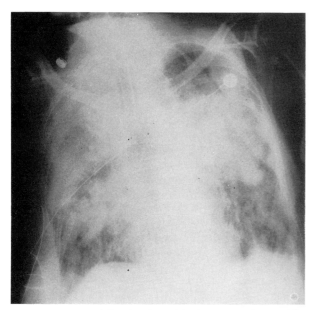

Figure 2–17. Interval deterioration of the lung parenchyma with marked bilateral pulmonary edema. These findings are indicative of the adult respiratory distress syndrome.

Adult Respiratory Distress Syndrome

General Information. The adult respiratory distress syndrome (ARDS) is an acute form of pulmonary congestion and edema resulting in acute respiratory failure. ARDS may also be referred to as shock lung, wet lung, stiff lung, or posttraumatic pulmonary insufficiency.

Diagnosis. ARDS is most common when poor vascular perfusion of the lungs exists. Postsurgical patients and patients with septicemia, pancreatitis, severe burns, severe pulmonary infections, oxygen toxicity, drug overdose, embolism, and major tissue trauma are at increased risk.

Radiographically, patients with ARDS show a widespread diffuse fluid *consolidation* of the lungs. This syndrome is characterized by dyspnea, tachycardia, cyanosis, hypoxemia, and obvious difficulty in lung ventilation (Fig. 2–17).

Treatment. Survival of patients with ARDS depends on the magnitude of initial injury and the degree of pulmonary congestion and edema. It may be necessary to intubate the patient and provide mechanical breathing assistance.

Pulmonary Edema

General Information. Pulmonary edema involves the replacement of air with fluid within the lung interstitium and alveoli. Edema fluid first collects in the lung interstitium. Alveolar filling usually occurs last and is associated with acute disease. Pulmonary edema may occur as a late result of a combination of events involving a long-standing condition or disease process. Congestive heart failure occurs when the

heart can no longer maintain sufficient arterial pressure to provide an adequate supply of oxygenated blood to the tissues. When airflow is inhibited, the osmotic pressure is decreased, resulting in passage of increased amounts of serous fluid through the capillaries and into the lung interstitium and alveoli. As this fluid consolidates within the tissue spaces, the patient experiences breathing difficulty. Breathing becomes progressively more labored, and the patient is obviously dyspneic. In the presence of chronic lung disease, pulmonary edema usually results from prolonged bronchial obstruction and interruption of airflow through the bronchi. Examples of chronic lung disease include asthma and emphysema.

Diagnosis. Pulmonary edema most frequently involves all lobes of both lungs. The PA chest x-ray reveals fluid *consolidation* that is most visible centrally near the hilum. The pattern subsequently becomes more diffuse as it spreads peripherally, leaving a relatively clear area around the edges of the lobes. This characteristic appearance resembles a butterfly or bat-wing pattern (Fig. 2–18).

Treatment. Treatment of pulmonary edema primarily involves an attempt to reduce the amount of extravascular fluid and to increase oxygenation of tissue by administering high concentrations of oxygen assisted by ventilation.

Cor Pulmonale

General Information. In its acute form, cor pulmonale is an emergency condition arising from a

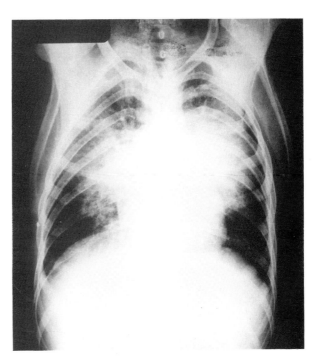

Figure 2–18. Pulmonary edema. A rather typical display of alveolar edema is present, with a fan-shaped distribution. This condition occurred as a result of renal failure.

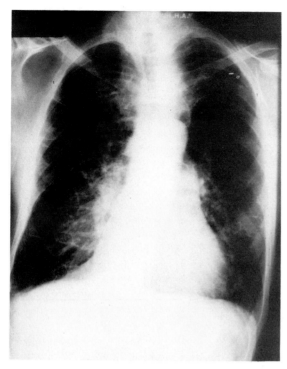

Figure 2–19. Cor pulmonale. There is multiple chamber enlargement, with evidence of poor pulmonary flow.

sudden dilatation of the right ventricle as a result of pulmonary embolism. Cor pulmonale may also progress in a chronic fashion, as when pulmonary arterial hypertension with right ventricular failure results from long-term obstructive lung diseases such as emphysema, silicosis, and fibrosis. These conditions greatly impair the blood flow through the pulmonary artery. This in turn impedes the flow of blood from the right ventricle, resulting in eventual dilatation and hypertrophy. Eighty-five percent of the cases of cor pulmonale are the result of COPD.

Diagnosis. The symptoms of cor pulmonale resemble those of congestive heart failure. The PA projection of the chest reveals an **enlarged** right ventricle with widespread pulmonary **edema** (Fig. 2–19).

Treatment. Treatment of cor pulmonale includes the administration of bronchodilators, heart stimulants such as digitalis, and diuretics such as furosemide (Lasix), to reduce fluid secretions. Lung ventilation reduces hypoxia and dyspnea.

Legionnaires' Disease

General Information. Legionnaires' disease is named for the outbreak of acute illness that occurred at an American Legion convention in Philadelphia, Pennsylvania, in 1976. The causative organism is *Legionella pneumophila*, which is a gram-negative bacillus that was isolated from the lungs of four patients who attended that convention, acquired the disease, and succumbed to it. This organism is now thought to be responsible for an estimated 7% of

pneumonia cases in the United States each year. The occurrence can be sporadic or of epidemic proportions. Middle-aged to elderly men who are smokers are those most susceptible. Patients acquiring this disease do not usually respond to the usual methods of treatment for pneumonia. Those who do survive can have permanent damage of the lungs, liver, and kidneys.

Diagnosis. Radiographically, legionnaires' disease most closely resembles bronchopneumonia. Anterior chest views usually reveal a **patchy** distribution of **infiltrate** throughout the lungs (Fig. 2–20).

Treatment. Treatment of this disease is similar to that for bronchopneumonia. Oxygen therapy and antibiotics are usually indicated, and supportive measures are provided to help the patient cope with nausea, vomiting, high fever, and renal failure.

Atelectasis

General Information. Atelectasis is a collapse of all or part of the lung due to failure of lung expansion or to resorption of air from the alveoli. Atelectasis may be acute or chronic and complete or incomplete.

Obstruction of a bronchus is the most common cause of atelectasis. Fetal atelectasis results when the lungs fail to expand fully at birth. Lack of full lung development or expansion is especially common in premature births and is most often associated with hyaline membrane disease. Atelectasis in the newborn results in dyspnea, cyanosis, elevated body

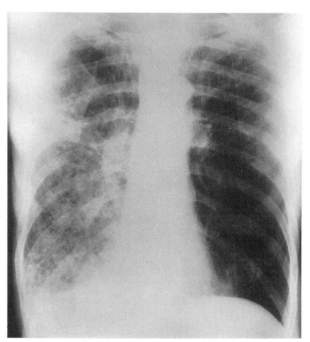

Figure 2–20. Legionnaires' disease. Acute disease is manifested by a patchy infiltrate involving all of the right lung and several areas of the left lung.

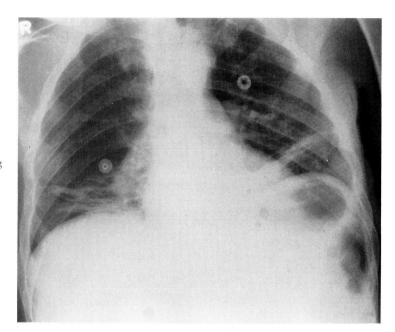

Figure 2–21. Plate-like atelectasis in both lung bases.

temperature, hypotension, and shock. Atelectasis may also be associated with lung *compression*. This compression results from pressure against lung tissue. Air, fluid, tumors, and enlarged lymph nodes all are known causes of atelectasis. Postoperative atelectasis is a complication associated with lack of lung expansion or aspiration following chest or abdominal surgery.

Diagnosis. Atelectasis often involves the smaller lobules of the lung. Characteristically common in the lobules is the presence of horizontal linear opacities, referred to as *plate-like atelectasis*. Plate-like atelectasis is associated with areas of infiltrate within the alveoli and often mimics pneumonia. In terms of fluid compression, both trauma and acute inflammatory disease are the usual offending agents (Fig. 2–21).

Fluid that accumulates within the pleural space and that is the result of a response to inflammation is referred to as *pleural effusion* (Fig. 2–22). When trauma is the causative factor, *hydrothorax* occurs. When blood is present in addition to the serous fluid, the condition is then referred to as *hemohydrothorax*. In order to correct this condition, the fluid must be removed. When the fluid is removed, the lung usually reexpands. Radiographically, atelectasis is identified as an area of *clear space* that is free of bronchial and vascular markings. The collapsed segment is usually located medially, and the space within the

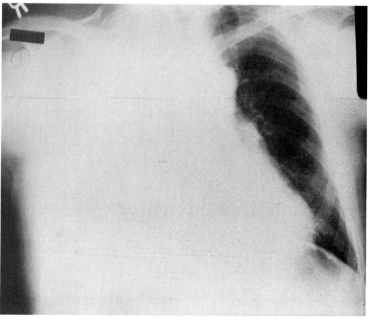

Figure 2–22. Massive effusion in the right pleural cavity.

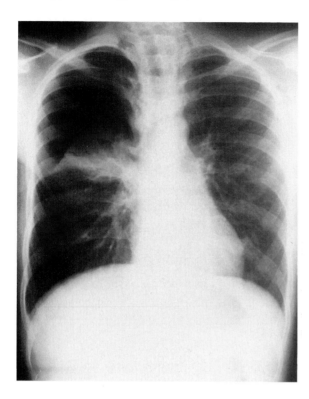

Figure 2–23. A 35 to 45% central collapse of the right upper lobe, secondary to respiratory tract infection, is shown. The patient is an 11-year-old girl.

thorax contains air (Fig. 2–23). Pneumothorax is the presence of air in the thorax. Atelectasis as a result of bronchial obstruction almost always involves fluid consolidation. In comparison, the lateral view of the chest demonstrates fluid consolidation better than a frontal view (Fig. 2–24). When a lobe collapses, other structures move to take up the space. Typically, the mediastinum and diaphragm may move toward the collapsed lobe. Of significance is the shifting of the

trachea when an entire lung collapses. *Tracheal shift* is caused by the difference in air pressure between the lung and pleural space. It is difficult to diagnose atelectasis when the collapsed segment lies behind an area of pleural effusion.

Treatment. The treatment of atelectasis is directed toward reexpanding the collapsed lung segment. Having the patient cough usually results in lung reexpansion. A detergent aerosol used with a mist-

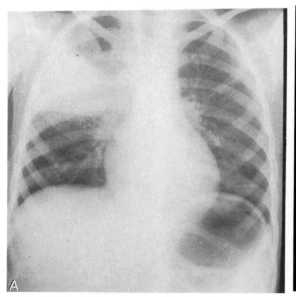
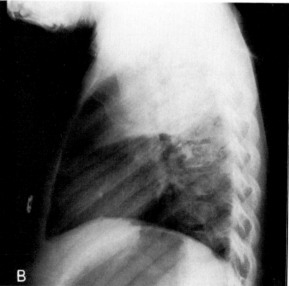

Figure 2–24. *A,* Posteroanterior chest film revealing right upper lobe pneumonia in a 4-year-old girl. *B,* Lateral chest film revealing fluid in all segments of the right upper lobe in a 4-year-old girl. The pneumonia shadow is sharply limited by the interlobar fissure between the mid and lower lobes.

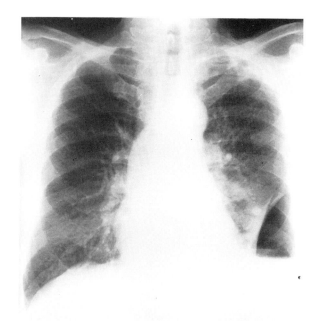

Figure 2–25. Hydropneumothorax in the left lung base. A pleural (lung) edge is noted adjacent to the pneumothorax.

producing apparatus may be administered. Thoracentesis is surgical puncture or tapping of the thoracic cavity. This is done to remove accumulations of fluid from the pleural cavity. The collapsed segment should reexpand with air after the compressing fluid is removed. Once the procedure is complete, the patient is positioned on his or her unaffected side to test the site of needle insertion. The wound should heal by itself.

Pneumothorax

General Information. Pneumothorax is the presence of air in the thorax. It can be caused by trauma, postoperative aspiration, interstitial lung disease such as emphysema, bronchopleural fistula, a ruptured esophagus, hyaline membrane disease, cystic fibrosis, and metastasis.

Diagnosis and Identification. Two visible radiographic signs are usually apparent on the PA chest radiograph when pneumothorax is suspected. The pleural edge is the line of visceral pleura forming the *lung edge*, which is separated from the chest wall by air. In addition, no vascular shadows are apparent in this area. The more the lung collapses, the more dense the appearance of the radiograph (Fig. 2–25). The detection of a pneumothorax may be difficult when the pneumothorax is extremely small. When a pneumothorax is suspected, the radiographer should include PA chest radiographs taken on *inspiration* and *expiration*. The expiration phase accentuates the pneumothorax because of the loss of negative pressure. In comparison, the film taken on *expiration* reveals more of the pneumothorax. This is important if the area of pneumothorax is small, because it could possibly be missed if a PA projection were taken only on inspiration. Because free air rises, it is imperative that erect positions be used (Fig. 2–26).

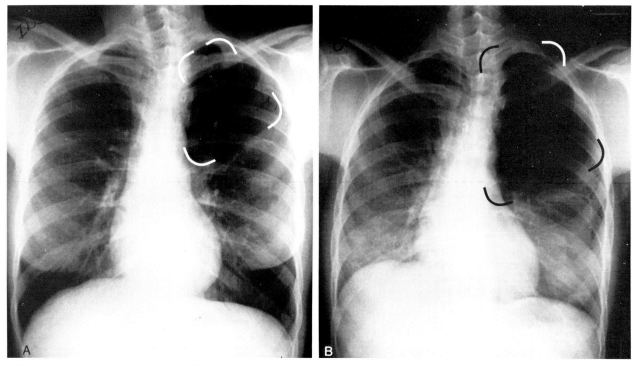

Figure 2–26. *A,* Spontaneous pneumothorax (brackets) demonstrated in the left upper lung on a posteroanterior chest film taken on inspiration. *B,* Spontaneous pneumothorax demonstrated in the left upper lung on a posteroanterior chest film taken on expiration. Note that the pneumothorax (brackets) is more apparent on expiration.

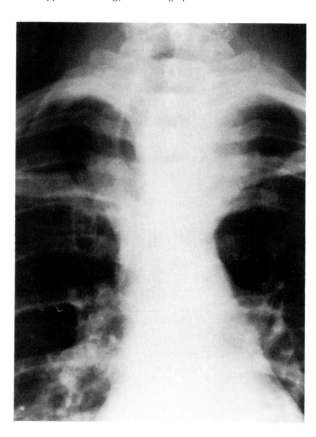

Figure 2–27. Deviation of the trachea. This is frequently seen on a posteroanterior chest film and indicates a tension pneumothorax.

Once the diagnosis of a pneumothorax has been confirmed, the next step is to determine whether or not any tension exists. In a *tension* pneumothorax, there is usually a shift of mediastinal structures toward the collapsed lobe. The trachea usually shifts toward the opposite side (Fig. 2–27). Tension pneumothorax is an especially dangerous form of pneumothorax characterized by air that escapes into the pleural cavity from a bronchus but that cannot reenter the bronchus. When this occurs, there is increased air pressure in the pleural cavity, causing progressive collapse of lung tissue. As a result, there is a marked impairment of venous return, which can severely compromise cardiac output and result in hypotension. The accuracy of patient positioning cannot be overemphasized. In evaluation of a potential tension pneumothorax and the displacement of midline structures, the coronal plane of the patient must be parallel to the film and not rotated.

Spontaneous pneumothorax usually affects healthy adults between the ages of 20 and 40 and is commonly associated with hyposthenic and asthenic body habitus. This type of pneumothorax is the result of rupture of subpleural emphysematous *blebs* or bullae. Blebs are blisters that form on the lung surface. There is no other indication of any abnormality or illness. The onset of spontaneous pneumothorax is sudden and dramatic. The patient usually complains of acute breathlessness accompanied by an acute, stabbing pain on either posterior side of the thorax. Many patients having these symptoms will be re-

ferred to the radiology department by their family physician without first being examined. Other such patients will frequently be treated in the emergency room. In either event, the radiographer must be alert to the importance of the patient's history and be sure to take PA inspiration and expiration chest radiographs.

Postoperative, traumatic, or *artificial* pneumothorax is a complication of thoracic surgery involving penetrating chest injuries such as gunshot or stab wounds or a bronchial biopsy. Rib fractures often result in a tear of the pleura, causing pneumothorax. In penetrating wounds, pneumothorax often coexists with hemothorax (Fig. 2–28). Pneumothorax may also be categorized as either *open* or *closed*. With open pneumothorax, air flows between the pleural space and the outside of the body. With closed pneumothorax, air reaches the pleural space directly from the lung. A complication of trauma is hydropneumothorax, an accumulation of serous fluid within the pleural cavity, which on the erect PA chest radiograph reveals horizontal *fluid levels* in the pleural cavity (Fig. 2–29). Pyopneumothorax, or pus in the thorax, is a complication when the penetrating wound is septic.

Treatment. Treatment is conservative unless increased pleural pressure (tension pneumothorax) is evident. A collapse of 30% or less of the lung usually does not require any treatment other than bed rest. If the patient's breathing is labored in the presence of sharp pain or if signs of physiological compromise

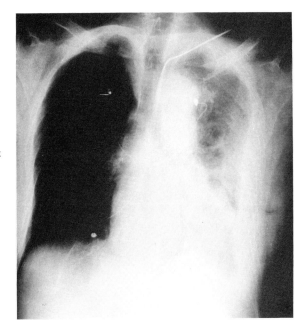

Figure 2–28. Moderate-sized pneumothorax following a translumbar aortogram in a 75-year-old woman.

are evident, further treatment is indicated. Most cases of pneumothorax require decompression of the lung by inserting a needle connected to a water seal drain into the pleural cavity. Approximately 50% of patients with tension pneumothorax will have a recurrence at some time. Recurrences are usually treated surgically.

Pneumonia

General Information. Pneumonia, an acute infection of the lung parenchyma, often impairs gas exchange. Three primary types of pneumonia have been identified: lobar, or bacterial pneumonia; lobular, or bronchopneumonia; and interstitial, or viral pneumonia or pneumonitis.

Overall, pneumonia is the sixth leading cause of death in the United States and is the leading secondary cause of death. Infants younger than 1 year and adults between the ages of 65 and 74 have the highest mortality rate. Despite the advances in antibiotic therapy, pneumonia currently accounts for 40% of hospital deaths. In 1985, 64,720 people succumbed to pneumonia. There were 7010 more pneumonia-related deaths in 1985 than in 1984. In 1983, the mortality rate, according to the Department of Health

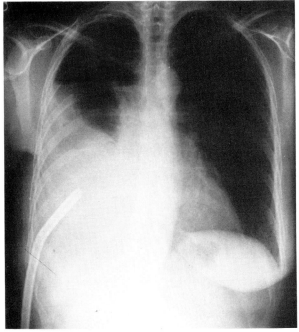

Figure 2–29. Right-sided hydropneumothorax postpneumonectomy in a 50-year-old woman.

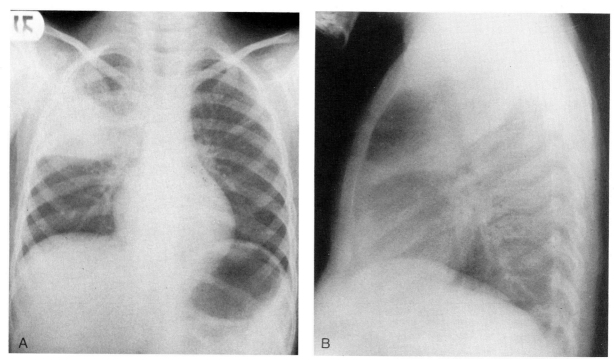

Figure 2–30. *A,* Right upper lobe pneumonia as seen on a posteroanterior chest film in a 4-year-old girl. *B,* Lateral view, revealing the involvement of all segments of the upper lobe.

and Human Services, was 27.9 deaths per 100,000 population based on a 10% sample of deaths.

Pneumonia may be caused by either bacteria or viruses. Ninety percent of all bacterial pneumonia is caused by the pneumococcus *(Streptococcus pneumoniae)* organism. Other offending agents include staphylococci and gram-negative enteric bacilli. These types of organisms are always present in the upper respiratory tract. They lie dormant until a person's resistance is lowered. Conditions such as the common cold, neoplastic diseases, alcoholism, or generalized poor health often lower the patient's ability to fight off these bacterial organisms.

Diagnosis. Lobar or bacterial pneumonia involves mostly the alveoli of an entire lobe without involving the bronchi. This disease invades the body via the nasal or oral passageways. It can occur unilaterally or bilaterally. When occurring bilaterally, it is referred to as double pneumonia. Characteristically, the alveoli become filled with inflammatory exudate so that air is prevented from entering. The onset of lobar pneumonia is usually acute and presents five cardinal symptoms: coughing, sputum production, pleuritic chest pain, chills, and fever. During this rapid onset, the pulse and respiration rates increase twofold.

Radiographically, lobar pneumonia presents a mass of consolidated *fluid* in one or more lobes. Depending on the concentration of alveolar exudate, the consolidation varies in opacification. In order to establish the degree of segmental involvement, it is essential that a lateral view be included in addition to the

standard anterior view of the chest (Fig. 2–30). If this condition is allowed to persist, complications are possible, such as lung abscess, empyema, pulmonary fibrosis, meningitis, and endocarditis.

Lobular or bronchopneumonia is a *patchy, irregular* distribution of disease that involves the inflammation of the bronchi and bronchioles with extension into the alveoli. Thus, bronchopneumonia involves all structures (bronchi, bronchioles, and alveoli) whereas lobar pneumonia involves only the alveoli. The symptoms of bronchopneumonia are more gradual in onset, less dramatic, and much milder than those of lobar pneumonia. Conditions such as bronchitis and pertussis may predispose to bronchopneumonia, because an inflammatory mucus exudate collects and obstructs bronchi. This is commonly referred to as *endobronchial* obstruction, and it often results in the continuation or recurrence of pneumonia that tends to be more severe than the initial event. Both lungs are usually involved, specifically the posterior and basal parts of the lower lobes. Radiographically, the patchy, irregular distribution is localized in one or more lobes around the bronchi (Fig. 2–31). Bronchopneumonia can be categorized into several subtypes: hypostatic, which is usually a secondary complication of heart disease and cerebral hemorrhage; aspiration, caused by inhalation of septic materials into the lung during surgery of the mouth, pharynx, or upper respiratory tract; postoperative, related to atelectasis caused by the plugging of bronchi by secretions or exudates; suppurative, characterized by necrosis and pus formation; and chemical, which is the result of inhaling poisonous or irritating gases.

Interstitial pneumonia (viral pneumonia or pneumonitis) is different from other forms of pneumonia in that it is caused by a virus and no exudate is present in the alveoli. Pneumonitis is often acquired secondarily as a complication of viral diseases such as measles, influenza, pertussis, chicken pox, psittacosis, and other infectious diseases. Viral pneumonia often occurs in epidemic proportions. Interstitial pneumonia is common in certain occupations such as farming. Farmer's lung is a form of pneumonitis resulting from the inhalation of dust from crop dust, moldy hay, or silage. Patients with farmer's lung generally complain of flu-like symptoms. Radiographically, the infection is distributed throughout *all* lobes but tends to be more central than peripheral. Viral pneumonia is more common but less severe than bacterial lobar pneumonia (Fig. 2–32).

Lipid pneumonia is caused by oil and fat substances that are introduced by aspiration of small droplets, producing peribronchial consolidation, which is essentially a foreign body reaction. Cod liver oil and olive oil may gain entrance to the lung during forced feeding, such as when vitamins are given to small children who resist. A form of aspiration pneumonia can also occur in the presence of a neuromuscular defect that impairs the swallowing mechanism, resulting in the aspiration of food contents into the lungs.

Treatment. Bacterial pneumonias are treated with the combination of antibiotics and bed rest. The specific viruses that cause pneumonia are unknown. Treatment of viral pneumonia is supportive and focuses on symptomatic relief. Patients are encouraged to remain in bed and to increase their intake of fluids.

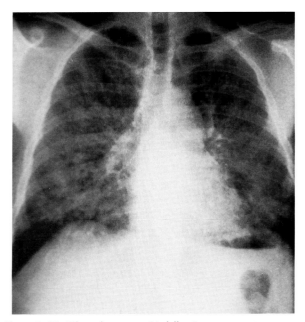

Figure 2–32. Bilateral pneumonitis following exposure to chicken pox and varicella virus. The patient is a 28-year-old man.

Pulmonary Embolism and Infarction

General Information. Pulmonary emboli usually originate in the deep veins of the lower extremities, pelvis, prostatic venous plexus, vena cava, and right atrium. Pulmonary embolism is most common in the elderly, persons with certain diseases, and following surgical procedures such as abdominal and pelvic operations. Patients with a history of pulmonary hypertension and pulmonary arteriosclerosis have an increased tendency to develop an embolism. Early postoperative ambulation helps prevent blood stasis in the deep venous system of the lower extremities and subsequent thrombi, which can break loose and travel to the lung as emboli. An embolus that blocks the pulmonary artery or one of its branches can produce an infarction and result in rapid death. This condition could be mistaken for a coronary occlusion. Pulmonary embolism is the most common pulmonary complication of hospitalized patients. It strikes an estimated 6,000,000 adults in the United States each year, resulting in more than 100,000 deaths. Although this condition may be asymptomatic, massive pulmonary obstruction and infarction are fatal more than 50% of the time. Aside from the thrombus, which is the most common embolic substance, emboli take other forms, including air, fat, metastatic neoplasms, brain tissue from severe head injuries, amniotic fluid, trophoblastic tissues in pregnancy, parasites, and foreign material such as talc, abused drugs, mercury, and iodized oil, such as that used in lymphangiography. Emboli are possible sequelae of fractures and severe burns.

Diagnosis. The first symptom of pulmonary embolism is usually dyspnea accompanied by chest pain.

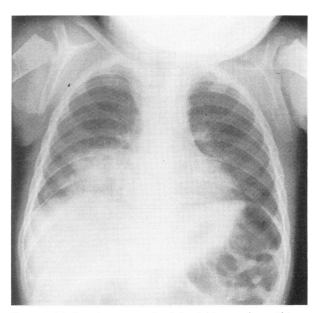

Figure 2–31. Bronchopneumonia of the right upper lung. This 16-month-old boy inhaled turpentine.

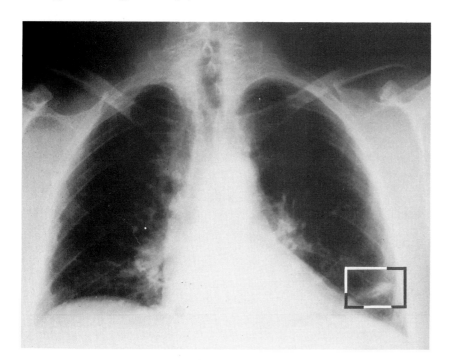

Figure 2–33. A wedge-shaped infiltrate (rectangle) in the left lower lung as the result of pulmonary emboli following a venogram.

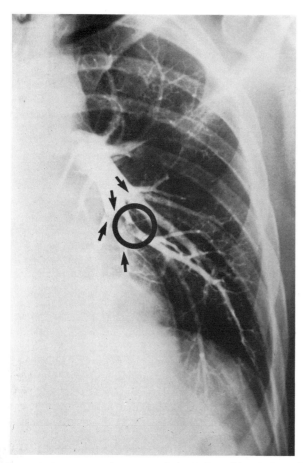

Figure 2–34. Large pulmonary embolus indicated by circle and arrows in the distal branches of the left lower pulmonary tree of a pulmonary angiogram.

It is not uncommon for the findings on the chest radiograph to be negative; however, densities similar to that of pneumonia with diffuse borders are common. Increased *radiolucency* distal to the embolus may be evident as a result of decreased perfusion of the vasculature. A characteristic *wedge-shaped* infiltrate also points to embolism. Pleural effusion may be evident on the affected side, as well as plate-like atelectasis (Fig. 2–33).

Small emboli usually do not produce any visible effect on chest radiographs unless they occur over a long period of time and cause pulmonary hypertension. Pulmonary angiography is useful in demonstrating pulmonary emboli when they are large and must be surgically removed (Fig. 2–34). Nuclear medicine lung-perfusion scans are used specifically to diagnose pulmonary embolism. One or more filling defects are usually seen on the scan, as well as other perfusion defects such as pneumonia, emphysema, and pleural effusion. The perfusion scan can rule out embolism so that other disease possibilities can be explored (Fig. 2–35).

Lung Abscess and Empyema

General Information. By definition, an abscess is a localized spherical lesion consisting of a collection of pus in a cavity formed by the disintegration of tissue. An abscess is caused by an organism that invades the tissue. Empyema is pus contained within a cavitary abscess. Empyema is a persistent purulent form of pleurisy that complicates bacterial pneumonia

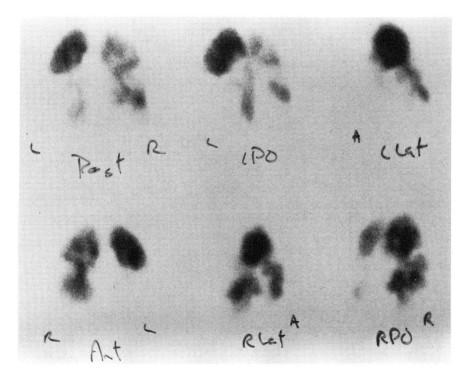

Figure 2–35. Multiple perfusion defects as seen on a nuclear lung scan. This 55-year-old man has a history of cancer.

and tuberculosis. It may also be the result of aspiration of oropharyngeal contents. Poor oral hygiene with dental gingival disease may also cause empyema.

Diagnosis. Infected lesions can be demonstrated radiographically on plain PA and lateral chest views and with linear tomography. It sometimes is difficult to differentiate an abscess from a lung tumor, but *tomography* helps make that distinction. Fluid consolidation in the lungs is a condition that can radically change or resolve itself in a short time. A lung tumor does not usually change quickly or resolve itself. Thus, tomography is quite useful in differentiating various types of lung pathology (Fig. 2–36).

Treatment. Preventing advancement of the disease is of prime importance. If an open wound ensues, warm moist applications help drain the pus from the wound. Various antibiotics are used to treat the infection.

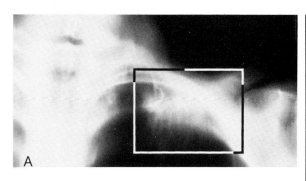
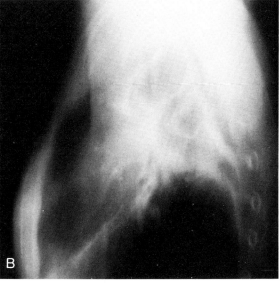

Figure 2–36. *A,* Anteroposterior linear tomogram revealing an empyemic process (rectangle) in the left lung apex of a 16-year-old. *B,* Several empyemic cavities seen on a lateral tomographic study of the left posterior lung. This occurred secondary to tuberculosis in this 40-year-old woman.

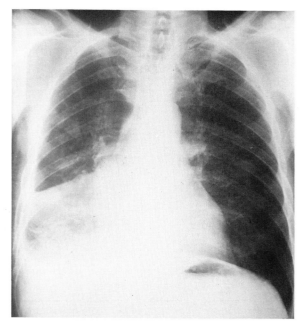

Figure 2–37. Right-sided pleural effusion in a 49-year-old man.

Pleural Effusion and Hydrothorax

General Information. Pleural effusion is an accumulation of an exudate or transudate in the pleural space or cavity as a consequence of various forms of inflammation, primary or secondary neoplasms, vascular infarction, collagen diseases, pneumoconioses, and organ failure. Hydrothorax is a collection of fluid in which no infection is present. It is frequently associated with trauma and pulmonary vascular diseases. Hemothorax is fluid containing blood and is commonly encountered with hydrothorax. Hemothorax is usually the result of blunt or penetrating chest trauma. It occurs in 25% of all cases of chest trauma. A mediastinal shift is frequently present on the chest radiograph. Pleural fluid that is a purulent exudate is known as pyothorax or empyema.

Diagnosis. The character of the pleural fluid—transudate, exudate, pus, or blood—cannot be differentiated radiographically because all pleural fluids have the same density as water and appear **white** or **opaque** on the radiograph. Depending on the stage of fluid accumulation, the visualization of the costophrenic angles varies from **blunted** to totally obliterated. When larger amounts of fluid are present, the fluid appears higher laterally than medially (Fig. 2–37). Characteristically, an air bronchogram is usually not associated with a pleural effusion. When air and fluid are observed simultaneously in the pleural space, hydropneumothorax is present (Fig. 2–38). Fluid that appears to change location when the body position is altered is referred to as free fluid. When there is no fluid shift with changes in body position, the fluid is said to be encapsulated or **loculated**. In the presence of encapsulated fluid, pleural thickening is seen elsewhere in the same side and frequently an **interlobar fissure**, a lens-shaped effusion, can be seen lying between the oblique or horizontal fissure (Fig. 2–39). In addition to the erect PA and lateral views of the chest, a lateral decubitus view is often necessary to differentiate pleural fluid from underlying pathology.

Treatment. Because pleural effusion can compress the lung and cause collapse and subsequent dyspnea, it is important that the fluid be removed by natural or surgical means. If the stimulus is removed, the fluid usually resolves itself and reabsorbs. However, when there are large amounts of fluid, a chest tube is inserted via thoracentesis and fluid is drained from the cavity. When empyema is present, the patient usually is given antibiotics by intramuscular injection.

Chronic Disorders

Chronic Obstructive Pulmonary Disease

General Information. COPD is a nonspecific chronic condition of persistent obstruction of bronchial airflow. It is often associated with long-term chronic respiratory disorders such as asthma, bronchitis, emphysema, tuberculosis, and pneumoconioses. COPD is the most significant pulmonary disorder in the United States and is the fifth leading cause of death. It is the second most common cause of hospital admission. According to the Social Security Administration, COPD is ranked second to heart disease as a cause of disability in men older than 40 years.

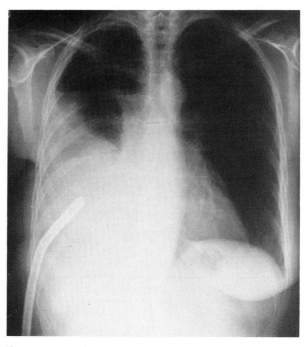

Figure 2–38. Hydropneumothorax postpneumonectomy in a 50-year-old woman.

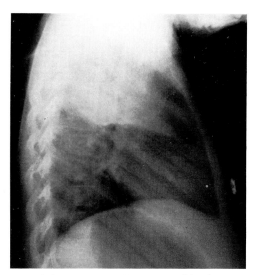

Figure 2–39. Lobar pneumonia in a 4-year-old girl. An interlobar fissure demonstrates involvement of the upper lobe.

COPD involves a combination of signs and symptoms, and there is no single specific cause. Factors such as smoking and inhalation of particulate matter have been identified. Employment situations such as mining and chemical industries may serve as environmental stimuli to provoke a significant variety of lung disorders that ultimately culminate in COPD. The offspring of affected persons are often more susceptible to lung diseases.

The advancement of this disease takes place before symptoms are apparent, so treatment is difficult and often unsuccessful. The early symptoms are dyspnea and a mild, persistent cough that is often disregarded as smoker's cough with sputum production. Eventually the individual becomes fatigued with even the least amount of physical activity.

Diagnosis. In addition to the physical symptoms of COPD, other diagnostic clues may be found on chest radiographs, which usually reveal *emphysema*. The cardiac silhouette is elongated, and the aortic arch is predominantly visible. The heart appears elongated on deep inspiration, with increased *radiolucency* noted bilaterally in the lower lung fields. The diaphragms are usually flattened rather than dome shaped (Fig. 2–40). The disease at this point is irreversible. An opaque bronchogram reveals dilated and ragged-appearing bronchi, especially in the lower lobes. This permanent dilatation is referred to as *bronchiectasis* (see Fig. 2–7). The patient's cough becomes progressively more productive of thick, mucus-laden sputum. The patient becomes less resistant to other forms of respiratory diseases. Bronchopleural infections are frequent, and other late effects such as pulmonary edema may develop, eventually leading to congestive heart failure.

Treatment. Because COPD occurs as a result of numerous insults to the respiratory system over a long period of time, the treatment usually consists of preventing further complications. In many cases, the symptoms can be only temporarily relieved, since the heart usually begins to fail. The heart begins to shut down because it can no longer compensate for decreased blood flow in the face of the accumulation of symptoms and the long-standing decreased airflow. The blood sent to the tissues is grossly inadequate. As lesser amounts of fluid are distributed to the lung parenchyma, serous fluid begins to leak through the vessel membranes, causing pulmonary edema. The edema compresses the already damaged lung tissue and makes it more difficult for the lungs to ventilate. Breathing becomes labored. Cardiac arrest ensues when the heart can no longer function.

Asthma

General Information. Bronchial asthma is a condition characterized by recurrent attacks of dyspnea with wheezing and difficulty in expiration due to spasmodic constriction of the bronchi. Three different types of asthma are identified: (1) *extrinsic* asthma is usually due to an allergic condition. The allergens are usually suspended in the air and often are in the form of pollen, dust, air pollution, and animal dander. Fifty percent of all cases of asthma are a result of an allergic sensitivity, affecting children and young adults. (2) *Intrinsic* or *nonallergic* asthma occurs secondary to existing bronchial infections, such as those involving the tonsils, adenoids, and paranasal sinuses. (3) *Mixed* asthma is a combination of both intrinsic and extrinsic types. Persons with any type of asthma are particularly sensitive to emotional

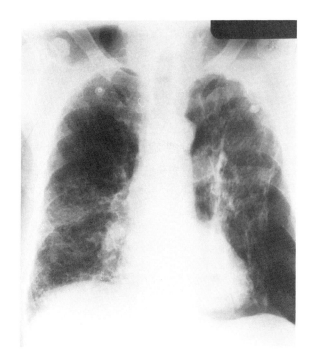

Figure 2–40. Diffuse interstitial scarring and bullous disease consistent with chronic obstructive pulmonary disease and emphysema in this 75-year-old man. A left pneumothorax is noted in the left base laterally and anteriorly.

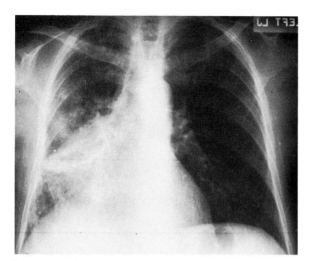

Figure 2–41. Chronic asthma in a 63-year-old woman. Areas of increased opacification are consistent with endobronchial obstruction.

stress, environmental changes in humidity and temperature, and exposure to noxious fumes or airborne allergens.

Diagnosis. Chest x-rays may be diagnostic during an attack, when the lungs are *hyperinflated* with trapped air. If mucus secretions are trapped, occluding bronchi, segmental atelectasis is usually apparent. Generally, when the bronchial lining thickens, areas of increased *opacification* are seen on the radiograph (Fig. 2–41). Allergy testing can identify those materials and foods to which the patient is sensitive.

Treatment. The treatment of asthma may involve the use of bronchodilators, antihistamines, and oxygen. Patients should know which allergens may provoke an asthma attack and must be aware of how stress and anxiety affect their condition.

Bronchitis

General Information. Chronic bronchitis is a clinical diagnosis determined on confirmation of a productive cough for a period of at least 3 months in 2 consecutive years. Bronchitis appears to be common in persons who smoke heavily for long periods, usually years. This condition produces widespread inflammation, with thickening of the bronchial walls and the secretion of mucus.

Diagnosis. The effects of chronic inflammation impede the passage of air through the bronchi. In more severe cases, bronchial obstruction occurs. A possible complication of bronchitis is bronchopneumonia. Chest radiographs may reveal *hyperinflation* and increased bronchovascular markings (Fig. 2–42).

Treatment. The most obvious treatment is the removal of the causative agent, smoking. Antibiotics are administered in the presence of infection. The patient may receive respiratory therapy, and medications can reduce spasm and increase airflow (bronchodilators). In more serious cases, oxygen may be administered.

Emphysema

General Information. Pulmonary emphysema is the most common chronic disease of the lungs and is a major cause of pulmonary disability. It is usually included as part of the syndrome associated with COPD. Pulmonary emphysema is an irreversible overaeration or dilatation of the air spaces accompanied by destruction of walls of the alveoli. Emphysema can be found at any location within the lungs, and it develops slowly over a period of years. It is associated with chronic inflammation such as that in heavy smokers. Emphysema is currently more prevalent in men than in women. Ventilation deficits can be detected as early as adolescence but are most often disabling between the ages of 50 and 80. Pulmonary emphysema can occur secondarily as a complication of other chronic respiratory illnesses, including asthma, bronchitis, and tuberculosis. It is one of the major causes of death in industralized countries. The mortality rate due to emphysema is doubling every 5 years, possibly because of increases in industrial air pollutants, exhaust fumes from automobiles, and smoking. The significant increase in disease, especially in women, is of great concern. It is thought that women are acquiring emphysema and other lung disorders more often as the result of increased cigarette smoking.

Diagnosis. Three types of pulmonary emphysema have been identified. In centrilobar emphysema, the alveoli occupying the central area become dilated and permanently expanded. This is more prominent in the upper lobes but may extend into all lung areas. Centrilobar emphysema is most commonly associated with bronchitis. The panolobar type is marked by enlarged lungs and a loss of vascular lung markings in the lower anterior segments. The paraseptal type is characterized by subpleural blebs and bullae.

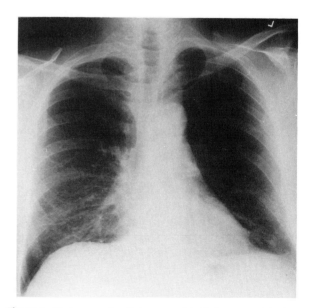

Figure 2–42. Increased radiolucency of both lungs consistent with chronic bronchitis, emphysema, and obstructive disease. The patient is a 56-year-old man.

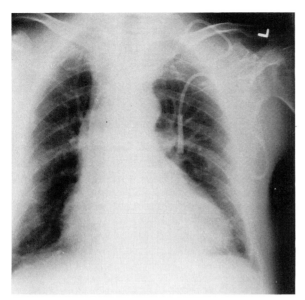

Figure 2–43. Flattening of both hemidiaphragms with emphysematous changes in a 57-year-old man. There is cardiomegaly, with vascular congestion. A transvenous catheter is seen entering the right atrium from the left.

PA and lateral chest radiographs most often reveal large, *oversized lungs* that are paper thin and compress with pressure. There are areas of increased blackening or radiolucency, compatible with *overinflation* and destruction of the distal bronchioles and alveoli. The pulmonary vessels present *tortuosity* and a *diminished* visibility. These are two important signs of pulmonary emphysema. The lung bases present a *flattened* appearance rather than the typical dome-shaped contour (Fig. 2–43).

As the lungs become less efficient, dyspnea usually results. A moist and persistent cough is evident because of the mixing of air and fluid in the alveoli. Rales can be heard. Because this alveolar dilatation involves large numbers of alveoli over a period of years, the patient may develop a barrel chest. Cardiac complications eventually ensue, with right ventricular hypertrophy and subsequent right heart failure or cor pulmonale.

Treatment. Aside from the elimination of smoking and other air pollutants, treatment is largely supportive. Bronchodilators can reduce bronchospasm and promote air movement through the bronchi. Antibiotics are administered for lung infection. Oxygen is administered as necessary.

Bronchiectasis

General Information. Bronchiectasis is a weakening of the wall of the bronchus due to chronic inflammation. The weakened wall becomes permanently dilated. It primarily affects the lower lobes of the lungs bilaterally. Because the lower segments are farthest away from the heart, they are most dependent on life-giving oxygen and thus are most susceptible to disease.

Bronchiectasis occurs in three forms: In the cylindrical or fusiform type, the bronchioles expand unevenly, show little change in diameter, and suddenly terminate in a squared-off fashion. Varicose bronchiectasis is characterized by abnormal, irregular dilatation and narrowing of the bronchi, which appear similar to varicose veins. Saccular or cystic bronchiectasis consists of many large dilatations at the end of the bronchi (Fig. 2–44).

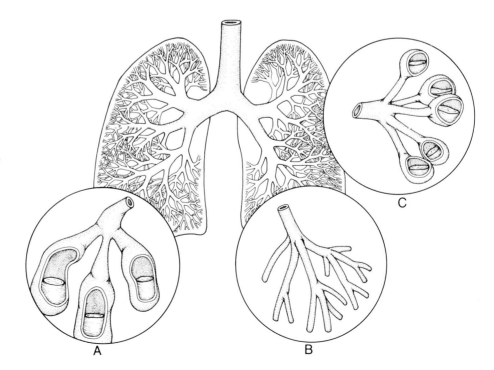

Figure 2–44. The three primary types of bronchiectasis: A = varicose; B = cylindrical or fusiform; C = saccular or cystic.

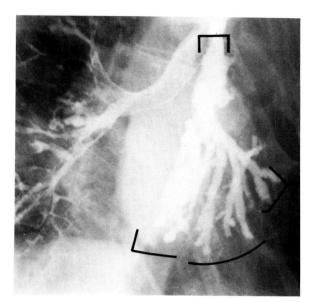

Figure 2–45. Oblique view of an opaque bronchogram reveals extensive dilatation of the left lower bronchi (brackets) consistent with bronchiectasis and long-term disease.

Bronchiectasis can affect both sexes and any age-group, but it is most prominent in persons with persistent chronic disease and inflammation. The dilatation is permanent (Fig. 2–45).

Diagnosis. The most apparent sign of bronchiectasis is a persistent cough that is accompanied by foul-smelling, mucopurulent secretions. Routine chest radiographs reveal *peribronchial thickening*, areas of atelectasis, and scattered cystic changes (Fig. 2–46).

Bronchoscopy is a surgical procedure for viewing the trachea and air passageways with a special endoscope that is passed into the trachea of a sedated patient. Bronchoscopy can determine the extent of disease and inflammation and makes possible a biopsy of tissue. This is often referred to as bronchial brushing. A minute bristle brush passed through a catheter is used to scrape tissue samples off of the bronchial wall. Bronchoscopy can also identify other lesions not previously recognized. Bronchography, a most definitive and reliable diagnostic procedure, often follows bronchoscopy. In bronchography, an oily positive contrast agent, frequently Dionosil, is instilled into the trachea. This is accomplished either by passing a catheter through the nose or mouth into the trachea or by percutaneous injection of contrast media through the intercricothyroid membrane. The medium is then aspirated into the lungs. Radiographs are obtained with the patient erect. Routine positions include PA, lateral, and both obliques. The radiopaque medium outlines the bronchial walls and reveals the location and extent of bronchiectasis (Fig. 2–47).

Treatment. Dilatation of the bronchi due to bronchiectasis is permanent, and there is essentially no curative treatment. The treatment is palliative, and

medications such as bronchodilators are used to help keep the air moving through the lungs. Postural drainage helps remove the secretions.

Tuberculosis

General Information. Even today pulmonary tuberculosis is still the most significant disease in many areas of the world, but no longer in the United States. The American Lung Association estimates that active disease afflicts nearly 14 of every 100,000 people. Tuberculosis is an infectious, inflammatory, and chronic disorder. It is most common in the lungs but may be found in most any organ or structure of the body. It is produced by various types of mycobacteria. Tuberculosis is transmitted by inhalation of infected droplets. In some areas of the world, this disease is transmitted by infected milk from dairy cattle. Within the body, the bacteria can remain dormant for many decades, only to reactivate when the patient's resistance is lowered.

The primary infection usually involves the middle or lower lung. The primary lesion consist of a small area of exudation in the lung parenchyma, which quickly spreads into the bronchopulmonary lymph nodes and gains entry into the bloodstream.

All school-age children receive the Mantoux or tine test, which consists of an intradermal injection or

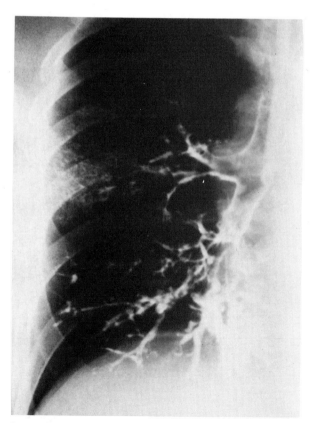

Figure 2–46. Bronchiectasis with peribronchial thickening.

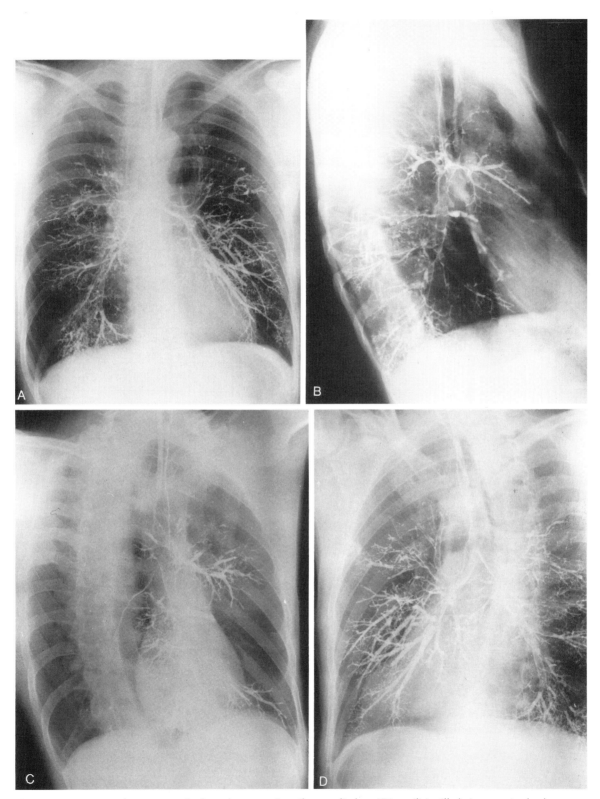

Figure 2–47. *A,* Normal posteroanterior bronchogram using oily propyliodone (Dionosil) instilled via a nasotracheal catheter. *B,* Normal left lateral bronchogram. *C,* Normal left anterior oblique view bronchogram. *D,* Normal right anterior oblique view bronchogram.

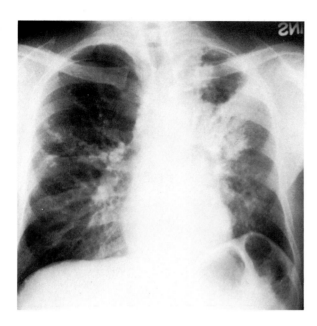

Figure 2–48. Widespread bilateral tuberculosis. Radiograph of a 56-year-old man taken up on inspiration.

penetration of a purified protein derivative of tuberculin. A raised indurated wheal 8 to 10 mm in diameter 48 to 72 hours after injection is considered a positive result. Because false positives are common, further testing is scheduled before a definitive diagnosis is made. False negatives can also occur in persons with certain viral disorders such as cancer.

Diagnosis. In addition to a positive reaction to tuberculin skin test and the presence of tubercular bacilli in sputum, diagnostic procedures include routine chest radiography, which typically reveals **nodular** lesions as well as patchy infiltrates, cavitation, fibrosis, and calcium deposits. Unfortunately, chest radiographs cannot always distinguish active from inactive disease. Tomography of the lungs helps distinguish an abnormal lesion from fibrotic scarring (Fig. 2–48).

Treatment. As compared with the 1950s and 1960s, when patients were placed in isolation in sanitariums for months and even years, now patients are treated with chemotherapy and oral medication over a 9- to 18-month period. This treatment requires only short-term hospitalization. Patients are not considered infectious after 2 to 4 weeks and can resume their usual life-style. In the past, the treatment of tuberculosis involved disfiguring types of surgery such as thoracoplasty. Materials such as paraffin wax and inflated plastic bags were inserted into the thoracic cavity (Fig. 2–49).

Pneumoconioses

General Information. Pneumoconioses are pulmonary changes taking place following the inhalation of a variety of dusts and particulate matter. These changes depend on the type and amount of dust inhaled, the size of the dust particles, and the duration of exposure. Some types of dust give rise to widespread nodules, even though there are no early symptoms. Silicosis is one condition in which the inhaled dust particles will eventually produce lung changes such as fibrosis of the lungs. Thus, some types of particulate matter are more dangerous than others. A small amount of asbestos can immediately give rise to pulmonary fibrosis.

There are four distinct types of pneumoconioses. Silicosis is the result of the inhalation of silica particles. This is the most common form of pneumoconiosis, and it occurs after 1 to 3 years of exposure in those operating sand-blasting equipment or working in deep tunnel projects. In the early stages, silicosis is usually asymptomatic. Silicosis has a favorable prognosis when fibrosis is not widespread. Respiratory distress and eventual cor pulmonale are the results of widespread pulmonary fibrosis.

Asbestosis is caused by inhalation of asbestos fibers. Individuals employed in the fireproofing and textile industries are often affected by this disease. Very small amounts of asbestos can cause pulmonary fibrosis. The earliest symptom of asbestosis is dyspnea on exertion, which usually is evident after about 10 years of exposure.

Berylliosis is caused by exposure to beryllium dust or inhalation of associated fumes. Beryllium can also be absorbed through the skin. It has been known to produce ulcers when beryllium was accidentally implanted in the skin.

Coal miner's disease is a progressive form of pneumoconiosis producing nodular pulmonary disease. Coal miner's disease is frequently referred to as black lung, miner's asthma, and anthracosis. Its incidence is highest in the anthracite coal mines in the eastern United States.

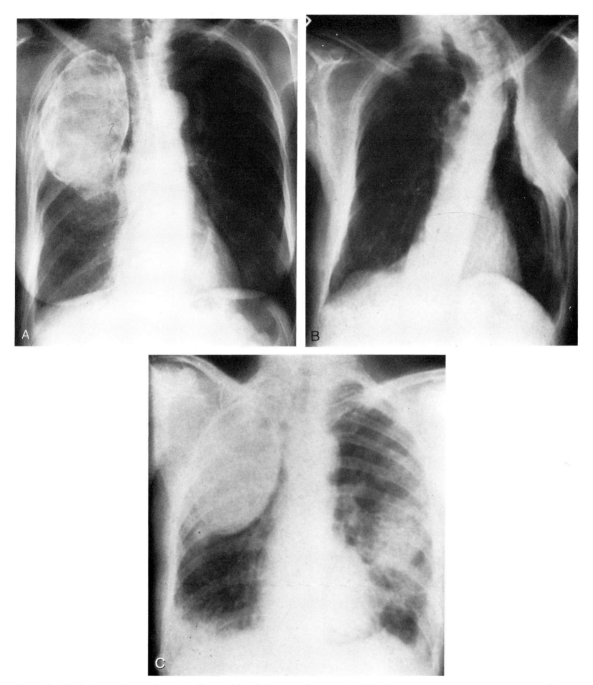

Figure 2–49. *A,* A paraffin pack or plumbage of the right upper lung cavity following pneumonectomy in a 60-year-old woman. *B,* Left thoracoplasty with some upper lobe scarring but no active disease in a 61-year-old woman. Also noted is levoscoliosis. *C,* An inflated plastic bag occupying the upper left cavity, with widespread tuberculosis apparent bilaterally.

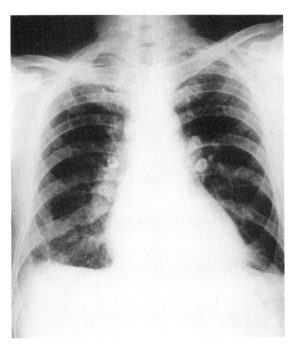

Figure 2–50. Eggshell calcification in both hilar regions consistent with silicosis.

Diagnosis. Diagnostic confirmation of silicosis is chiefly accomplished via routine chest radiography. Nodules result when alveolar macrophages ingest silica particles, which they are unable to process. PA and lateral chest radiographs typically reveal small, discrete *nodular* lesions distributed bilaterally throughout the lungs, with concentration in the upper lobes. The hilar lymph nodes may be enlarged and exhibit *eggshell* calcifications (Fig. 2–50).

In asbestosis, the clinical manifestations appear before the lung changes are noted on the radiographs. The radiographs often reveal fine, irregular, and linear diffuse infiltrates. Extensive fibrosis results in a *honeycomb* or ground-glass appearance. There is also evidence of pleural thickening and calcification, with obliteration of the costophrenic angles. In the later stages, the heart appears enlarged and presents a classic shaggy heart border (Fig. 2–51).

The chest radiographs of a patient having berylliosis usually show pulmonary edema, as evidenced by *patchy diffuse infiltrates* with prominent peribronchial markings.

In coal miner's pneumoconiosis, numerous small *opacities* less than 10 mm in diameter are most prominent in the upper lung fields. In advanced stages of this disease, cavitary lesions may be identified (Fig. 2–52).

Treatment. The primary goal in treating all forms of pneumoconioses is to relieve the apparent respiratory symptoms, minimize hypoxia, and prevent infections. Daily treatments with bronchodilating mists and aerosols, steam inhalation, and chest physical therapy, which involves controlled coughing and postural drainage, all are excellent methods of treatment. However, success of these supportive methods depends on the extent of disease.

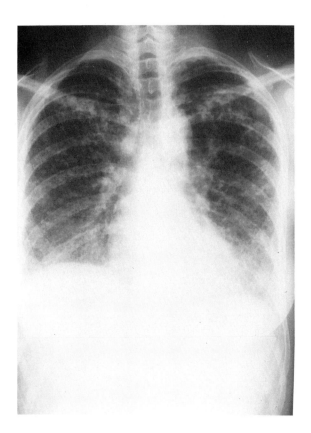

Figure 2–51. Extensive bilateral infiltrate with a ground-glass appearance and a shaggy heart border consistent with asbestosis. The patient is a 40-year-old woman.

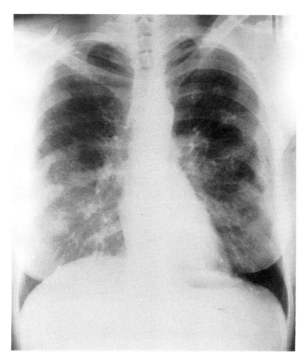

Figure 2–52. Multiple opacifications bilaterally, consistent with pneumoconiosis.

Fungal Diseases

Histoplasmosis

General Information. Histoplasmosis is an infection caused by a yeast-like organism, which can be detected in sputum, bone marrow, and lymph node biopsy samples. This condition is known by several names, including Ohio Valley disease, Central Mississippi Valley disease, Appalachian Mountain disease, and Darling's disease. Histoplasmosis assumes three forms. The primary acute form is the most common and is typically benign. It is characterized by a mild respiratory tract illness that includes headaches, fever, general malaise, anorexia, cough, and chest pain, which resolves spontaneously.

The progressive disseminated form causes hepatomegaly, generalized lymphadenopathy, anorexia, weight loss, fever, and numerous other symptoms.

The chronic pulmonary cavitary type is the most serious, usually mimics tuberculosis, and involves a productive cough, dyspnea, and occasional hemoptysis.

Diagnosis. Routine chest radiographs typically reveal pulmonary *calcifications* that are multiple, uniformly round, small, and totally benign. The chronic form may produce cavitary lesions that may resemble those of tuberculosis (Fig. 2–53).

Treatment. Primary acute histoplasmosis acts like a mild respiratory tract illness and usually requires minimal treatment. The progressive and chronic forms are more severe and require a treatment plan that may include chemotherapy, surgical lung resection, and supportive oxygen therapy. Patients having the more severe forms may require long-term hospitalization. Individuals working in fields should be encouraged to wear face masks to minimize inhalation of contaminated particulate matter.

Coccidioidomycosis

General Information. This fungal infection is also referred to as San Joaquin Valley fever and is found in the southwestern United States, especially between the San Joaquin Valley in California and southwestern Texas. It is most prevalent in the warm, dry months and in open dusty areas. This disease is most common among migrant farm workers who inhale soil contaminated by dried bird droppings. Respiratory tract infections are the result of this inhalation. Symptoms such as cough, pleuritic chest pain, fever, sore throat, chills, malaise, and headache are typical. This condition usually resolves in a few weeks without incident.

Diagnosis. Routine chest radiographs usually reveal a diffuse bilateral *infiltrate* and pleural *effusion.* The symptoms along with the occupational history usually provide the basis for diagnosis.

Treatment. Treatment of coccidioidomycosis is very conservative, and bed rest usually relieves the symptoms.

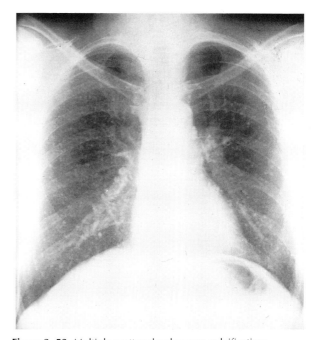

Figure 2–53. Multiple scattered pulmonary calcifications representing a miliary distribution. Findings are consistent with a previous granulomatous process, such as histoplasmosis in this 51-year-old man.

Self-Assessment Quiz

For each of the following questions, select the one best response and circle the letter that precedes it.

1. Among the leading causes of death, chronic obstructive pulmonary disease ranks
   a. second
   b. third
   c. fourth
   d. fifth

2. Which chest position is used to separate anatomical structures that are superimposed?
   a. anterior
   b. posterior
   c. oblique
   d. AP

3. The air-bronchogram sign becomes visible when areas of fluid consolidation collapse, contrast each other, and render the bronchi visible.
   a. true
   b. false

4. The silhouette sign is the loss of visualization of normal anatomy that should be present on a routine anterior view of the chest.
   a. true
   b. false

5. The collection of thick mucus, reduced airflow, and trapping of bacteria all are signs of
   a. hyaline membrane disease
   b. croup
   c. cystic fibrosis
   d. azygos vein fissure

6. Cystic fibrosis is an inherited condition that affects
   a. the lungs
   b. the bile ducts
   c. the pancreas
   d. all of the above

7. Hyaline membrane disease is a condition typically found in premature infants.
   a. true
   b. false

8. An insufficient quantity of surfactant may result in a condition known as
   a. hyaline membrane disease
   b. cystic fibrosis
   c. emphysema
   d. croup

9. Crib death is otherwise known as
   a. hyaline membrane disease
   b. sudden infant death syndrome
   c. pertussis
   d. histoplasmosis

10. Azygos vein fissure is considered to be a congenital normal lung variant.
    a. true
    b. false

11. A bark-like cough produced by inflammation, edema, and spasm is characteristic of the disorder known as
    a. croup
    b. atelectasis
    c. emphysema
    d. asthma

12. When airflow is inhibited, the osmotic pressure is decreased, resulting in serous fluid passing through the capillaries and into the lung interstitium and alveoli. This statement correctly describes
    a. atelectasis
    b. pulmonary edema
    c. pyothorax
    d. pleural effusion

13. Cor pulmonale is a condition that results in
    a. enlargement of the right ventricle
    b. pulmonary arterial hypertension
    c. failure of the right side of the heart
    d. all of the above

14. Radiographically, legionnaires' disease resembles
    a. atelectasis
    b. pneumothorax
    c. bronchopneumonia
    d. pneumonitis

15. Atelectasis is correctly described as
    a. the overexpansion of alveoli with air
    b. air in the thorax
    c. a collapse of all or part of the lung
    d. pus or blood in the lung

16. The most common cause of atelectasis is
    a. trauma
    b. infection
    c. obstruction of a bronchus
    d. pneumonia

17. Fluid accumulating within the pleural space is called
    a. pulmonary edema
    b. pneumothorax
    c. atelectasis
    d. pleural effusion

18. The term *lung edge* is used in conjunction with
    a. pneumothorax
    b. pneumonia
    c. pulmonary edema
    d. pleural fluid

19. When pneumothorax is suspected, the radiographer needs to
    a. take PA and lateral chest views
    b. include both lateral views
    c. take only a routine PA chest film
    d. include PA chest radiographs taken on inspiration and expiration

20. A tension pneumothorax may be associated with a shift of the trachea.
    a. true
    b. false

21. Subpleural or emphysematous blebs or bullae are findings associated with
    a. congestive heart failure
    b. cardiomegaly
    c. spontaneous pneumothorax
    d. pneumonia

22. Among the leading causes of death in the United States, pneumonia ranks
    a. second
    b. third
    c. fourth
    d. fifth
    e. sixth

23. Lobar pneumonia mostly involves lung alveoli of an entire lobe and is an acute disease caused by a
    a. bacterial organism
    b. virus

24. A patchy, irregular distribution of lung disease may be described as lobular or
    a. viral pneumonia
    b. pneumonitis
    c. bronchopneumonia
    d. pneumothorax

25. Interstitial pneumonia is also known as
    a. pneumonitis
    b. atelectasis
    c. viral pneumonia
    d. both pneumonitis and viral pneumonia

26. Aspiration pneumonia is which type of pneumonia?
    a. Viral
    b. Bronchopneumonia

27. A characteristic wedge-shaped infiltrate of the lung may indicate the presence of a pulmonary embolism.
    a. true
    b. false

28. Pus contained within a cavitary abscess is termed
    a. hemothorax
    b. pneumothorax
    c. hydrothorax
    d. pyothorax

29. Which of the following respiratory disorders may be associated with chronic obstructive pulmonary disease?
    a. asthma
    b. bronchitis
    c. emphysema
    d. tuberculosis
    e. all of the above

30. A permanent dilatation of the distal lower bronchi is termed
    a. bronchiectasis
    b. broncholysis
    c. bronchopneumonia
    d. emphysema

31. The most common chronic disease of the lungs is
    a. bronchitis
    b. emphysema
    c. atelectasis
    d. bronchiectasis

32. Hyperinflation or the overdistension of alveoli with air is called
    a. atelectasis
    b. bronchiectasis
    c. emphysema
    d. pneumothorax

33. Flattened lung bases, increased blackening or radiolucency, and a barrel chest all are indications of
    a. atelectasis
    b. emphysema
    c. pneumonia
    d. pneumothorax

34. Tuberculosis is still the most significant disease in many areas of the world.
    a. true
    b. false

35. Emphysema is the direct opposite of atelectasis.
    a. true
    b. false

36. The inhalation of dust and particulate matter is correctly described as
    a. asbestosis
    b. pneumoconiosis
    c. berylliosis
    d. silicosis
    e. all of the above

37. A benign lung disease that is caused by a yeast-like organism and is common in the farming industry is known as
    a. asbestosis
    b. histoplasmosis
    c. tuberculosis
    d. bronchiectasis

Study Questions

1. Describe the different forms of emphysema.

2. Describe the radiographic appearance of lobar pneumonia, bronchopneumonia, and interstitial pneumonia.

3. What is the significance of lung diseases in terms of patient morbidity and mortality?

4. What occupations are more apt to predispose to the development of chronic lung disease?

5. In addition to routine chest radiography, what diagnostic methods may be employed to image chest pathology?

6. What are the most common congenital disorders that affect the lungs? How successful are the current methods of treatment?

Three

Alimentary Tract

Related Terminology

achalasia
achlorhydria
adynamic ileus
aganglionic
anastomosis
atresia
Billroth II
cardiospasm
celiac disease
cobblestone sign
coiled spring sign
Crohn's disease
double bubble sign
epiphrenic diverticulum
esophageal varices
esophagogastrectomy
gastrojejunostomomy
guaiac
Hirschsprung's disease
hose-pipe sign
incarceration
intussusception
malabsorption syndrome
Meckel's diverticulum
Menetrier's disease
paraesophageal hernia
peptic ulcer
pulsion diverticulum
pyloric stenosis
saw-tooth pattern
Schatzki's ring
single bubble sign
stepladder sign
string sign
traction diverticulum
trefoil cap
Trendelenburg's position
ulcerative colitis
vagotomy
Valsalva's maneuver
vasopressin
volvulus
Zencker's diverticulum

Objectives

Upon completion of Chapter 3, the radiographer will be able to

- Identify the radiographic manifestations of the listed diseases of the alimentary tract.

- Describe the cardinal symptoms and signs of the most common alimentary tract disorders.

- Describe the purposes of the various radiographic methods in the demonstration of alimentary tract anatomy.

- Describe the current medical and surgical treatment for the listed disorders of the alimentary tract.

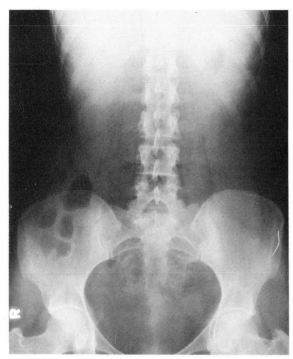

Figure 3–1. Normal flat plate of the abdomen.

Imaging of the Alimentary Tract

Flat Plate of the Abdomen

The plain film of the abdomen, flap plate, or kidney-ureter-bladder workup (KUB) is often considered a preliminary film that precedes most radiography of the alimentary tract. The flat plate of the abdomen is taken to assure the proper positioning of the patient and the inclusion of the kidneys, ureters, and urinary bladder on the radiograph. The preliminary film indicates whether or not the exposure factors are appropriate. The soft tissues should reveal the lateral abdominal wall and peritoneal fat layer. Shadows of the psoas muscle, lower border of the liver, and kidneys should be apparent. Congenital disorders, normal variants, and gross abnormalities must be ruled out before administering any contrast agent by any route. Other considerations include unexplained calcifications; pregnancy; gaseous patterns; and enlargement, displacement, duplication, or absence of any organs. The radiograph must be correctly identified with right or left markers. In order to assure proper location of abdominal organs, the film is taken on complete but not forced exhalation. Forced exhalation will result in increased involuntary motion (Fig. 3–1).

Upright or Erect Abdomen

The erect abdominal study is frequently employed with the flat plate of the abdomen as part of an obstructive or free-air series. This position is often difficult to attain if the patient is severely ill. It is recommended that, when possible, the patient be placed erect for a few minutes prior to film exposure. This allows time for the air to rise and better demonstrates air-fluid levels in dilated bowel loops, which are manifestations of many acute abdominal conditions. Free air, when present, is situated beneath the diaphragm. Fluid consolidations, such as pleural effusion or hydrothorax, can be determined with an erect view of the abdomen. The erect abdominal study should be identified with an appropriate lead marker. The diaphragms must be included on all erect views of the abdomen. For obese patients, it may be necessary to place the film crosswise and take two separate exposures to ensure visibility of the diaphragms as well as the abdomen (Fig. 3–2).

Lateral Decubitus Abdomen

The left lateral decubitus position is attained with the patient lying down on the left side. The side that is down always denotes the side of interest. This is accomplished with the patient's back in contact with the film of an upright radiographic table, chest unit (chest technique), or grid cassette. As is the case with other abdominal positions, the iliac crest is centered

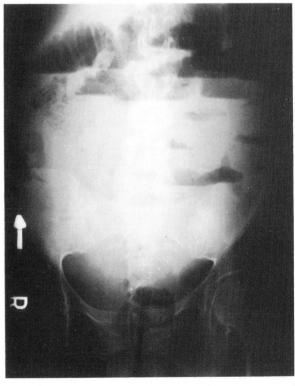

Figure 3–2. Upright abdomen with fluid levels indicating a small bowel mechanical obstruction due to invading carcinoma in a woman, age 53. Note that the diaphragms are not visible. Upright position must always reveal the diaphragms.

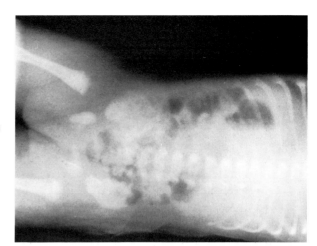

Figure 3–3. Lateral decibutus film of the abdomen revealing a normal bowel pattern in a neonate.

to the midpoint of the film, which for adults is 14 × 17 inches. The lateral decubitus position is often used when the patient cannot assume the upright position. Of interest are air-fluid levels and intestinal gas patterns. For the immobile patient, ventral or dorsal decubitus positions may be employed (Fig. 3–3).

Contrast Agents

Barium sulfate is the most frequently used contrast medium for the alimentary tract. In most cases, previously prepared individual containers of flavored barium are used. The advantage of these single units of barium lies in the consistent quality of the preparation. In the 1960s, it was not uncommon for radiographers to have their own "soda fountain" in the barium kitchen. The consistency of the barium varied, and so did the level of contrast on the radiograph. Various contrast preparations are available for studies that require a change in consistency. Esophotrast is a contrast agent that is thick enough to facilitate performing an esophagram. Typical barium has one part barium to one part water. Thick barium usually has a consistency equal to four parts barium to one part water. It is commercially prepared for easy administration. Barium is a high-density medium that coats the mucosal lining of the alimentary tract and makes possible the diagnosis of many diseases.

Air is frequently used in combination with barium to present a double-contrast image. Double-contrast studies of the stomach have long been employed in demonstrating early gastric carcinoma. Double-contrast examinations of the colon are most useful and are superior to physical examination of the colon for detecting small polypoid lesions and early mucosal ulcerations associated with inflammatory bowel disease. Water-soluble contrast agents such as Gastrografin are employed when perforation of the viscera is suspected. Barium sulfate does not absorb and could result in a potentially septic condition of the abdomen (Fig. 3–4).

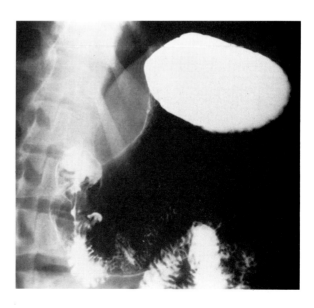

Figure 3–4. Double-contrast upper gastrointestinal series. Except for a small diverticulum at the second portion of the duodenum, the anatomy is otherwise normal.

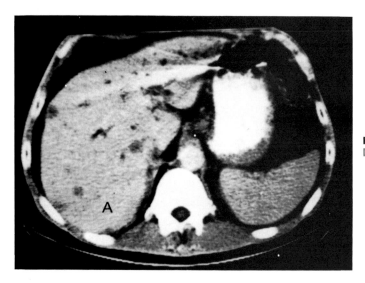

Figure 3–5. Multiple liver metastases (A, dark areas on the liver) in a 63-year-old man.

Computed Tomography and Ultrasonography

Although the diagnostic applications of computed tomography (CT) and ultrasonography are somewhat limited in the alimentary tract, both modalities are useful in demonstrating retroperitoneal masses and metastasis. CT is especially useful in demonstrating metastases of the liver, kidneys, and pancreas and many other types of pathology (Figs. 3–5 and 3–6).

Nuclear Medicine

Radioisotope scans of the alimentary tract are used almost exclusively for the diagnosis of Meckel's diverticulum and gastrointestinal bleeding (Fig. 3–7).

Disease Processes

A wide range of diseases and conditions afflict the alimentary tract. This chapter reviews the most common congenital and inflammatory disorders of the esophagus, stomach, small intestine, and colon. Growth disturbances affecting the alimentary tract will be discussed in Chapter 8.

The Esophagus

The Normal Esophagus

The esophagus is a hollow tubular structure that is approximately 10 inches in length. It articulates proximally with the pharynx and distally with the stomach

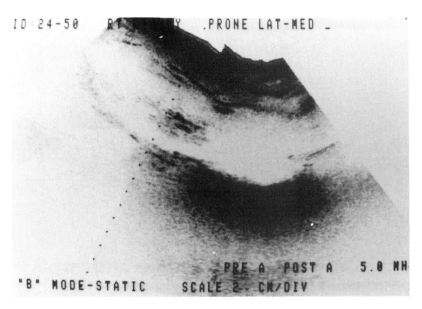

Figure 3–6. Sonogram of a hypertrophic kidney and a small cyst in a 30-year-old woman.

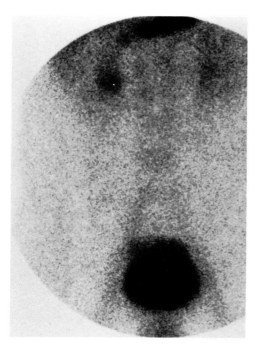

Figure 3–7. Isotope scan of the small intestine. There is no gastro-intestinal bleeding or Meckel's diverticulum. The intestinal mucosa reveals a "hot spot" in the area of the terminal ileum if a Meckel's diverticulum is present.

barium-filled esophagus situated between the verte-brae and the heart (Fig. 3–8).

Congenital Disorders

Esophageal Atresia and Tracheoesophageal Fistula

General Information. Esophageal atresia is an ab-normal condition characterized by the incomplete development of the esophagus. In most of such cases, the esophagus is atypically short and terminates in a blind pouch. Esophageal atresia is almost always associated with a fistulous tract that communicates with the trachea. Tracheoesophageal fistula occurs in approximately 1 of every 800 live births. It occurs equally often in both sexes and is associated with hydramnios, a condition in which there is an excess of amniotic fluid. Approximately one-third of affected infants are born prematurely. Tracheoesophageal fis-tula may be present with other developmental atre-sias. Frequent locations of atresia include the biliary tract, intestine, and anus. Congenital heart and gen-itourinary defects are also common. Esophageal atre-

at the cardiac orifice. Radiographic interpretation of the esophagus is accomplished with the assistance of a barium meal. The esophagus may be examined as a part of an upper gastrointestinal series, using thin barium, or independently of other structures, with a thick barium meal. The most common patient com-plaint is *dysphagia,* which is difficulty swallowing. Many abnormal conditions produce dysphagia, in-cluding a swallowed foreign body, neuromuscular defects, hiatus hernia, and carcinoma. The role of the esophagram is to rule out organic disease.

During fluoroscopy, the patient's esophagus is viewed in the erect, horizontal, and Trendelenburg's positions. Fluoroscopic spots are taken immediately after swallowing barium, and various combinations of breathing and positioning maneuvers are performed to demonstrate any obvious pathology that would not otherwise be detected. Delayed films are taken on conclusion of the fluoroscopic procedure. For the additional films, the patient swallows thick barium. The patient assumes the erect or recumbent position, according to the wishes of the radiologist. The routine positions for an esophagram include prone (postero-anterior [PA] projection), right anterior oblique po-sition (PA projection), and right lateral position. For each exposure, the patient swallows two mouthfuls of barium and then suspends respiration on inhalation until the exposure is terminated. The radiographs should visualize the entire barium-filled esophagus. For the right anterior oblique (RAO) position, the patient should be obliquely rotated approximately 35 to 40 degrees. This position will demonstrate the

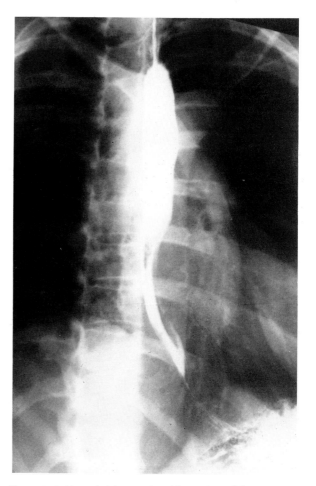

Figure 3–8. Normal right anterior oblique view of the esophagus.

A

7.7%   0.8%

86.5%   4.2%

0.7%

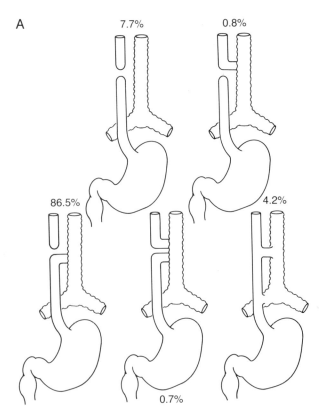

Figure 3–9. *A*, The five types of esophageal atresia and tracheoesophageal fistula. The percentages reflect the frequency of occurrence. *B*, Esophageal atresia in a neonate. The esophagus ends in a blind pouch. *C*, Gastrografin is seen in the right bronchi following aspiration in this neonate.

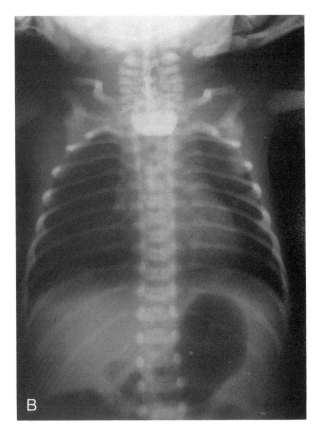

B

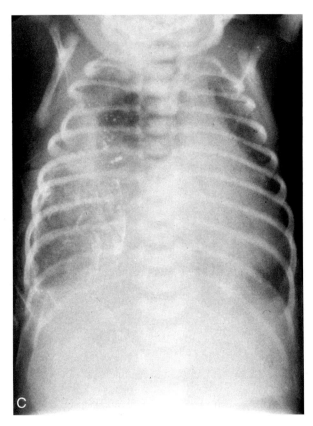

C

sia and tracheoesophageal fistula are serious surgical emergencies in newborns and require immediate diagnosis and correction. Five different forms of these conditions exist, with varying frequency.

Diagnosis. Of the five types shown in Figure 3–9A, the third type is the most common form (86.5%). The newborn infant appears to swallow normally but soon coughs, becomes dyspneic and cyanotic, and may stop breathing. Saliva is aspirated into the lungs via the fistula, and bile and gastric reflux are apparent. Fluid in the lungs is apparent on the chest radiograph, resembling bronchopneumonia. The right upper lung is most affected. Gas is apparent in a distended stomach and intestine. Acute respiratory distress and copious drooling are the cardinal signs of this disorder. In addition to noting the findings on the chest radiograph, the physician will encounter an obstruction when attempting to pass a nasogastric catheter.

Treatment. Immediate surgery is necessary to save the infant's life. The actual surgical procedure will depend on the type of anatomical deformity present. Because fistulas are common postoperatively, repeat chest films with Gastrografin are performed about 10

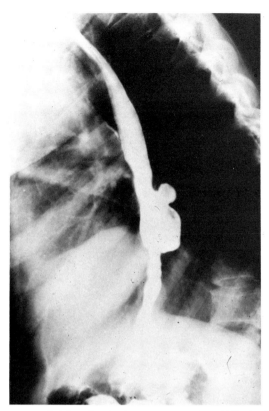

Figure 3–11. Pulsion diverticulum (arrows) in the middle third of the esophagus, as seen on the lateral view in a 51-year-old man.

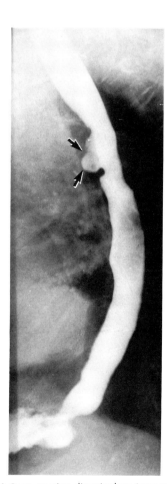

Figure 3–10. A 2-cm traction diverticulum (arrows) in the proximal one-third of the esophagus, as seen on the lateral view in a 79-year-old woman.

days after surgery and again after 1 and 3 months. These follow-up films will also evaluate the effectiveness of the surgical repair.

Diverticula

General Information. Esophageal diverticula are outpouchings of one or more layers of the esophageal wall. When congenital, they are due to a weakness in the muscular wall of the esophagus. Diverticula can also occur secondary to adjacent inflammation. There are three types of esophageal diverticula. ***Traction*** diverticula often occur secondary to scarring from an adjacent inflammatory disease process and are usually triangular, with the apex of the triangle pulled toward the diseased area. Traction diverticula are the most common type and can be observed radiographically in the middle third of the esophagus. The usual cause of traction diverticulum is an external lesion such as achalasia (Fig. 3–10).

A ***pulsion*** diverticulum is a protrusion or sac formed by a congenital weakness of the muscle membrane through the muscularis membrane of the esophagus. Pulsion diverticula can be observed just above the cardiac sphincter or just above the diaphragm. Zencker's diverticulum is a pulsion type that is exclusive to the area just above the cardia and is the result of increased intraesophageal pressure and muscle weakness (Fig. 3–11).

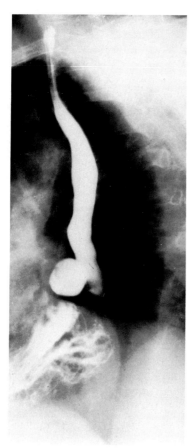

Figure 3–12. Epiphrenic (pulsion) diverticulum situated just above the diaphragm, as seen on the lateral view of the esophagus in a 62-year-old man.

Epiphrenic diverticula, another pulsion type, as the name implies, are found just above the diaphragm (Fig. 3–12).

Esophageal diverticula are more common in men than in women. Zencker's diverticula are more common in men older than 60 years, whereas epiphrenic diverticula are more common in middle-aged men.

Diagnosis. Typically, patients having diverticula are asymptomatic unless the lesions are large. Traction diverticula in the proximal segment may accumulate food and secretions, resulting in mechanical obstruction. This condition is especially uncomfortable when the patient is recumbent. It may be further complicated by aspiration of food contents into the bronchi, resulting in aspiration bronchopneumonia.

Radiographically, an esophageal diverticulum is very apparent as an outpouching or herniation. A Zencker's diverticulum is often wider than that of the esophagus. The esophagus narrows as it joins the diverticulum. Traction diverticula have a wide base and assume the shape of a funnel or triangle in the middle third of the esophagus. Epiphrenic diverticula, being lower, usually compress the distal esophagus.

Treatment. For most diverticula, treatment is conservative as well as palliative. Bland diet, chewing food thoroughly, and drinking significant amounts of water after eating are ways to control the effects of diverticula. Surgical removal of large diverticula may be necessary. The inability to swallow or difficulty swallowing is the primary reason for surgery. When eating, the person with a large diverticulum must be careful to take small bites of food, chew the food well, and swallow only small quantities of food in order to avoid choking and discomfort.

Inflammatory Disorders

Esophageal Varices

General Information. Esophageal varices are *dilated, tortuous veins* of the distal esophagus. They are usually a direct complication of portal venous hypertension and portal vein thrombosis, which may result from cirrhosis of the liver. When the pressure in the portal venous system substantially rises, blood backs up into the spleen and flows through collateral channels to the venous system, bypassing the liver. As a result, the veins of the distal esophagus enlarge and often rupture, resulting in gross hematemesis requiring immediate treatment to restrain hemorrhage and prevent shock.

Patients with obstructive liver disease and alcoholics with cirrhosis are the most frequent victims of this disorder. Cirrhosis patients who hemorrhage have a low survival rate. Seventy percent of patients with esophageal varices will not survive 1 year from the time of onset.

Diagnosis. Hemorrhage is the usual first sign of esophageal varices. Patients require emergency treatment. A free-air abdominal series is almost always indicated. The radiographer must exercise caution when preparing for the upright chest and abdomen films, for the patient has suffered a significant blood loss and will frequently faint when being elevated into the erect position from a recumbent position. Esophageal varices appear as *lucent*, tortuous *wavelike* filling defects that deform the mucosal pattern so that the folds are no longer parallel. The filling defects are the result of the enlarged collateral veins. The varices are best demonstrated after passage of the main bolus. Valsalva's maneuver will further dilate the collateral veins and enlarge the filling defects (Fig. 3–13).

Other means of diagnosis include endoscopy, which can identify the exact site of hemorrhage. Angiography presents another means of diagnosis, but because of the patient's blood loss and poor condition, the added risk is questionable. In terms of diagnostic comparison, angiography is not as accurate as endoscopy.

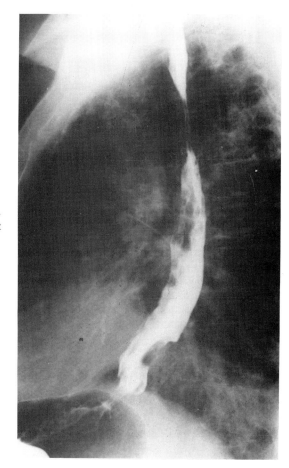

Figure 3–13. Multiple filling defects of the greater length of the esophagus, consistent with extensive esophageal varices. The patient is a man, age 75.

Treatment. Vasopressin may be infused into the superior mesenteric artery via angiography or may be infused by intravenous drip to stop hemorrhage. Vasopressin is a hormone secreted by the hypothalamus and stored in the posterior pituitary for release when necessary. It can also be produced artificially for clinical use. Vasopressin functions to stimulate contraction of the muscular walls of vessels, reducing hemorrhage.

Surgical bypass procedures (shunts) redirect blood flow and thereby decrease venous pressure in the liver. After surgery, the patient must be carefully monitored for additional hemorrhage, hypotension, compromised oxygen supply, and altered states of consciousness. Emergency shunts have a mortality rate of between 25 and 50%.

Hiatal Hernia

General Information. Hiatal hernia is a common condition that affects approximately one-half of the population. It is characterized by herniation or pro-trusion of the stomach through an incompetent cardiac sphincter in the left hemidiaphragm. Hiatal hernia may be congenital or acquired. Although the exact cause is unknown, it is thought that the site of the defect is the phrenoesophageal membrane, which firmly anchors the distal esophagus to its proper position.

Two primary types of hiatal hernia have been identified: a *direct* or *sliding* hiatal hernia and a *paraesophageal* or *rolling* hernia. In a paraesophageal hernia, the fundus herniates through the diaphragm but the esophageal junction often remains competent below the junction. A rolling hernia does not affect the esophagus directly, and the cardiac portion remains intact. A large paraesophageal hernia will remain above the diaphragm in the erect position and may be seen on a PA chest film. When all of the stomach slides above the diaphragm, the condition is referred to as intrathoracic stomach. A direct or sliding type is the most common and represents 90% of all hiatal hernias. Most are asymptomatic and do not require treatment. Occasionally, patients with large sliding hernias complain of severe pain in the

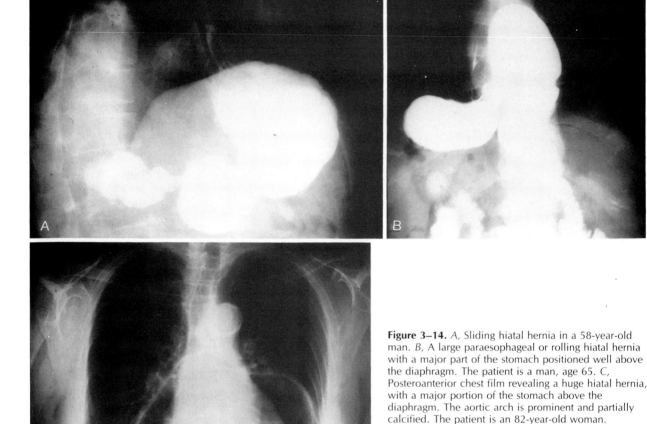

Figure 3–14. *A,* Sliding hiatal hernia in a 58-year-old man. *B,* A large paraesophageal or rolling hiatal hernia with a major part of the stomach positioned well above the diaphragm. The patient is a man, age 65. *C,* Posteroanterior chest film revealing a huge hiatal hernia, with a major portion of the stomach above the diaphragm. The aortic arch is prominent and partially calcified. The patient is an 82-year-old woman.

chest and abdomen with difficulty breathing. This condition may mimic a heart attack (Fig. 3–14).

Diagnosis. The initial symptom a patient experiences is a feeling of fullness in the chest, especially after meals. In almost all cases, the patient suffers recurring regurgitation or reflux of gastric contents and acids into the distal esophagus, resulting in cardiospasms and esophagitis or heartburn. In patients with a direct or sliding hiatal hernia, the stomach fundus moves into the chest at the esophagogastric junction.

The routine upper gastrointestinal series will detect most hiatal hernias. Routine fluoroscopic spots are taken in a number of positions, with the patient erect as well as recumbent. The radiologist uses Trendelenburg's position and Valsalva's maneuver for demonstration of a hiatal hernia. The use of both methods together is 50 to 60% accurate in demonstrating hiatal hernia.

A radiographic confirmation of a sliding hiatal hernia is accomplished with the demonstration of a *Schatzki's ring*, which is thought to be the site where the esophagus and stomach join. This ring is a circular involuntary sphincter that opens and closes with the passage of food and liquid from the esophagus into the stomach (Fig. 3–15).

Treatment. The most frequent complication of a sliding hernia is hemorrhage. Ulceration, hemorrhage, obstruction, incarceration, volvulus, and intrathoracic gastric dilatation are the complications of a rolling hernia. Because gastric reflux is a common symptom, sliding hernias must be differentiated from angina pectoris, biliary disease, diverticulitis, and peptic ulcer.

Most treatments for hiatal hernia are conservative and include dietary considerations. Spicy foods should be avoided because they contribute to excess acid formation and precipitate reflux esophagitis.

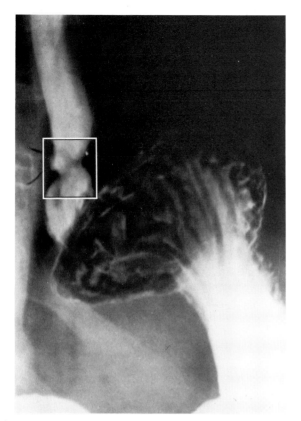

Figure 3–15. A small central hiatal hernia with mild reflux when in the supine position. Schatzki's ring defect is present, as well as a small active ulcer at the base of the distal esophagus (rectangle). The patient is a 50-year-old woman.

Correct eating habits must be observed. Patients should remain erect after meals or take a walk. Reclining after eating tends to cause discomfort, especially after heavy meals. Patients should also avoid clothing that is constricting. Antacids are used to decrease inflammation of the mucosa.

Gastroesophageal Reflux

General Information. Gastroesophageal reflux is the primary cause of inflammation of the esophagus. This condition can be both acute and chronic. It is described as the backward flow or reflux of gastric and sometimes duodenal contents into the esophagus, usually past the sphincter and into the distal esophagus. Gastroesophageal reflux or esophagitis may occur in the absence of vomiting or belching. It is thought to occur when the cardiac sphincter is incompetent and the pressure in the stomach is greater than in the esophagus.

Persistent episodes of this type are referred to as esophagitis, cardiospasm, or heartburn. The site of discomfort is located just beneath the sternum and is often associated with hiatal hernia. In addition to being linked with poor eating habits and a hyper-

sthenic body build, reflux is associated with postoperative complications of pyloric surgery, long-term nasogastric intubation, excessive intake of alcohol, smoking, use of atropine and morphine, and increased intraabdominal pressure.

Diagnosis. The most frequent radiographic indication of gastroesophageal reflux is **peptic strictures** at the lower end of the esophagus. There is also a strong relationship with hiatal hernia. Peptic strictures are characteristically short and have smooth outlines with tapering ends (Fig. 3–16).

Treatment. The patient's symptoms are similar to those in hiatal hernia. Thus, the treatment is also similar. Careful attention to dietary habits is critical to recovery. Complications including severe pain, ulceration, and hemorrhage will ensue if patients do not make necessary adjustments in their eating habits.

Achalasia

General Information. Achalasia is a neuromuscular disorder in which the gastroesophageal sphincter fails to relax, resulting in a functional obstruction. The esophageal body is atonic and becomes progressively dilated, often to great proportions. The patient complains of progressive dysphagia and a full feeling in the sternal region.

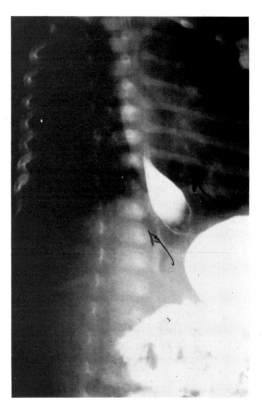

Figure 3–16. Slight achalasia and gastroesophageal reflux after injecting 10 ounces of barium in a 1-month-old boy.

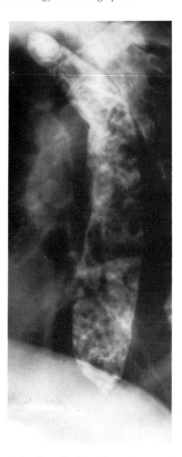

Figure 3–17. A significantly dilated esophagus with a smoothly tapered distal end. This is compatible with achalasia. The patient is a 69-year-old man.

Diagnosis. Radiographically, achalasia presents as a smooth, tapered narrowing of the distal esophagus. In its proximal and middle regions, the esophagus is extremely dilated, contains food residues, and lacks peristalsis (Fig. 3–17).

Treatment. The treatment of achalasia is conservative. The patient is put on a low-bulk, bland diet and is advised to avoid large meals, chew food thoroughly, to eat slowly, and to drink plenty of fluids with meals. To reduce the possibility of aspiration, the patient is urged to sleep with the head and shoulders elevated.

The Stomach and Duodenum

The Normal Stomach and Duodenum

Radiography of the stomach and duodenum is accomplished via an upper gastrointestinal series, which is one of the most routine procedures in diagnostic radiology. The single-contrast method uses prepared barium as the primary contrast agent. The purpose of this procedure is to detect ulcerations, tumors, inflammations, or anatomical malposition of these organs. The upper gastrointestinal series also is used to monitor the healing pattern of ulcers. With treatment and patient cooperation, the ulcer should decrease to about one-half of its initial size after about 3 weeks. A lesion that does not decrease may represent a more serious condition such as metastasis.

When the double-contrast method is desired, the patient is given some form of a gas-producing substance followed by a small amount of barium. For the double-contrast method, both contrast agents are first given to the patient while he or she is in the erect position. This is followed by lowering the patient into the recumbent position and then rotating or turning the body from side to side. The gaseous medium facilitates the expansion of the stomach, and the rotational movements promote coating of the mucosal lining. In some cases, the radiologist may wish to minimize peristalsis. This is accomplished by administering glucagon or any other anticholinergic agent. Glucagon relaxes the gastric muscularis and allows for greater distension of the stomach. The advantage of the double-contrast method is enhanced visualization of small lesions that may be obscured with conventional single-contrast radiography of the stomach and duodenum (Fig. 3–18).

Following fluoroscopy, several overhead radiographs are taken of the patient in the recumbent position. If there is any delay between the ending of fluoroscopy and the beginning of radiography, the patient is given additional barium to drink because the stomach begins to empty and enough barium must be present to provide adequate demonstration of the mucosal lining of the stomach and duodenum.

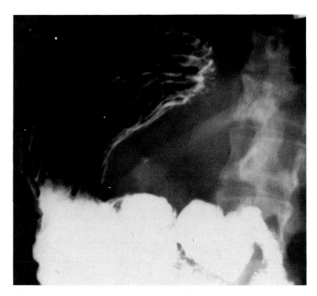

Figure 3–18. Normal right anterior oblique view of the stomach with the use of glucagon.

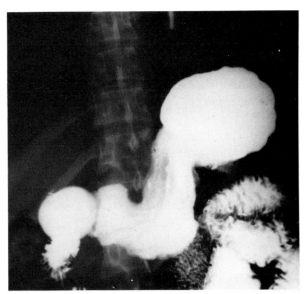

Figure 3–19. Normal posteroanterior view of the stomach and duodenum.

There will be some difference from hospital to hospital, but radiography of the stomach and duodenum usually involves the following patient positions: PA, RAO, lateral, and left posterior oblique (LPO). The exact positioning of the patient and the placement of the cassette are strongly influenced by the body habitus. In general, a hypersthenic patient has a stomach that is higher and lies in a more transverse presentation. This sometimes requires the cassette to be placed crosswise in the Bucky tray. A patient with a sthenic, hyposthenic, or asthenic body type has a stomach that is J-shaped, and the cassette is situated lengthwise. Because the diaphragms in these patients are more dome-shaped, the stomach is situated lower to the left of the spine than in the hypersthenic patient. All exposures should be suspended at the end of exhalation

The PA stomach position demonstrates the entire stomach and duodenal bulb. The PA should be performed first, because the stomach will change location somewhat when the patient is rotated into the next position. The movement of the stomach is again based on the body habitus (Fig. 3–19).

From the PA position, the patient is adjusted into a RAO position. The large majority of patients are of the sthenic or average body build and require an average obliquity of between 40 and 70 degrees. Obliques of less than 40 degrees and more than 70 degrees are recommended for the opposite extremes, hyposthenic and hypersthenic body types. The stomach descends 2 to 3 inches when the patient is moved from the PA to the RAO position. The RAO best demonstrates the pyloric canal and duodenal bulb. The duodenal bulb and loop should be observed in profile (Fig. 3–20).

On completion of the RAO, the patient is adjusted into the right lateral position. This position is used to demonstrate both the anterior and posterior bor-

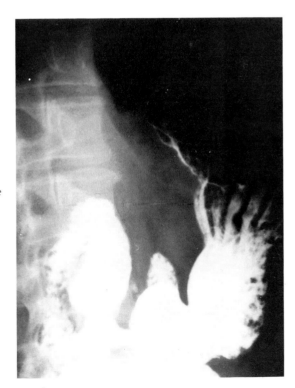

Figure 3–20. Normal right anterior oblique view of the stomach and duodenum.

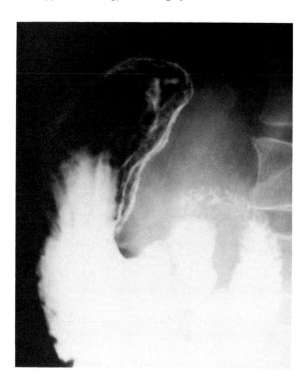

Figure 3–21. Normal lateral view of the stomach.

ders of the stomach, the pyloric canal, and the duodenal bulb and loop (Fig. 3–21).

The patient is then rotated from the lateral position to the LPO position. The stomach ascends so that the fundus conforms to the dome of the left hemidiaphragm. The LPO position reveals the gastric fundus. The pyloric canal and duodenal bulb lack opacification because of the effect of gravity (Fig. 3–22). At the conclusion of the stomach overheads, the option exists for continual observation of the barium as it passes through the small intestine. This is accomplished by taking periodic films of the abdomen over a 3-hour period. The barium should reach the terminal ileum in 2½ to 3 hours.

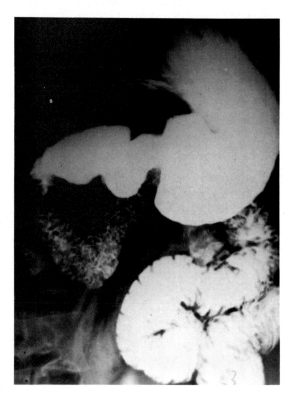

Figure 3–22. Normal left posterior oblique view of the stomach and duodenum.

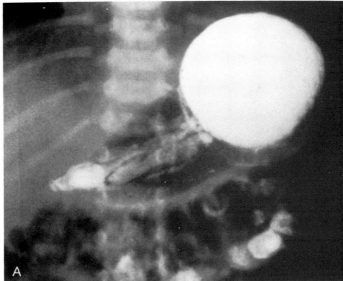

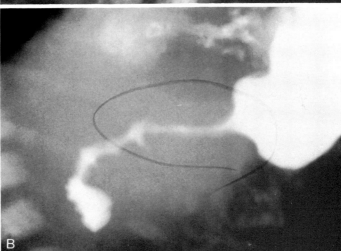

Figure 3–23. A, Gross distension of the stomach of a neonate after administration of contrast medium, with no evidence of gastric emptying due to pyloric stenosis. B, Evidence of hypertrophic narrowing of the pyloric canal in a neonate. The narrowed pyloric canal is referred to as the string sign.

Congenital Disorders

Hypertrophic Pyloric Stenosis

General Information. Pyloric stenosis is a narrowing of the pyloric canal producing pyloric obstruction. It is caused by **hypertrophy** or thickening of the pyloric muscle. This anomaly is the second most frequent congenital disorder of the gastrointestinal system. Pyloric stenosis occurs in approximately 0.4% of all live births and typically affects the firstborn male. Nine out of 10 affected infants are boys. The manifestations of pyloric stenosis may occur anytime from age 2 weeks to 2 months.

Diagnosis. The initial sign of pyloric stenosis is vomiting, first mild, then increasingly severe and projectile. Vomiting can occur both during and after feedings. The infant cries because of hunger, cramping, and constipation. A muscular mass about the size of an olive may be palpable. The abdomen appears distended. When pyloric stenosis is suspected, the

radiologist may opt to further thin the barium mixture or to use a water-soluble contrast agent such as Gastrografin. Prepared barium is often too thick to pass through the narrowed and elongated pyloric channel. The radiological demonstration of a hypertrophied pyloric canal is referred to as a **string sign** (Fig. 3–23).

Treatment. Pyloric stenosis is usually corrected by surgery. The procedure, a pyloromyotomy, involves incising and splitting the longitudinal and circular muscles of the pylorus.

Inflammatory Disorders

Hypertrophic Gastritis (Menetrier's Disease)

General Information. Chronic hypertrophic gastritis is a long-term disorder of varying severity. Some of the predisposing factors include chronic alcoholism, malnutrition, trauma, recurring acute gastritis,

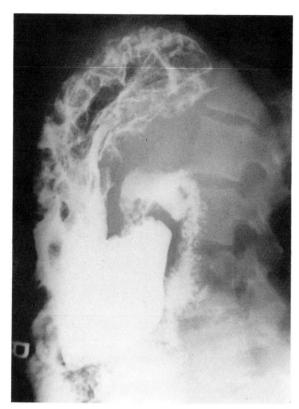

Figure 3–24. Giant hypertrophic gastritis, otherwise known as Menetrier's disease.

smoking, excessive intake of analgesics, and functional neuroses. This condition is a profound form of gastritis with marked epithelial hyperplasia and is most common in males in the age-group between 40 and 60 years.

Diagnosis. Menetrier's disease is characterized by the enlargement of the gastric folds of the proximal and middle portions of the stomach (Fig. 3–24). The normal mucosal folds are about 1 mm in diameter; the abnormal folds are approximately 7 mm in diameter.

Treatment. The treatment of Menetrier's disease is similar to that of chronic gastritis. If the lesion is due to a functional disorder, a vagotomy may be indicated. If significant damage to the mucosa is apparent in the form of an ulceration, a partial or total gastrectomy may be the treatment of choice.

Peptic Ulcers

General Information. Peptic ulcer is a chronic injury of the gastric and duodenal mucosa due to the effects of hydrochloric acid and proteolytic enzymes. Gastrin, a gastrointestinal hormone released during digestion and emotional stress, activates the acid-secreting glands. Drugs such as aspirin and steroids, smoking, and poor dietary habits commonly precipi-

tate peptic ulcers. Predisposing genetic factors are thought to be associated with the occurrence of this disorder. The pylorus and duodenum are particularly affected by hydrochloric acid and proteolytic enzymes because of their horizontal position.

Peptic ulcer is one of the most common causes of chronic ill health in the western world and is a frequent cause of an acute abdomen, which may merit immediate attention in the hospital emergency room. It is believed that as much as 10% of the general population may be affected by peptic ulcer at any one time. In 1985, 6600 people died as a result of the disease. Peptic ulcer is twice as common in men as in women. The primary reason for the higher incidence in men is the low incidence of peptic ulcer in women approaching menopause. In general, duodenal ulcers are two to three times more common than gastric ulcers. In men, duodenal ulcers are seven times more common than gastric ulcers. Duodenal ulcers are most common between the ages of 20 and 50, whereas gastric ulcers are most common between 40 and 60.

Diagnosis. Duodenal ulcers typically are found in patients with blood type O and are the most common form of ulcer. Duodenal ulcers usually occur in the first portion of the duodenum, referred to as the cap or bulb. The occurrence in the duodenal bulb is about 95%. Pain is the cardinal symptom. This gnawing-hunger type of pain is usually relieved by eating. During an upper gastrointestinal series, the radiologist always asks the patient to describe the pain and whether or not the pain is relieved by eating. These questions are also appropriate for the radiographer to ask when taking a history prior to the examination. In addition to the type of pain, the location and duration of pain are also important. Radiographically, the duodenal ulcer appears as a collection of barium and mucosal folds that are edematous and radiate to the edge of the ulcer. The ulcer usually protrudes from the surface of the bulb. When the ulceration is active, spasms are often present, and the ulcer does not fill with barium (Fig. 3–25).

Duodenal ulcers recur with regularity, and scarring and fibrosis are usually evident. This fibrosis often causes the bulb to resemble a *cloverleaf* on an upper gastrointestinal study. This finding is referred to as a *trefoil cap* and is difficult to differentiate between an ulceration and a pseudodiverticulum. Recheck upper gastrointestinal studies are performed to evaluate the level of healing. Endoscopy may be used to determine the exact site of hemorrhage with new disease. The biopsy also is used to rule out carcinoma.

In addition to ulceration, the complications of duodenal ulcer include perforation, hemorrhage, and stenosis. Perforation occurs about 5% of the time, and when it does occur, there is a release of acid pepsins into the peritoneal cavity, producing irritation of the peritoneum. The spillage of acid pepsins

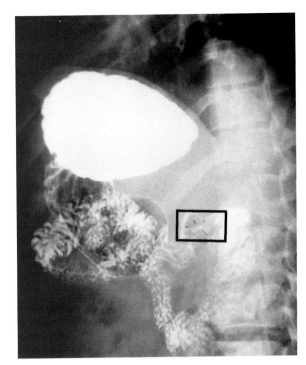

Figure 3–25. A 3.8-mm linear ulcer (rectangle) collecting in the duodenal bulb along the posterior surface in a 25-year-old man.

accounts for the pain and for the board-like rigidity (reflex) of the abdomen. Hematemesis, another complication, is bloody, dark red vomitus that resembles coffee grounds. The darkened appearance of the blood is due to its alteration by gastric acids. Melena is the passage of dark, tar-like stools. Duodenal

obstruction usually occurs secondary to inflammatory changes.

Gastric ulcers can appear almost anywhere in the stomach. The area of the lesser curvature is the most frequent ulcer site (Fig. 3–26). The pyloric antrum and the fundus are the next most common areas of

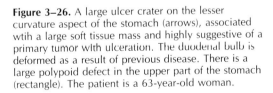

Figure 3–26. A large ulcer crater on the lesser curvature aspect of the stomach (arrows), associated wtih a large soft tissue mass and highly suggestive of a primary tumor wlth ulceration. The duodenal bulb is deformed as a result of previous disease. There is a large polypoid defect in the upper part of the stomach (rectangle). The patient is a 63-year-old woman.

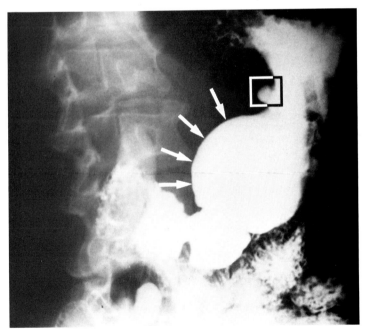

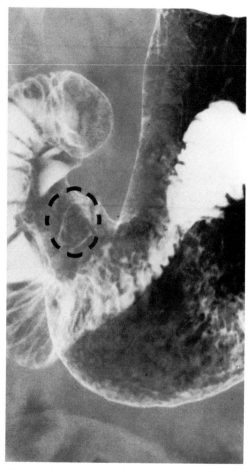

Figure 3–27. Benign ulcer, distal pyloric antrum, on the anterior wall (dotted circle) in a 39-year-old woman.

ulcers often recur as gastric carcinoma. Fifty percent of cases of gastric carcinoma occur in the pyloric antrum, and approximately 25% occur in the lesser curvature.

Treatment. For the most part, treatment of duodenal ulcers is very conservative. Patients are encouraged to eat several small meals instead of the usual three larger meals per day. Their diet should not contain spicy foods or foods that are hard to digest, and they should totally abstain from alcoholic beverages. Smoking is discouraged, as is the intake of drugs such as analgesics and steroids. In acute situations, the patient is urged to rest in bed. Stomach discomfort should be soothed with gastric sedatives and antacids. As much as possible, the patient should avoid emotional stress. When the mucosa is chronically irritated, ulcers recur. A *vagotomy* is a surgical procedure for the purpose of removing the source of gastric acid by abolishing the neural stimulation of cells located within the gastric mucosa. The vagotomy results in a diminished response of these cells to stimuli such as emotional stress, spicy foods, and so on.

The treatment of benign gastric ulcers is similar to that of duodenal ulcers, in that it is for the most part conservative. However, when complications such as hemorrhage, perforation, or obstruction are present, chronic recurrent disease or malignancy is a diagnostic consideration. The presence of hemorrhage sub-

ulceration (Fig. 3–27). The greater curvature and cardia are often least involved with ulcers (Fig. 3–28).

Gastric ulcers most often affect patients with type A blood and are somewhat related to patient age. In older adults, the lesions are fairly common in the proximal half of the stomach. Young adults rarely have lesions in the proximal stomach. Gastric ulcers are the end result of many chronic conditions such as alcoholism, drug abuse, burns, and uremia. Ulcers can occur from the long-term placement of a gastric tube. Gastric ulcers are most often diagnosed by endoscopy rather than by barium studies.

Radiographically, the gastric ulcer appears as an *outpouching* or niche when viewed tangentially and as a circular collection of barium when seen face on. An ulcer may not always be visible because of the variable filling and emptying of the stomach. Once an ulcer is identified, it should be determined which body positions will demonstrate the lesion to best advantage.

The complications are similar to those of duodenal ulcers, but a major difference exists in that gastric

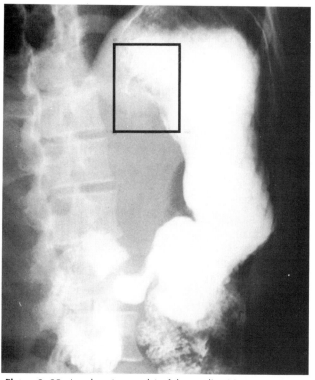

Figure 3–28. An ulcer (rectangle) of the cardia, 21 × 10 mm. The patient is a 34-year-old man.

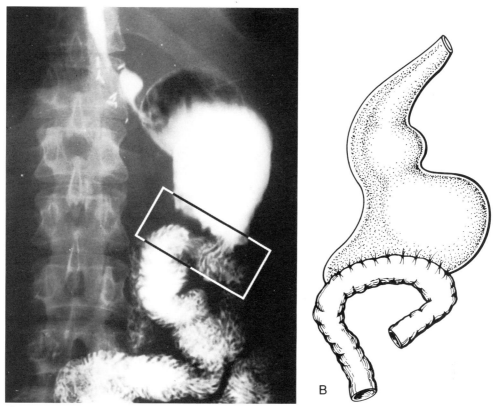

Figure 3–29. *A,* Billroth II gastrojejunostomy (rectangle) in a 58-year-old man. *B,* Illustration of the Billroth II gastrojejunostomy.

stantially increases the possibility of a large lesion. The primary surgical treatment is referred to as ***gastrectomy***. Surgical removal of the whole stomach is called total gastrectomy. Excision of a portion of the stomach is partial or subtotal gastrectomy. When a subtotal gastrectomy is performed, the remaining stomach is anastomosed to a loop of the jejunum. This procedure is known as a ***gastrojejunostomy.*** The jejunum is commonly anastomosed with the remaining gastric body. A gastrojejunostomy is often indicated for an ulcerative lesion of the lesser curvature of the stomach. However, with low-lying ulcers of the pyloric antrum, the chances of recurrence and malignancy are unusually high. The pyloric antrum contains the glands that secrete gastrin, a hormone that stimulates the acid-secreting glands. Forty to seventy percent of gastric carcinomas are found in the gastric antrum. The gastrectomy becomes necessary because of probable complications such as hemorrhage, obstruction, and perforation. A major postgastrectomy complication is stenosis. The gastrojejunostomy assures the integrity and continuity of that portion of the digestive tract. The most frequent type of subtotal gastrectomy is the ***Billroth II*** procedure (Fig. 3–29). This procedure includes the surgical removal of the pyloric antrum and distal portion of the gastric body, with closure of the duodenum and anastomosis of the jejunum to the remaining gastric

body. This popular procedure is not without complications. A repeat upper gastrointestinal series is performed to assure the continuity of the anastomosis and to rule out the presence of leaking. The patient experiences other complications as the result of the rapid dumping of food into the jejunum, resulting in nausea and epigastric fullness. When a total gastrectomy is performed, continuity is restored via anastomosis between the end of the esophagus and duodenum.

The Small Intestine

Congenital Abnormalities

Meckel's Diverticulum

General Information. Meckel's diverticulum is a failure of the embryonic connection with the yolk sac to disappear. It is the second most common developmental abnormality of the alimentary tract and affects approximately 2% of the population, primarily males. In its typical presentation, a blind tube, similar to the appendix, opens into the distal ileum near the ileocecal valve.

Diagnosis. Meckel's diverticulum is usually asymptomatic. It is frequently encountered in postmortem

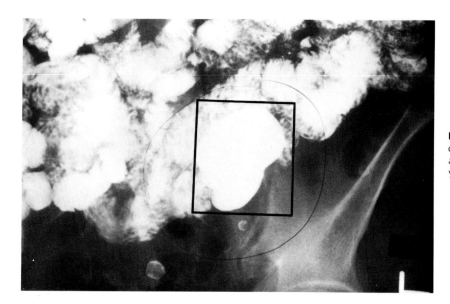

Figure 3–30. A distended Meckel's diverticulum (rectangle), 6 × 4 cm, arising from the terminal ileum in a 52-year-old man.

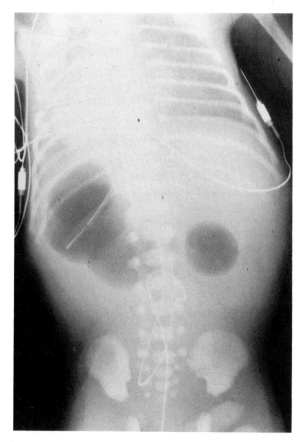

Figure 3–31. Apparent bowel obstruction in a neonate weighing 4 pounds 2 ounces; 25 ml of air was injected into a nasogastric tube, revealing no movement of air into the bowel. The stomach and proximal duodenum are greatly distended with air. This is referred to as the double bubble syndrome and is indicative of duodenal obstruction. Surgery revealed that two parts of the fetal pancreas grew around the descending duodenum.

(autopsy) examinations. Although it varies in size, it is usually about the size of a small finger. The most frequent aspect of the lesion is inflammation, resulting in abdominal pain, especially near the umbilicus. Bloody dark red feces (melena) may also be noted. Meckel's diverticulum is most often seen on routine radiography of the small intestine as a barium-filled *outpouching* of the distal ileum. Although serious complications are the exception rather than the rule, they can include bowel obstruction, intussusception, and volvulus (Fig. 3–30).

Treatment. Surgical resection of the involved portion of the terminal ileum and antibiotic therapy are the most frequent methods of treatment.

Duodenal Atresia

General Information. Duodenal atresia is a congenital abnormality characterized by the absence of a lumen between the stomach and duodenum. Without immediate surgical correction this condition is incompatible with life.

Diagnosis. Duodenal atresia results in a separate gaseous distension of the stomach and proximal duodenum, referred to radiographically as the *double bubble* sign (Fig. 3–31).

Treatment. This condition must be treated surgically. The procedure involves creating an opening of the duodenum that then is in communication with the pyloric canal.

Inflammatory Disorders

Celiac Disease

General Information. Celiac disease is one of the more common diseases included in the *malabsorption*

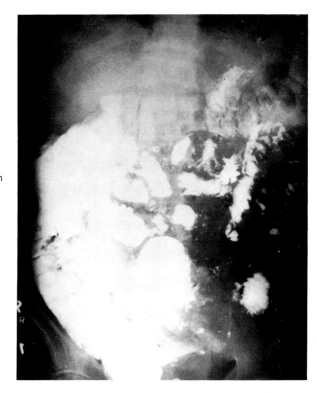

Figure 3–32. Celiac disease in a 44-year-old man. There is protracted barium passage with bowel dilatation and thickening of the mucosal folds. There is also clumping, and barium appears to be broken up into segments.

syndrome. This condition is characterized by a failure of the small intestine to absorb necessary food constituents, allowing the nutrients to accumulate in the stool and leading to weight loss and steatorrhea (fat in the stool). Celiac disease may be due to an alimentary tract defect, a mucosal abnormality, or lymphatic obstruction. A mucosal defect of the jejunum is the most common cause, marked by atrophy and declining function of the jejunal villi. Celiac disease is also known as *sprue bowel* and *gluten-induced enteropathy.* It is essentially a sensitivity to certain cereal grains, usually wheat. It is also possible that patients with celiac disease may produce an intramucosal enzyme that prevents gluten absorption. This disease is thought to be hereditary because it occurs in familial clusters. Females are afflicted twice as frequently as males. It occurs in approximately 1 in every 3000 individuals, usually Caucasian siblings of northwestern European ancestry

Diagnosis. Patients lose weight. The stool is usually large, foul smelling, bulky, frothy, and pale and contains large amounts of fat. Recurring diarrhea and abdominal cramping alternating with constipation are common. In severe cases of malnutrition, there may be edema and abdominal distension. Because of this malabsorption, a deficiency is noted in vitamins B, D, and K, and levels of sodium, potassium, and chlorides are low. Diagnosis may be confirmed with a jejunal biopsy and elimination of gluten from the diet. The biopsy may reveal an absence of villi and the presence of ulcerations and perforations. Radio-

graphic barium studies of the small intestine reveal *protracted* barium passage (Fig. 3–32). The bowel is *dilated,* and the mucosal folds are thickened. In place of the normal continuous flow of barium, there may be clumping or flocculation so that the barium is broken up into multiple segments. The barium-filled loops of bowel may appear less opaque than normal because of dilution by excessive fluid.

Treatment. In order for treatment to be successful, a gluten-free diet must be maintained for the remainder of the lifetime. Aggressive vitamin therapy is initiated. In place of wheat, rice flour is substituted.

Regional Enteritis (Crohn's Disease)

General Information. Regional enteritis, or Crohn's disease, is one of two major bowel disorders classified as inflammatory. This is a chronic disorder primarily affecting the *terminal ileum* (50%), but it can affect any part of the intestine (30%). This condition affects *all* layers of the bowel wall. It may also involve the regional lymph nodes and the mesentery. Regional enteritis is most prevalent in adults between the ages of 20 and 40, with the peak onset at age 27. It is two to three times more common in Jews and least common in blacks. The actual cause of this disease is unknown.

Approximately 5% of patients with Crohn's disease have one or more relatives who are similarly afflicted. In the acute stage of this disease, the patient has significant right lower quadrant pain, cramping, flat-

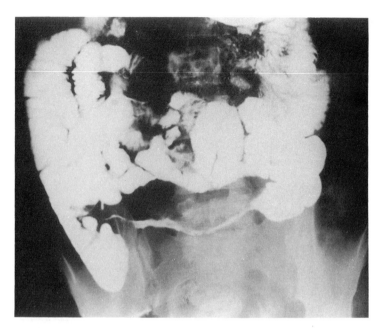

Figure 3–33. Ulcerative changes and severe narrowing of the terminal ileum, which measures 13 cm. Severe narrowing of the terminal ileum is referred to as the string sign and is consistent with regional enteritis or Crohn's disease. The patient is a 21-year-old woman.

ulence, nausea, and diarrhea. At this point, these symptoms may mimic acute appendicitis. Bleeding may vary from minimal to massive.

Diagnosis. Several distinguishing features are present on radiographs of the barium-filled intestine. The diseased loops of bowel appear to lie separately, displaced from other parts because of the inflamma-

tory lesions. These multiple affected areas are referred to as skip lesions. Perhaps the most demonstrative signs on the barium follow-through are *strictures* and an abnormal appearance of the mucosa. The strictures vary in length and present the characteristic *string sign* (Fig. 3–33). The bowel proximal to a stricture is usually dilated. Ulcerations that are

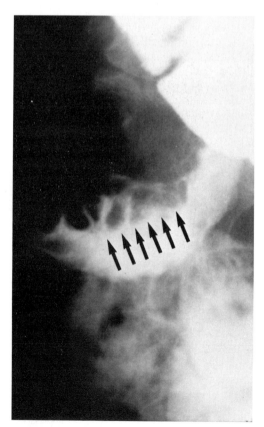

Figure 3–34. Regional enteritis in a 26-year-old man. Note the 8-cm nodular, spiculated, mucosal pattern (arrows), referred to as the cobblestone pattern.

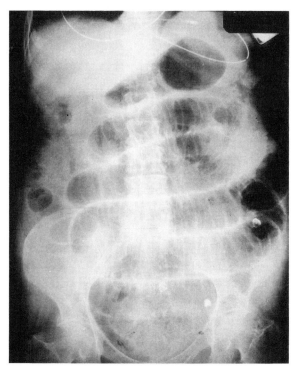

Figure 3–35. Air-distended small intestine ileus in a 53-year-old woman. This is referred to as the stepladder sign and is indicative of a small bowel obstruction.

peristalsis and often results from neural stimulation of the bowel. This is referred to as **adynamic** or **paralytic** ileus. Adynamic ileus is common as a postoperative complication. Ileus can also occur as the result of spasm, when it is referred to as **dynamic** ileus. Mechanical obstruction may be caused by adhesions, volvulus, and hernias. The patient complains of abdominal pain, and the abdomen is distended. Vomiting and diarrhea are also common signs. It is interesting to note that nausea is not usually present. The intestinal obstruction must be relieved so that the vascular supply to the bowel wall is not interrupted.

Diagnosis. In addition to the symptoms and signs described above, the absence of nausea is interesting and is characteristic of this particular bowel condition, unlike many others. X-rays of the abdomen reveal the presence and location of intestinal gas or fluid. In a small bowel obstruction, the bowel loops often reveal a characteristic **stepladder** pattern (Fig. 3–35).

Treatment. Abdominal distension is relieved by decompression. To intubate the patient with a Miller-Abbott tube, the tube is passed into the site of obstruction (Fig. 3–36). If the tube is unable to bypass the obstruction, surgery is necessary to remove the obstruction and prevent a bowel infarction. The exact extent of surgery depends on the condition of the bowel and the exact cause of the obstruction.

present and combined with edema present another classic sign referred to as the **cobblestone** appearance (Fig. 3–34). There is also thickening of the bowel wall, which lessens the appearance of the mucosal folds to the extent that the folds may be absent. This condition may further be complicated with fistulous connections to other structures such as other bowel loops, the bladder, or the vagina. Sigmoidoscopy or colonoscopy may demonstrate patchy areas of inflammation, which differentiate Crohn's disease from ulcerative colitis. Colonoscopy also includes a biopsy, which is most cases yields a definitive diagnosis.

Treatment. The treatment of regional enteritis is based on the symptoms present. Antiinflammatory drugs and other medications are given according to the severity of the condition. Physical rest and a restrictive diet are most important in minimizing the advancement of this disease. In the presence of stenosis, the patient is not allowed to eat fruits and vegetables. If this condition involves malabsorption, a low-fat diet is indicated. Surgery is indicated when the bowel is perforated and when massive hemorrhage is present or to correct fistulous tracts and intestinal obstructions. About 70% of patients with Crohn's disease require surgery.

Intestinal Obstruction or Ileus

General Information. Ileus is an intestinal obstruction that frequently occurs because of the lack of

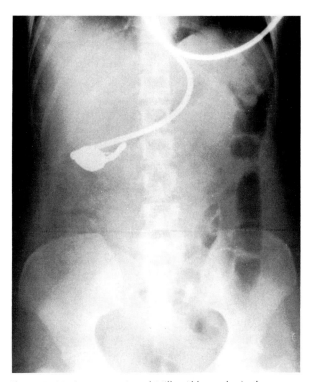

Figure 3–36. A mercury-tipped Miller-Abbott tube in the stomach of a 35-year-old woman. The lack of intestinal gas or bowel shadow indicates a closed-loop obstruction.

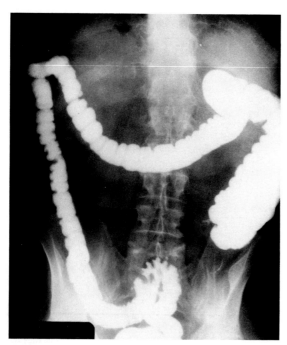

Figure 3–37. Anterior view of a filled colon.

The Large Intestine

The Normal Large Intestine

The large intestine or colon is primarily demonstrated radiographically by a procedure commonly referred to as a barium enema. Barium enters the colon via gravity, through a rectal tube. Barium sulfate, the primary contrast medium, is often combined with air for a double-contrast study. This is often referred to as an air-contrast colon examination. In the single-contrast method, the colon is filled to the point of distension. The radiologist takes several spot views of the colon with the patient in various positions. After this part of the examination, the radiographer takes either a supine or prone radiograph of the opacified colon. High kilovoltage, between 100 and 120 kVp, is necessary to demonstrate the barium-filled colon. The normal anatomy of the opacified colon is shown in Figure 3–37.

Following the filled film, the patient is instructed to go to the washroom and evacuate the barium. Once the initial evacuation is complete, the patient feels immediate relief from abdominal cramping and will usually return to the dressing room. If an air contrast study is to be performed, the patient returns to the fluoroscopic room and is again placed on the radiographic table. Air is then injected into the colon via a rectal tube. Additional fluoroscopic views are taken by the radiologist, and several views are taken by the radiographer with the patient in the anteroposterior (AP), PA, and lateral decubitus positions. The patient then returns to the washroom and com-

pletes the evacuation of barium. The postevacuation film is usually taken after the second evacuation of the colon. It reveals the contraction of the colon and the mucosa lined with barium (Fig. 3–38).

Congenital Disorders

Intussusception

General Information. Intussusception is a *telescoping* or *invagination* of a part of the bowel into an adjacent distal portion. Of these cases, 95% are reported in children, and 87% before the age of 2 years. Of these children, 70% are between the ages of 4 and 11 months. In children there is no underlying cause, whereas in adults intussusception occurs in relation to polyps, carcinoma, and Meckel's diverticulum. It has been suggested that pediatric intussusception may be linked to viral diseases. It appears that seasonal peaks, coinciding with peak incidence of respiratory tract infections, seem to correlate with the incidences of intussusception and other bowel disorders. The telescoping of the bowel into itself—the intussusception—is propelled along the bowel by peristalsis, pulling more bowel along with it. This in effect produces edema, hemorrhage, and possible obstruction. If this condition is not treated within 24 hours, the bowel will become gangrenous because its

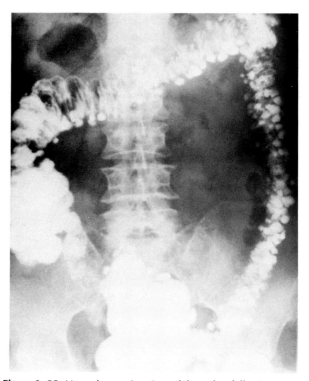

Figure 3–38. Normal posterior view of the colon following evacuation.

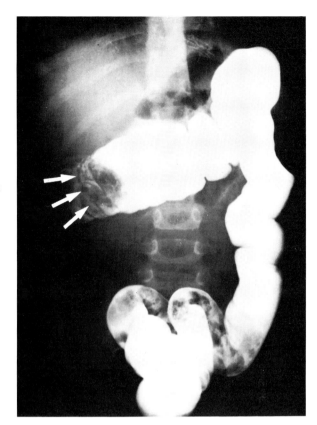

Figure 3–39. Colocolic intussusception in a pediatric patient. The cecum, ascending colon, and hepatic flexure have telescoped into the transverse colon. Note the coiled spring sign (arrows).

blood supply is cut off. This may be a life-threatening situation.

Diagnosis. Four clinical effects are usually evident: (1) Intermittent and severe periods of abdominal pain; afflicted children scream in pain and often draw their legs up to their abdomen; (2) vomiting of stomach contents initially and bile later; (3) abnormal stools, which resemble currant jelly and contain a mixture of mucus and blood; and (4) a tender and distended abdomen. A sausage-shaped mass is palpable in the abdomen. The barium enema is most useful in demonstrating this condition. It usually reveals a characteristic sign referred to as the *coiled spring sign* disclosing a major filling defect (Fig. 3–39). In most cases, the ileum telescopes into the colon. Frequently, the barium enema can save the infant from having major abdominal surgery because the procedure itself reverses the condition. In adults, because intussusception is frequently caused by tumor, surgery is unavoidable. Plain radiographs (without barium) in the upright position can demonstrate a soft tissue mass or a complete or partial obstruction. In the event of obstruction, the loops of bowel will be dilated. A white blood cell (WBC) count of up to 15,000 indicates bowel obstruction. A WBC count greater than 15,000 may indicate a strangulated bowel. A WBC count greater than 20,000 may indicate a complete bowel infarction.

Treatment. A special type of barium enema referred to as hydrostatic reduction is performed by the radiologist, who drips a barium solution into the rectum for approximately 3 feet and traces the progress with fluoroscopy. If this procedure is successful, the barium flows into the ileum and reduces the mass. If the hydrostatic reduction is unsuccessful, then surgery is indicated. During surgery, manual reduction is first attempted. If the reduction is unsuccessful, then a bowel resection will usually be needed. Consideration must be given to events of bowel strangulation or the presence of gangrene.

Hirschsprung's Disease

General Information. Hirschsprung's disease occurs as a result of an absence of ganglion cells in the rectosigmoid region (95% of the time). Peristalsis is lacking, and, as a result, the normal evacuation of stool is impaired and large amounts of feces are retained in the sigmoid colon. Hirschsprung's disease is also referred to as *congenital aganglionic megacolon.* This condition is thought to be a familial congenital defect and occurs in 1 in 2000 to 1 in 5000 births. It mostly affects infant males, at a rate six to seven times more frequently than females, and is most prevalent in Caucasians. Hirschsprung's disease is also common in patients with Down's syndrome and

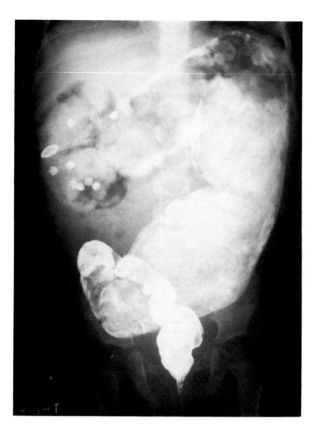

Figure 3–40. Anteroposterior projection of the abdomen taken 4 hours after a barium enema in a girl, age 1½ years. Note the eight metallic objects in the right side of the colon. The patient apparently chewed the buttons off her gown.

anomalies of the urinary tract. The clinical manifestations of this disease usually appear shortly after birth. Signs of obstruction are observed as early as 24 to 48 hours after birth.

Diagnosis. As a result of improper evacuation of feces, significant amounts of gas are present, distending the abdomen. The child is constipated, and there may be repeated episodes of obstruction. The rectal biopsy and the barium enema are the primary means of diagnostic confirmation. The appearance of a grossly *dilated sigmoid* colon, containing massive amounts of feces and a *narrowed* segment just below the dilatation are the cardinal signs (Fig. 3–40). Patients with Hirschsprung's disease should be examined without the usual bowel preparation, which would remove the evidence of the narrowed bowel segment just distal to the dilatation. The radiologist should be careful not to allow too much barium to pass through the narrowed segment. This would only serve to make evacuation that much more difficult.

Treatment. Surgical resection of the aganglionic segment usually relieves this condition. An infant can die within 24 hours without treatment. The initial treatment may be a temporary colostomy, until the infant is older (10 months) and is better able to withstand surgery. It is essential to maintain the fluid electrolyte balance until the condition is corrected.

Mechanical Disorders

Intestinal Obstruction

General Information. Obstruction is any hindrance to the passage of the intestinal contents. Causes may be mechanical, neural, or both. Rather than a disease entity, obstruction is a manifestation produced by many causes. Intraluminal obstruction may be caused by intussusception and impactions from feces, barium, food, and so on. Obstruction of the bowel wall may be due to congenital factors (atresia, stenosis, imperforate anus, Meckel's diverticulum), traumatic causes (hematoma, stricture), inflammation (Crohn's disease, diverticulitis), and neoplasms. Extrinsic compression may be caused by adhesions, hernia, anomalous vessels, abscesses, hematoma, neoplasms, and volvulus. Eighty percent of all intestinal obstructions are the result of adhesions, hernias, and carcinoma. In the small intestine, 90% of the obstructions are the result of incarcerated hernia and adhesions.

Diagnosis. The most characteristic symptoms include abdominal pain, vomiting, and abdominal distension. The most important event occurs when the patient exhibits signs of a strangulated bowel and subsequent peritonitis, with extreme tenderness and rigidity of the abdomen. Routine AP, upright, and

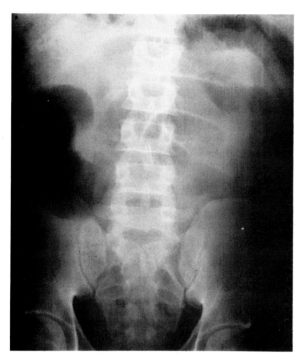

Figure 3–41. A distended air-filled colon with a closed loop of sigmoid colon, consistent with volvulus. The patient is a 46-year-old woman.

ticulosis is most apparent in the lower descending and rectosigmoid colon.

Diagnosis. Although this condition is essentially asymptomatic, the patient often experiences a change in bowel habits, alternating between constipation and diarrhea. Diverticulosis is often an incidental finding on a barium enema, when diverticula are usually *filled* with barium. Barium-filled diverticula can be singular or multiple or can occur in clusters (Fig. 3–42).

Treatment. Diverticulosis usually does not require treatment since it is asymptomatic. When bowel symptoms are present, a bland diet, stool softeners, and occasional doses of mineral oil may be indicated. The patient is made aware of the proper diet to minimize any problems.

Volvulus

General Information. Volvulus is simply a loop of bowel *twisting* upon itself. This condition may result from a rotational abnormality, an ingested foreign body, or possibly an adhesion. In some cases, the cause is never found. This condition is more common in certain geographic areas, with Yugoslavia and Bulgaria having the highest incidence. Dietary factors are thought to be related to this phenomenon. Volvulus usually occurs in a segment of intestine that is

decubitus views of the abdomen show the presence and location of intestinal gas or fluid. In small bowel obstruction, a characteristic *stepladder* appearance is noted. In the upright position, characteristic air bubble signs are apparent and often are indicative of obstruction. The *single bubble* sign is suggestive of pyloric stenosis. The *double bubble* sign is suggestive of duodenal atresia. In colon obstruction, a barium enema demonstrates a distended air-filled colon or closed loop of sigmoid colon with significant distension, as seen with volvulus (Fig. 3–41).

Treatment. As is the case with small bowel obstruction, the usual treatment involves the decompression of the intestine with a Miller-Abbott tube. The replacement of fluids and electrolytes and the surgical removal of the obstruction are also usual.

Diverticulosis

General Information. Diverticulosis is defined as a pouch- or sac-like herniation of the mucous membrane lining through a defect in the muscularis portion of the bowel wall. The diverticula are multiple and widely scattered throughout the colon of elderly persons. Diverticula become more prevalent in men after age 40. The hernial protrusions occur in the absence of inflammation, are asymptomatic, and are mainly associated with aging. A low-fiber diet contributes to the weakening of the bowel wall. Diver-

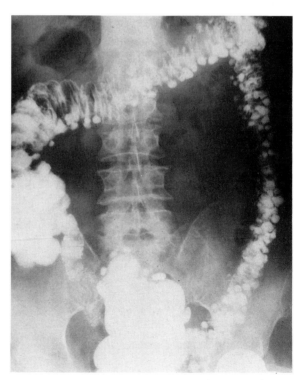

Figure 3–42. Scattered diverticula (diverticulosis) throughout the colon of an 88-year-old woman.

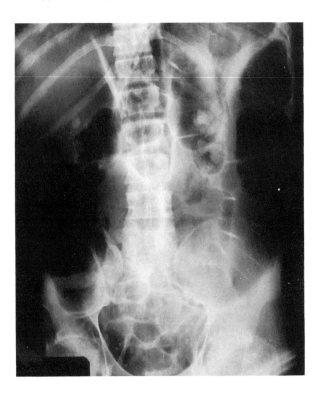

Figure 3–43. A characteristically bean-shaped and enormously distended loop projecting up from the pelvis, similar to an inverted U, which is consistent with the sigmoid volvulus.

long enough to twist. The most common site, the sigmoid colon, usually is affected in elderly patients. Volvulus in children is most common in the small intestine. Other frequent sites are the cecum and stomach. Volvulus represents 4% of all intestinal obstructions. It seems to have a higher incidence in patients with cystic fibrosis.

Diagnosis. The cardinal signs and symptoms that characterize volvulus and that can be determined on a physical examination include vomiting and marked abdominal distension following the sudden onset of severe abdominal pain. In the absence of immediate treatment, strangulation of the twisted bowel loop, ischemia, infarction, perforation, and life-threatening peritonitis may ensue. Routine AP, lateral, and decubitus radiographs of the abdomen usually reveal obstruction with gas distension, *absence* of haustral sacculations, and abnormal air-fluid levels of the sigmoid colon or cecum. The barium enema reveals a smooth, tapered narrowing because of twisting of the colon, with significant dilatation of the bowel proximal to the twist. There characteristically is a *bean-shaped*, enormously distended loop of sigmoid projecting up from the pelvis, similar to an inverted letter U. When the cecum is affected, its distended appearance is observed below the diaphragm, usually in the left hypochondrium. Of added importance is the WBC count. If the count exceeds $15,000/mm^3$, strangulation of the bowel is apparent. When the count is greater than $20,000/mm^3$, an infarction is

usually found. In either case, surgery is indicated (Fig. 3–43).

Treatment. Generally, the treatment varies according to the location and the severity of the volvulus. Sigmoid volvulus can be reduced by deflating the bowel and expelling the gas by careful insertion of a sigmoidoscope. To confirm the presence of a vascular occlusion, especially of the aorta and inferior mesenteric artery, an abdominal flush arteriogram and selective catheterization can be performed.

Inguinal Hernia

General Information. Inguinal hernia, or rupture, as it is commonly called, occurs when part of an internal organ protrudes through an opening in the containing wall of its cavity. Although many types of hernia are possible, inguinal hernia is the most common, accounting for 75% of all hernias. Preventive repair of inguinal hernias is the most common abdominal operation. With an inguinal hernia, one or more loops of bowel enter the groin and become trapped. In the event of twisting, the blood supply may be compromised or totally cut off, producing an infarct in the intestine. Bowel infarction is a potentially life-threatening situation. Inguinal hernias are more common in men because of a congenital defect that results when the peritoneum is transported to the inguinal region as the testes descend from the abdomen into the scrotum. Lifting, coughing, straining, and acci-

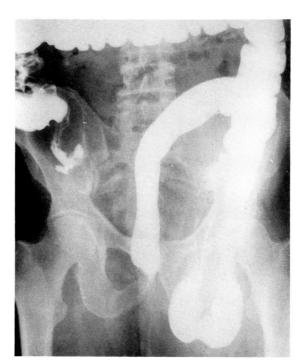

Figure 3–44. Indirect inguinal hernia in a 39-year-old man.

dents are the most common causes of inguinal hernia. Obesity is a contributing factor because of increased pressure in the abdomen. In the elderly, inguinal hernias occur as a result of generalized weakness in the bowel wall in the absence of a congenital hernial sac. Two distinct types of inguinal hernia are possible. A *direct* inguinal hernia occurs when the protruding sac pushes directly outward through the weakest part of the abdominal wall. An *indirect* inguinal hernia occurs when the protruding sac pushes directly downward at an angle into the scrotal sac. The indirect type is the more common form of inguinal hernia.

Diagnosis. Following the incident in which a rupture has occurred, a lump appears when a patient stands or strains. The lump disappears in the recumbent position. Depending on the severity and tension, pain varies from constant to intermittent (during physical activity). In an infant, inguinal hernia often coexists with an undescended testicle or a hydrocele. While the patient is standing and performing Valsalva's maneuver, the lump can be palpated. A barium enema is performed to rule out bowel obstruction (Fig. 3–44).

Treatment. The treatment depends on whether the hernia is reducible or irreducible. When reducible, the hernia can be pushed back by manipulation into its proper location. An irreducible hernia is also referred to as an *incarcerated* hernia. This means that the hernia is so occluded that it cannot be manipulated back into place. An irreducible inguinal hernia usually requires surgical repair.

Inflammatory Disorders

Diverticulitis

General Information. Small outpouchings of colonic mucosa and submucosa that herniate between the main muscle bundles are called diverticula. A person in whom diverticula are present is said to have diverticulosis. With the added complication of inflammation, the patient is described as having diverticulitis. Diverticulosis is asymptomatic and is largely due to the aging process, but diverticulitis is promoted by the accumulation or lodging of feces in the pouches. Spreading of this inflammation to surrounding tissue is common and is referred to as peridiverticulitis. This chronic inflammatory process causes thickening of the bowel wall and adjacent tissues, with constriction of the lumen of the bowel. Other manifestations of this disease often mimic carcinoma.

Diagnosis. Diverticulitis is most frequently encountered in the distal colon. The primary sign of this disease is *hemorrhage*, which occurs in response to the inflammation. The patient experiences a colicky pain with either constipation or diarrhea, possibly with blood in the stools. Radiographically, the barium enema demonstrates the barium *outlining* but not filling the diverticula, which are filled with impacted feces, and a characteristic *saw-tooth* pattern. In cases of acute diverticulitis, a barium enema may cause the bowel to rupture, so this barium enema

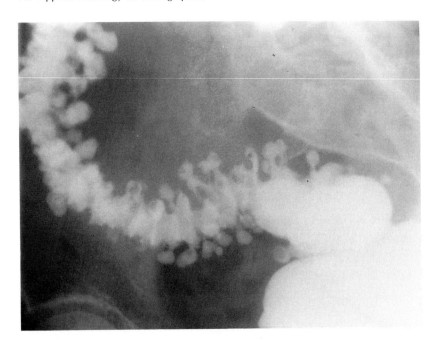

Figure 3–45. Characteristic saw-tooth pattern consistent with diverticulitis in a 62-year-old woman.

study requires caution. Because this condition is largely inflammatory, colonic spasm is often noted on the radiographs (Fig. 3–45).

Treatment. The treatment of diverticulitis involves minimizing the inflammation and treating the infection. Patients are placed on a high-residue diet, and antibiotics and antispasmodics are administered. When the condition does not respond to the usual course of treatment, there is a possibility of several complications such as perforation, peritonitis, obstruction, or fistula. A colon resection removes the involved segment of colon.

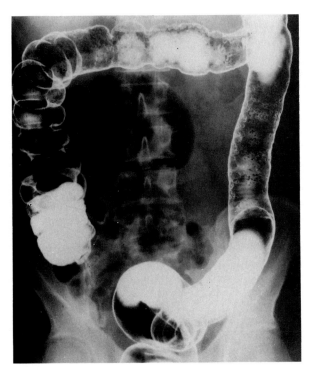

Figure 3–46. Air contrast of colon revealing multiple ring-shaped filling defects, presumably representing pseudopolyposis in view of this 43-year-old man's history of ulcerative colitis. Also noted is the lack of haustral sacculations of the descending colon. This is referred to as the stovepipe sign, another indication of ulcerative colitis.

Ulcerative Colitis

General Information. Ulcerative colitis is a diffusely distributed *mucosal* disease of the colon. Because ulcerative colitis affects the mucosa and submucosa of the rectosigmoid region whereas Crohn's disease affects *all layers* of the bowel wall, especially the terminal ileum, these two conditions are easy to differentiate. Ulcerative colitis is most common in young adults and has a higher incidence in patients who are Jewish and persons in higher than average socioeconomic groups. There is some suggestion that the incidence is higher in persons with a prior family history of the illness and in persons allergic to milk and substances that release inflammatory histamines in the bowel. It is thought that emotional stress plays an important role, coinciding with the onset of this disorder. The cardinal signs in the acute stage of onset include ulceration and excessive bloody diarrhea with pus and mucus. The disease usually begins at the anus and ascends into the rectosigmoid region. In the most severe cases, the total colon may be involved (50%). Ulcerative colitis is characterized by remissions and relapses and has the capability of recurring over a lifetime. When it occurs chronically, some complications include irregular ulcerations, anorexia, weight loss, electrolyte imbalance, toxic megacolon, stricture, perianal fistula, and carcinoma. Carcinoma is most common in the fourth decade of life, in about 10% of those patients who have had ulcerative colitis for more than a 10-year period. This form of carcinoma is highly malignant and is most common in patients whose initial onset of ulcerative colitis occurred early in life. Only 20% of patients having this carcinoma will survive a 5-year period.

Diagnosis. Diagnosis can be accomplished by means of a sigmoidoscopic examination. This is usually followed by colonoscopy and biopsy. Barium enemas are performed to determine the extent of the disease and complications. In the early stages of the disease, the bowel wall appears shaggy or finely serrated. In the later stages, a more ragged and marginal ulceration may become evident. There usually is shortening and thickening of the mucosa with loss of the haustral sacculations, giving the bowel a *hose-pipe* appearance (Fig. 3–46). In 2 to 5% of the cases, there is toxic megacolon. The barium enema assists the physician in distinguishing ulcerative colitis from Crohn's disease, as well as from amebic and bacillary dysentery.

Treatment. The treatment of ulcerative colitis is largely conservative. Eighty-five percent of the time the emphasis of treatment is in controlling inflammation, replacing the nutritional loss, and helping patients gain weight and strength. Periodic sigmoidoscopic examinations are done to detect malignancy, especially if this is a long-standing disease. Surgery is usually a last resort and will be performed in the event of toxic megacolon. The surgical procedure performed is a proctocolectomy with ileostomy.

Self-Assessment Quiz

For each of the following questions, select the one best response and circle the letter that precedes it.

1. When adjusting the patient for a left lateral decubitus position, which side of the patient's body is in contact with the surface of the table or cart?
   a. right
   b. left

2. Free air in the abdominal cavity can be demonstrated with the patient in which of the following positions?
   a. AP erect
   b. prone
   c. lateral decubitus
   d. AP supine
   e. AP erect and lateral decubitus

3. Which of the following are contraindicated when a perforated viscus is suspected?
   a. barium sulfate
   b. Esophotrast
   c. Gastrografin
   d. Barotrast
   e. barium sulfate, Esophotrast, Barotrast

4. CT and ultrasonography are useful modalities for demonstrating metastases of abdominal viscera.
   a. true
   b. false

5. The most common patient complaint in the presence of esophageal disease is
   a. pain
   b. pressure
   c. dysphagia
   d. nausea

6. A congenital absence of a lumen is known as
   a. atresia
   b. a fistula
   c. stenosis
   d. coarctation

7. An abnormal path or tract leading from one organ to another is called
   a. atresia
   b. a fistula
   c. stenosis
   d. coarctation

8. Esophageal atresia is frequently associated with
   a. tracheoesophageal fistula
   b. foramen ovale
   c. imperforate anus
   d. volvulus

9. An outpouching of one or more layers of the esophageal wall describes
   a. a diverticulum
   b. a hernia
   c. an ulceration
   d. an invagination

10. The terms *Zenker's* and *pulsion* refer to types of
    a. hiatal hernias
    b. diverticula
    c. ulcerations
    d. anastomoses

11. The terms *epiphrenic* and *traction* refer to types of
    a. colonic diverticula
    b. ulcerations
    c. esophageal diverticula
    d. tumors

12. Esophageal varices are dilated, tortuous
    a. arteries
    b. veins

13. Esophageal varices are usually a complication of
    a. gastric distension
    b. hiatal hernia
    c. portal venous hypertension
    d. biliary atresia

14. Vasopressin is a hormone that causes arteries to
    a. dilate
    b. constrict

15. The terms *sliding* and *rolling* pertain to
    a. esophageal atresia
    b. hiatal hernia
    c. esophageal varices
    d. inguinal hernia

16. Cardiospasms, esophagitis, and heartburn are terms usually associated with
    a. hiatal hernia
    b. diverticulitis
    c. portal venous hypertension
    d. pyloric stenosis

17. Achalasia is a neuromuscular disorder of the esophagus that results in progressive esophageal
    a. constriction
    b. dilatation

18. In the incidence of congenital disorders of the alimentary tract, hypertrophic pyloric stenosis ranks
    a. first
    b. second
    c. third
    d. fourth

19. The cardinal sign of congenital pyloric stenosis is
    a. excessive drooling
    b. anorexia
    c. projectile vomiting
    d. diarrhea

20. Peptic ulcers can be found in the
    a. stomach and duodenum
    b. stomach only
    c. duodenum and terminal ileum
    d. duodenum only

21. The most frequent site of gastric ulcer is the
    a. duodenum
    b. pylorus
    c. lesser curvature
    d. greater curvature

22. The Billroth II procedure may also be described as
    a. gastrojejunostomy
    b. colon resection
    c. gastroesophagectomy
    d. colostomy

23. Meckel's diverticulum is the leading congenital defect of the alimentary tract.
    a. true
    b. false

24. Meckel's diverticulum can be found anywhere in the small and large intestine.
    a. true
    b. false

25. The double bubble sign is associated with
    a. duodenal atresia
    b. imperforate anus
    c. esophageal atresia
    d. gastritis

26. Celiac disease is also known as
    a. the double syndrome
    b. gastritis
    c. the malabsorption syndrome
    d. spastic colon

27. Which of the following is a synonym for Crohn's disease?
    a. hypertrophic gastritis
    b. peptic ulcer
    c. regional enteritis
    d. spastic colon

28. The portion of the bowel that is primarily affected in persons with Crohn's disease is the
    a. cecum
    b. duodenum
    c. terminal ileum
    d. sigmoid colon

29. Which of the following best describes a distended bowel?
    a. nausea
    b. hematemesis
    c. double bubble sign
    d. ileus

30. A telescoping of the bowel into itself is termed
    a. intussusception
    b. volvulus
    c. atresia
    d. incarceration

31. The stepladder sign is a radiological sign that may indicate bowel
    a. herniation
    b. obstruction
    c. metastases
    d. hemorrhage

32. Congenital megacolon is otherwise known as
    a. Meckel's disease
    b. Crohn's disease
    c. Hirschsprung's disease
    d. diverticulosis

33. Diverticulosis is typically
    a. a disease of the elderly
    b. an asymptomatic disorder
    c. a type of polyp
    d. an asymptomatic disorder of the elderly

34. A twisting of the bowel upon itself is termed
    a. intussusception
    b. atresia
    c. volvulus
    d. stenosis

35. An indirect inguinal hernia occurs when the protruding sac pushes directly
    a. outward through the weakest part of the abdominal wall
    b. downward at an angle into the scrotal sac

36. Feces accumulate within the outpouchings of the colon in the condition known as
    a. diverticulitis
    b. diverticulosis

37. Ulcerative colitis is a diffusely distributed mucosal disease.
    a. true
    b. false

38. The cardinal sign in the acute stage of ulcerative colitis is
    a. hemoptysis
    b. hematemesis
    c. ulceration with bloody diarrhea
    d. black tarry stool

39. The hose-pipe appearance is a typical sign of
    a. ulcerative colitis
    b. Crohn's disease
    c. bowel obstruction
    d. volvulus

Study Questions

1. Explain the importance of the plain film of the abdomen.

2. Describe the different types of hiatal hernias.

3. Explain the use of Valsalva's maneuver and Trendelenburg's position as they relate to radiography of the upper gastrointestinal tract.

4. Describe a major sign or symptom of each of the following disorders:
   Pyloric stenosis
   Esophageal atresia
   Tracheoesophageal fistula
   Hirschsprung's disease

5. Describe the comparative features of ulcerative colitis and Crohn's disease.

6. Which organs are involved in the Billroth II surgical procedure? Why is this procedure done?

7. What is the significance of each of the following?
   String sign
   Coiled spring sign
   Double bubble sign
   Stepladder sign
   Schatzki's ring
   Trefoil cap

8. Describe three mechanical disorders of the colon.

Four

The Hepatobiliary System

The Liver
Inflammatory Disorders

The Gallbladder
Inflammatory Disorders

The Pancreas
Congenital Disorders
Inflammatory Disorders

Related Terminology

bilirubin
cholecystitis
cholelithiasis
hemolytic
jaundice
Laennec's cirrhosis
mucoviscidosis
pancreatitis
viral hepatitis

Objectives

Upon completion of Chapter 4, the reader will be able to

- List the primary congenital and inflammatory disorders of the liver, gallbladder, and pancreas.

- List the modalities that are used to image the liver, gallbladder, and pancreas.

- List and describe the routine positions used in radiography of the gallbladder and bile ducts.

- Describe the various forms of cholangiography.

- Explain the rationale and methodology of cholecystography.

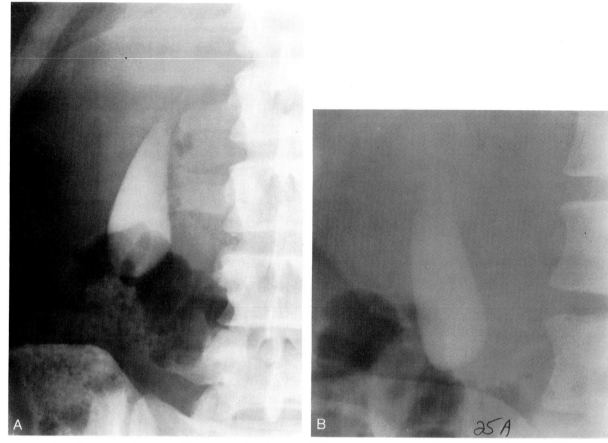

Figure 4–1. *A,* Posteroanterior view of the normally functioning gallbladder. *B,* Left anterior oblique view of the normally functioning gallbladder.

The liver, gallbladder, and pancreas are accessory organs of digestion. The clinical features of diseases involving these accessory organs often are clearly evident. In other cases, however, the symptoms may be less specific and may resemble those of other abnormal abdominal conditions. Because the pathological conditions are so varied, numerous methods of diagnostic imaging are employed. The referring physician often requests diagnostic procedures in a sequential combination. A *cholecystogram,* for example, is performed in conjunction with an upper gastrointestinal series.

In the presence of vague symptoms, it is not uncommon for the physician to order examinations of the colon, small intestine, and urinary tract in addition to the upper gastrointestinal and gallbladder series. These procedures are usually performed over a 2- to 3-day period, depending on whether the first dose of contrast medium permits visualization of the gallbladder.

Oral cholecystography most often is ordered to assess the degree of gallbladder function. Calculi within the gallbladder or the bile ducts are often detected visibly or by presumption when the gallbladder does not visualize. An opaque stone in the common bile or cystic duct can be determined by its position relative to the normal gallbladder. A cholecystogram usually consists of plain films of the gallbladder with the patient in the posteroanterior (PA) and left anterior oblique (LAO) positions (Fig. 4–1).

To demonstrate layering or stratification of gallstones, the right lateral decubitus position is used (Fig. 4–2). Upright posterior oblique spot views may be taken by the radiologist (Fig. 4–3). Many x-ray departments give patients a fatty meal following the fluoroscopic spots. After about 20 minutes, anterior

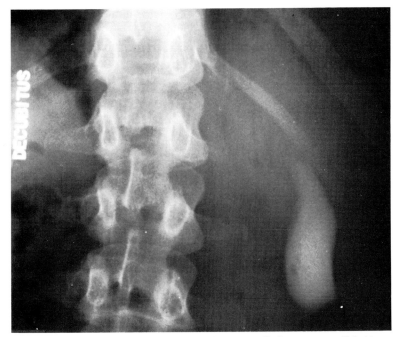

Figure 4–2. Right lateral decubitus view of the normally functioning gallbladder.

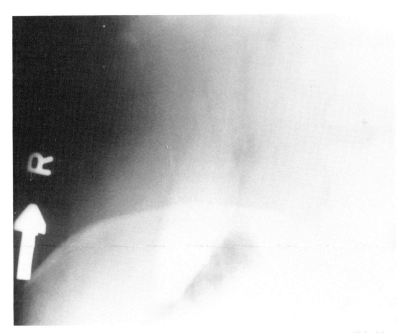

Figure 4–3. Upright posterior oblique view of the normally functioning gallbladder.

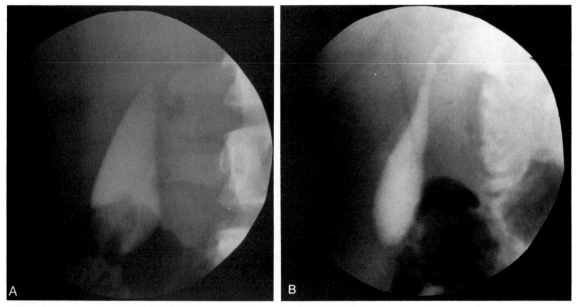

Figure 4–4. *A,* Normally functioning gallbladder before a fatty meal. *B,* Normally functioning gallbladder after a fatty meal.

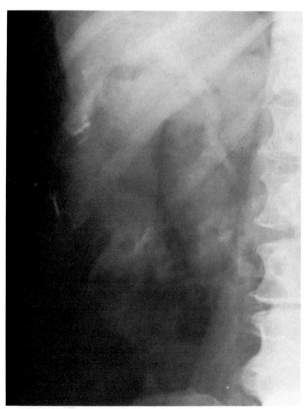

Figure 4–5. Normal right posterior oblique intravenous cholangiogram with excellent visualization of the hepatic and common bile ducts.

views should reveal a **contracted** gallbladder that has emptied as a result of the ingested fatty meal. When ingested, fat causes the release of the hormone **cholecystokinin**, which stimulates gallbladder contraction (Fig. 4–4).

Intravenous cholangiography is indicated in situations in which oral cholecystography is not possible. The patient may have recurring cholecystitis following previous cholecystectomy or may be allergic to the oral contrast medium. The bile ducts are visualized in the posterior and posterior oblique positions about 20 to 30 minutes after injection. Like the oral method, the intravenous method is usually unsuccessful in patients with severe liver disease or obstructive jaundice (Fig. 4–5).

A **cholecystectomy** is the surgical removal of the gallbladder and cystic duct. Because of the high probability of calculi in the bile ducts, an operative or surgical cholangiogram is routinely performed. This usually involves an x-ray of the bile ducts after they are injected with contrast medium. This surgical radiograph is interpreted by the radiologist as soon as possible. When further stones are identified, the surgeon may perform a common duct exploration. If the potential for further calculi exists, a T-tube may be inserted for a later postoperative T-tube cholangiogram. The T-tube cholangiogram is also useful for demonstrating strictures of the common bile duct and assessing neoplastic obstruction (Fig. 4–6).

Percutaneous transhepatic cholangiography is primarily indicated to diagnose obstructive jaundice,

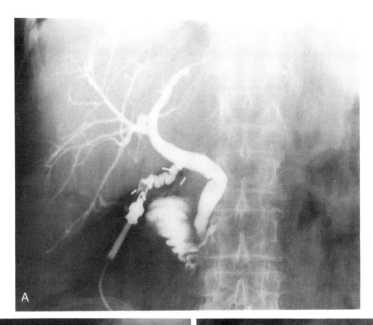

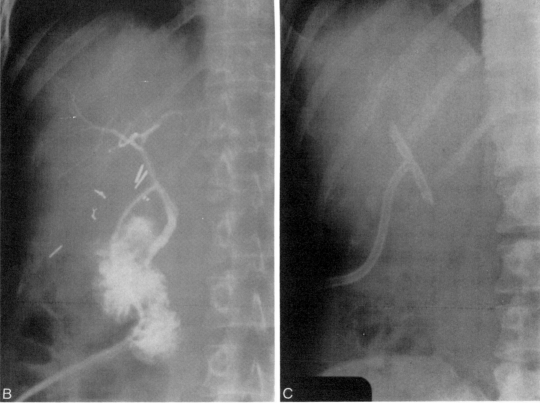

Figure 4–6. *A,* Surgical cholangiogram taken after removal of the gallbladder in a 46-year-old woman. No additional stones were located in the bile ducts. *B,* Negative postoperative T-tube cholangiogram with excellent visualization of the T-tube and bile ducts in a 44-year-old woman. *C,* Scout film for location of the T-tube in a 42-year-old woman.

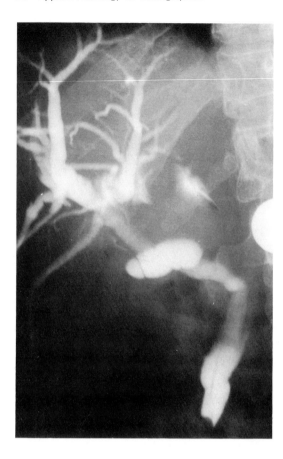

Figure 4–7. A 7-mm meniscus-shaped filling defect in the common bile duct at the ampulla of Vater, most compatible with a common duct stone with mild to moderate dilatation. The patient is a woman, age 71.

but only when all other methods of cholangiography are not possible (Fig. 4–7).

Splenoportography is performed to determine the existence of portal hypertension and to differentiate between intra- and extrahepatic portal obstruction.

An injection takes place percutaneously into the splenic pulp, with resulting visualization of the portal system (Fig. 4–8).

Hepatic angiography is accomplished via a pressurized injection into the celiac trunk or selectively

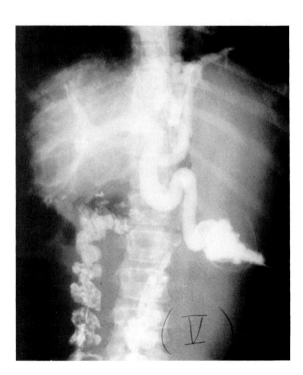

Figure 4–8. Negative splenoportogram of a 12-year-old girl.

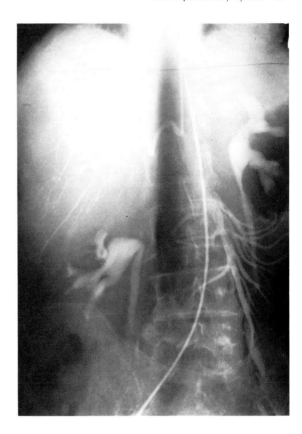

Figure 4–9. An essentially normal selective hepatic arteriogram with prominence of the portal venous system. A ptotic right kidney is seen in this 76-year-old woman.

into the hepatic artery. This procedure is designed to demonstrate both primary and metastatic tumors as well as vascular lesions (Fig. 4–9).

Endoscopic retrograde cholangiopancreatography (ERCP) involves the cannulation of the ampulla of Vater, common bile duct, or pancreatic duct under fluoroscopic control. This is currently the preferred method for investigating obstructive jaundice (Fig. 4–10).

Ultrasonography has dramatically improved the

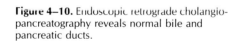

Figure 4–10. Endoscopic retrograde cholangiopancreatography reveals normal bile and pancreatic ducts.

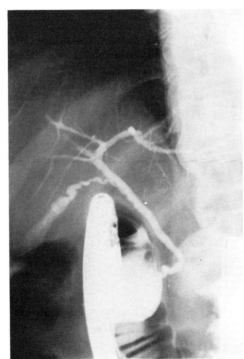

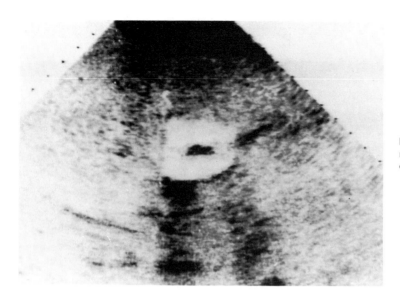

Figure 4–11. Sonogram revealing cholelithiasis and metastasis of the liver and pancreas in a 48-year-old woman.

detection of nonopaque calculi in the gallbladder. Recent developments in sonographic imaging have led to improved differentiation between solid lesions, cysts, and normal tissue (Fig. 4–11).

Computed tomography (CT) is especially useful for differentiating primary and metastatic tumors from cystic lesions (Fig. 4–12).

Radioisotope liver scans demonstrate cold areas or areas of diminished uptake (Fig. 4–13).

Because so many diagnostic imaging methods are available, it seems reasonable to use the noninvasive procedures first. The more sophisticated procedures such as percutaneous transhepatic cholangiography and angiography should be reserved for special applications. CT and ultrasonography are the best methods for demonstrating liver masses, cysts, and abscesses. Ultrasonography is best for differentiating solid masses from cysts. Although CT and ultrasonog-

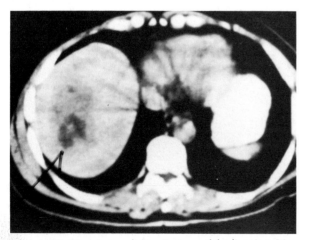

Figure 4–12. CT scan revealing metastases of the liver in a 36-year-old woman.

raphy basically are used for the same purpose, ultrasonography is far less expensive than CT.

The Liver

Inflammatory Disorders

Viral Hepatitis

General Information. Viral hepatitis is a common primary disease of the liver. Approximately 70,000 cases are reported annually in the United States. It is characterized by destruction of specific liver cells referred to as hepatocytes. Viral hepatitis also results in necrosis, autolysis, jaundice, and hepatomegaly. This disease occurs in three forms: (1) Type A is the most common form and is highly contagious. Ingestion of contaminated water, milk, or food is the usual cause. It is more common in children and young adults of low socioeconomic status. (2) Type B, serum hepatitis, can occur at any age and is often acquired via contaminated blood. Skin punctures from used needles are a hazard to the radiographer, and blood for transfusion can be contaminated, posing another risk. Accidental skin punctures are most common among laboratory technicians, blood bank workers, and dentists. However, radiographers working in angiography are also vulnerable because they are assisting the radiologist in close quarters. When handling needles and other used surgical items, it is advisable to wear gloves to prevent potentially contaminated blood from entering a skin wound. Acquired immunodeficiency syndrome (AIDS) can be accidently transmitted via this method. Type B is especially common among homosexuals, presumably because of oral and anal sexual contact. (3) Type C, or type non-A/non-B is the result of a yet unidentified

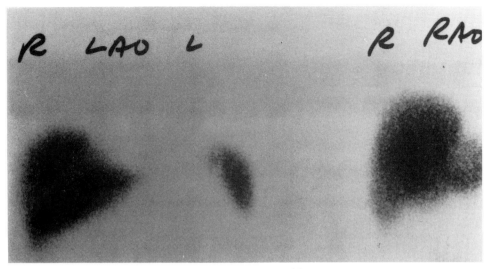

Figure 4–13. A negative radioisotope liver scan of a 52-year-old woman.

virus that bears no resemblance to types A or B. Type A usually has an acute onset and a reasonable prognosis. Type B has a more gradual onset and a higher mortality rate in the elderly.

Diagnosis. The patient's history usually differentiates type A from type B. Various blood types reveal abnormalities consistent with this disease. Detection of an antibody to type A confirms the diagnosis. An abnormal prothrombin time may indicate severe liver damage. Serum glutamic-oxaloacetic transaminase

(SGOT) is an indicator of liver damage when present in excessive amounts. Serum glutamic-pyruvic transaminase (SGPT) also indicates liver damage and cellular necrosis, which are often present when the patient has jaundice. Serum bilirubin is another indicator of liver dysfunction. Its value is excessive in all forms of hepatitis. Serum alkaline phosphatase is also elevated. The plain flat plate of the abdomen often reveals hepatomegaly (Fig. 4–14). The radionuclide scan usually reveals patchy areas of hepato-

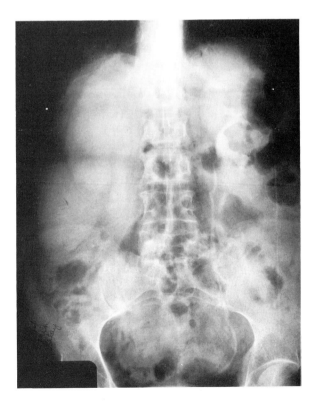

Figure 4–14. Intravenous pyelographic study reveals hepatomegaly, which is consistent with chronic hepatitis and/or cirrhosis. Nonopacification of the right collecting system is noted in this 84-year-old woman.

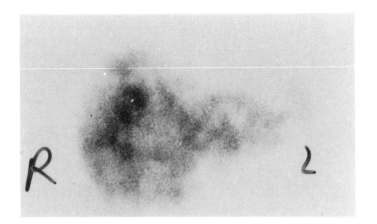

Figure 4–15. Radioisotope liver scan reveals an area of hepatocellular necrosis in a 61-year-old man. This is consistent with cirrhosis.

cellular necrosis (Fig. 4–15). Under the guidance of fluoroscopy, a liver biopsy can be taken to confirm the finding of necrosis. Ultrasonography differentiates the cellular densities. CT is also used to assess the level of necrosis.

Treatment. The primary treatment for hepatitis is bed rest, especially in the early stages of the disease. The patient's diet should contain ample calories and protein. Medications may be administered for nausea and vomiting, and eating several small meals daily may help to combat anorexia.

Cirrhosis

General Information. Cirrhosis is a chronic liver disease that is characterized by diffuse destruction and necrosis of hepatocytes with fibrotic regeneration (fibrous connective tissue repair). When fibrotic tissue is present, liver function is altered. The changes in structure lead to an alteration of blood and lymph flow, resulting in insufficiency. Cirrhosis is twice as common in men as in women and is especially evident in chronic alcoholics who are malnourished and usually older than 50 years. The mortality rate is high, and many patients die within 5 years after the initial onset. There are several types of cirrhosis; however, our discussion centers on those types encountered in diagnostic imaging.

Alcoholic cirrhosis, sometimes referred to as Laennec's cirrhosis, accounts for about 30 to 50% of all types of cirrhosis. More than 90% of patients with cirrhosis have a history of alcoholism. Most of the liver damage is the result of malnutrition. The lack of dietary protein precipitates fibrosis.

Biliary cirrhosis is the result of any disease that ultimately reduces or blocks the flow of bile through the ducts. Biliary cirrhosis accounts for 15 to 20% of all cases of cirrhosis.

Postnecrotic cirrhosis is the result of chronic, long-term hepatitis. This type of cirrhosis accounts for about 10 to 30% of all cases of cirrhosis.

Diagnosis. The clinical signs and symptoms of cirrhosis are similar in all forms of the illness, especially in the early stages. Most of the symptoms involve the gastrointestinal system and include anorexia, indigestion, nausea, vomiting, diarrhea, or constipation. The patient may complain of dull abdominal cramping. The symptoms become more serious and apparent in the later stages and include portal venous hypertension and hepatic insufficiency. Obvious difficulties are apparent in other body systems. Fluid accumulates in the abdomen and limits thoracic expansion. Fluid accumulating in the abdominal cavity, termed acites, interferes with the gas exchange and results in hypoxia. With liver dysfunction, there is an accumulation of toxic wastes such as bilirubin and ammonia, resulting in central nervous system depression. This is referred to as hepatic or portal encephalopathy, and it results in lethargy, impaired speech, paranoia, stupor, and possibly an eventual comatose state. Due to hematological changes affecting blood clotting, the patient experiences bleeding tendencies such as spontaneous epistaxis (nosebleeds), subcutaneous pinpoint hemorrhages (petechiae), and bleeding gums. The skin appears extremely dry, and the patient complains of pruritus (itching). Hepatomegaly is apparent on a plain radiograph of the abdomen. Jaundice may be apparent and is the result of the excessively high serum bilirubin. A major complication of cirrhosis is esophageal varices, which result from portal venous hypertension. The elevation of pressure in the portal vein causes blood to back up into the spleen and flow through collateral circulation to the venous system, bypassing the liver. This pressure causes these collateral veins to enlarge and subsequently rupture. Varices are varicose/collateral veins located at the distal esophagus (Fig. 4–16). When the veins rupture, hemorrhage ensues, usually resulting in massive hematemesis. This hemorrhage is usually the first sign of portal venous hypertension. Exact diagnosis of esophageal varices is provided through an endoscopic examination, which locates the exact site of

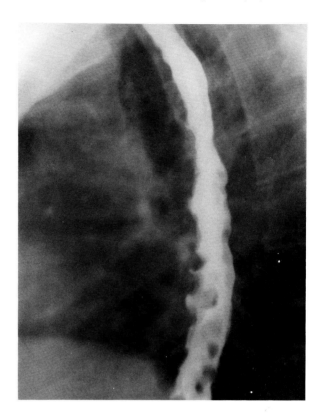

Figure 4–16. Esophagogram reveals multiple filling defects of the greater length of the esophagus, which is consistent with varices. The patient is a 75-year-old man.

hemorrhage. Angiography carries with it a high risk and is not considered to be as accurate as endoscopy. The liver biopsy provides the most accurate diagnosis of cirrhosis. A radionuclide liver scan usually reveals abnormal thickening and a liver mass. Splenoportal venography reveals the portal venous system. Percutaneous transhepatic cholangiography is capable of differentiating intrahepatic from extrahepatic obstruc-

tive jaundice and reveals any other liver pathology (Fig. 4–17).

Treatment. The success of treatment depends on how much damage the liver has suffered and the degree of involvement of other vital organs. Thus, the treatment is designed to remove or alleviate the underlying causes of cirrhosis as well as treat the complications. Much of the treatment is dietary. A

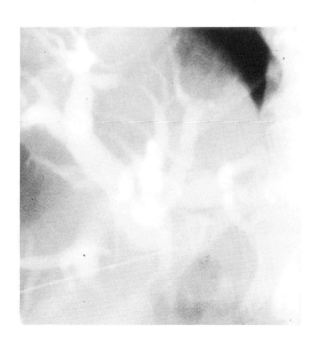

Figure 4–17. Percutaneous transhepatic cholangiogram of a 57-year-old woman reveals an obstruction of the high origin of the common bile duct.

diet that is high in calories and moderate to high in protein is indicated. Sodium is greatly restricted, and the patient is encouraged to get professional counseling. Medications are administered with extreme caution, since the damaged liver may not be able to carry out its vital function in detoxifying poisons. Diuretics are vital but must be monitored carefully. The patient must be checked periodically for bleeding.

The Gallbladder

Inflammatory Disorders

Cholecystitis/Cholelithiasis

General Information. Cholecystitis is an inflammation of the gallbladder that can be both an acute as well as a chronic disorder. In acute cholecystitis, the cystic duct usually is obstructed by mucus or calculus. As the liver bile accumulates in the gallbladder, it becomes increasingly concentrated and eventually irritates the wall of the gallbladder. As

this inflammation increases, bacteria become more evident.

As a result, chronic cholecystitis almost always develops in association with gallstones. Patients with chronic disease present symptoms such as belching, fullness after meals, nausea, heartburn, and an inability to eat normal-sized meals. The symptoms are usually aggravated by the ingestion of fatty foods. Chronic cholecystitis can also be caused by pancreatitis, carcinoma of the gallbladder, or obstructive jaundice but most frequently is the result of gallstones.

Cholelithiasis, or stones in the gallbladder, is a common condition affecting about 20 million people in the United States. It annually accounts for one billion dollars in medical expenses. Gallstones are most common in affluent countries. Cholelithiasis is more common in women, and obese individuals are at increased risk. Cholelithiasis has been reported to afflict more than 80% of American Indian women, who have poor absorption of bile acids and decreased ability to convert cholesterol into bile acids. Cholelithiasis is the fifth leading cause of hospitalization in adults and is responsible for 90% of all gallbladder

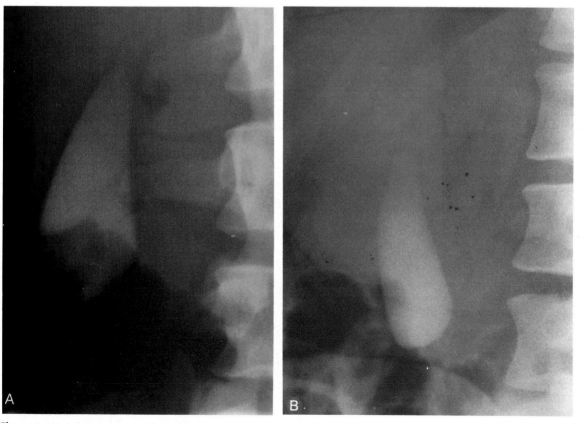

Figure 4–18. *A,* Posteroanterior view of the normal gallbladder. *B,* Left anterior oblique view of a normal gallbladder.

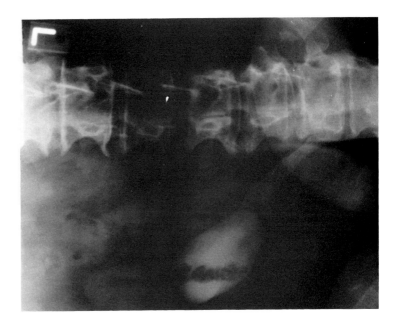

Figure 4–19. The right lateral decubitus position reveals a layering of gallstones in a 36-year-old woman.

and bile duct disorders. One of every 10 patients with gallstones will eventually have common bile duct involvement. Calculi obstructing the hepatic or common bile ducts may lead to obstructive jaundice. Although the incidence of gallstones increases with age, many of the more serious cases are middle-aged patients, who suffer from an acute form of cholecystitis and eventually require surgical intervention. Older patients in general have chronic symptoms and are treated conservatively.

Diagnosis. The typical method of diagnosis is predicated on the patient's signs and symptoms and the results of a cholecystogram in conjunction with the ingestion of an oral iodinated contrast agent. The most common contrast agent is supplied in tablet form. The patient swallows six to eight tablets, one at a time with water, following the evening meal. The evening meal should be light and must not include any foods containing fat. Instructions about the amount of hydration depend on the patient's condition.

The purpose of the cholecystogram is to determine the ability of the gallbladder to fill, concentrate bile, and empty. If the cholecystogram is successful, the contrast agent has filled the gallbladder, rendering it visible. Diminished visibility of the gallbladder may be indicative of disease. To differentiate between a slowly functioning and nonfunctioning gallbladder, a repeat or double-dose gallbladder examination is performed the following day. The patient is given the same dose of tablets, with the same instructions to follow. The gallbladder x-rays are repeated the next morning. If there is little or no difference in opacification of the gallbladder, there is a good chance that the gallbladder is diseased. Studies using oral contrast agents for cholecystography have documented a 98% accuracy in diagnosis. In other words, if the gallbladder is not adequately visualized after two doses of contrast media, it is presumed to be diseased. Surgically, this has been proved to a level of 98% accuracy.

The gallbladder series usually begins with the patient positioned in the PA and LAO positions. The PA is taken on a 10 × 12-inch cassette, and the LAO often uses an 8 × 10-inch cassette (Fig. 4–18). Another popular routine view is the right lateral decubitus. For this position, patients lie on their right side on a cart with their abdomen in contact with the surface of the upright table or chest board. The central ray is directed horizontally to the gallbladder region. This position is used to demonstrate *layering* or *stratification* of gallstones. This phenomenon is the result of the inability of the contrast agent to mix with bile, resulting in a layering or stratification that may resemble floating gallstones (Fig. 4–19). If the gallbladder visualizes, the radiologist will take upright fluoroscopic spots with the patient being rotated from the anteroposterior (AP) position into various degrees of obliquity in the left posterior oblique (LPO) position. In some hospitals, patients ingest a fatty meal after fluoroscopy. The fatty meal is often cream or some dairy product derivative. After about 20 to 30 minutes, a PA film is then taken of the gallbladder. The radiologist compares the film of the filled gallbladder with the film after the fatty meal. The latter should reveal a smaller gallbladder, which contracted and emptied in response to the fatty meal. These additional films are warranted when

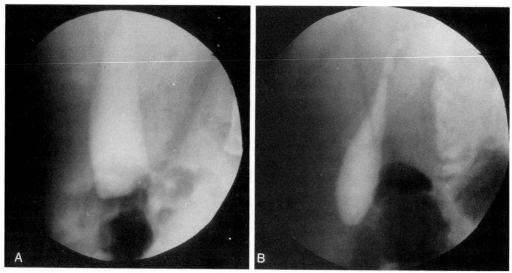

Figure 4–20. *A,* Film of a normal gallbladder before a fatty meal. *B,* Film of a normal gallbladder after a fatty meal, revealing a contracted gallbladder, which emptied in response to the ingestion of fat.

stones are suspected. Stones lodged in the neck of the gallbladder and in the cystic duct are usually better visualized after a fatty meal (Fig. 4–20).

In addition to cholelithiasis, there are other reasons for nonvisualization. Patients may be unable to tolerate the oral contrast agent. If they vomit the contents before the tablets are absorbed, the gallbladder will not be seen. Liver dysfunction, pancreatitis, ductal obstruction, gallbladder disease, and elevated serum bilirubin are examples of conditions that can prevent the gallbladder from visualizing.

Alternate methods of visualizing the gallbladder and bile ducts may need to be considered. The intravenous cholangiogram (IVC) is especially effective in visualizing cholecystitis and can demonstrate inflammation of the affected tissues. The IVC may also be considered for a patient who has cholecystitis in spite of previous surgery to remove the gallbladder. In such cases, it is presumed that stones may have developed somewhere in the bile ducts. For an IVC, the patient is injected with a contrast agent via a drip infusion. Approximately 20 to 30 minutes after the injection, radiographs are taken of the patient in the supine and right posterior oblique (RPO) positions. IVC is often combined with tomography for demonstration of the bile ducts (Fig. 4–21).

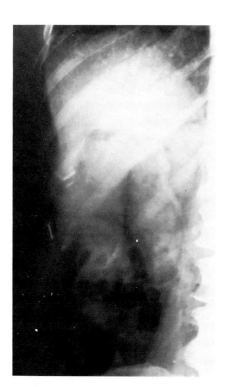

Figure 4–21. Intravenous cholangiogram revealing normal hepatic and common bile ducts in a 53-year-old woman in the right posterior oblique position.

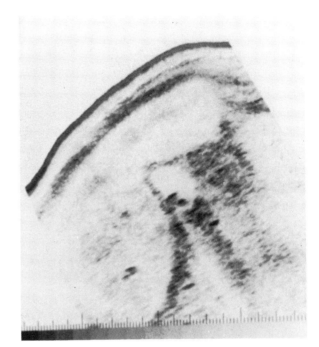

Figure 4–22. Multiple echogenic densities of the gallbladder consistent with cholelithiasis. The patient is a 48-year-old woman.

Most recently, ultrasonography has been used for the purpose of demonstrating stones that consist solely of cholesterol, are not opaque, and cannot be seen in the gallbladder using conventional imaging methods (Fig. 4–22).

Percutaneous transhepatic cholangiography was once the only means of demonstrating the bile ducts when obstructive jaundice was in evidence. However, this procedure carries a much higher risk than ERCP, which is now replacing it. ERCP permits improved direct visualization of the common bile duct and pancreatic ducts. It is particularly effective, even in the presence of jaundice (Fig. 4–23).

Gallstones can be detected in two ways. They are often asymptomatic and are observed on radiographs as incidental findings. Calcified gallstones may appear on radiographs of the ribs, abdomen, and gastrointestinal tract. Generally, the radiologist dictating the report usually requests a follow-up to correlate the findings based on the patient's clinical history. Although the condition may not present symptoms at this time, the patient is counseled about proper

Figure 4–23. Dilatation of the main pancreatic duct at its origin, with tortuosity of the pancreatic duct throughout its course, as seen on endoscopic retrograde cholangiopancreatography of a 61-year-old man. The overall finding is consistent with chronic pancreatitis.

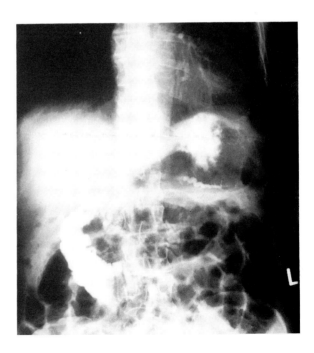

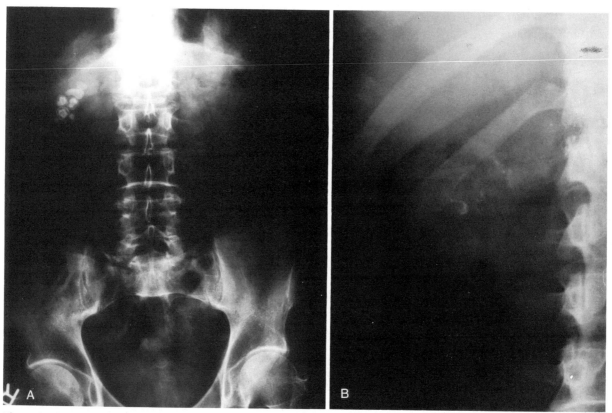

Figure 4–24. *A,* Several calcified gallstones of varying sizes and shapes visualized in the right upper quadrant in a 46-year-old woman. *B,* The gallbladder did not visualize after the administration of two doses of contrast medium in this 52-year-old man.

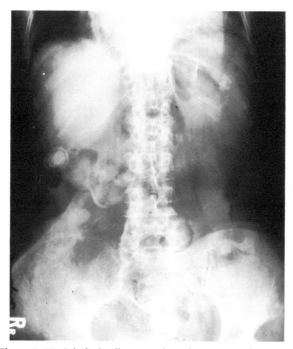

Figure 4–25. Calcified gallstone in the right upper quadrant on a flat plate of the abdomen in a 90-year-old woman. This stone consists of three to four combined elements.

dietary habits. In acute cases, a large calculus may obstruct ductal passageways and result in nonvisualization of the gallbladder (Fig. 4–24).

Gallstones usually are composed of one or more of three bile constituents: calcium *bilirubinate,* calcium *carbonate,* and *cholesterol.* About 10% of the time, a gallstone is said to be pure. A pure gallstone consists almost entirely of one of the three listed substances. Pure gallstones are formed in the presence of an excessive amount of the stone-forming substance. The most frequent type of gallstone is the *mixed* gallstone. Mixed stones account for about 80% of all stones and contain a mixture of varying proportions of all three substances. The mixed gallstone usually forms in the gallbladder as part of a metabolic disorder. The solvents and bile acids are absorbed faster than the calculus-forming substances they hold in solution. Mixed stones are almost always multiple and sometimes are evident in huge numbers. They vary in size from 0.1 cm to 2 cm in diameter and are usually very hard with rough surfaces. *Combined* gallstones are most frequently encountered in patients with cholecystitis. These stones are often incidental findings on the kidney-ureter-bladder (KUB) workup, when they are seen to be composed of a calcified nucleus with a lucent exterior layer (Figs. 4–25 and 4–26).

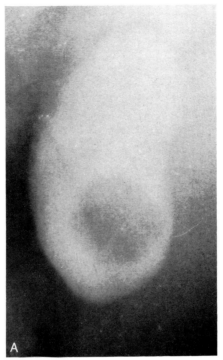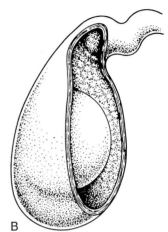

Figure 4–26. *A,* Oral cholecystogram reveals a functioning gallbladder despite the presence of a single large radiolucent gallstone in a 47-year-old woman. *B,* Illustration of a single large nonobstructing gallstone.

Cholesterol stones are usually solitary, soft, and light in weight. Their formation is most likely due to a metabolic dysfunction. The solitary cholesterol stone is too large to enter or obstruct ductal passageways and is usually nonopaque. Calcium bilirubinate stones are formed by precipitation of bile pigment in the gallbladder and are associated with an increased concentration of bilirubin in the bile, such as in patients with hemolytic jaundice or pernicious anemia. Calcium bilirubinate stones are typically radiolucent (Fig. 4–27). Calcium carbonate stones occur the least frequently. They usually cause total obstruc-

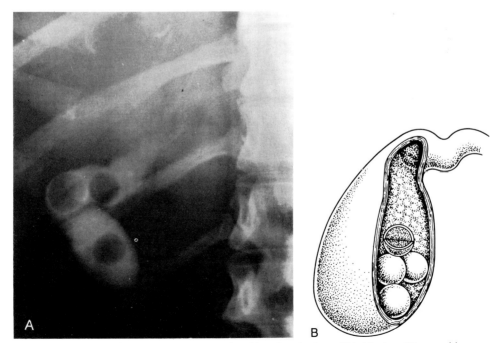

Figure 4–27. *A,* Three large gallstones observed within a functioning gallbladder in a 28-year-old woman. *B,* Illustration of a gallbladder containing four stones.

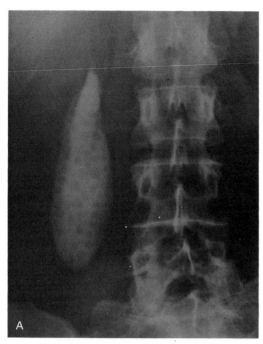
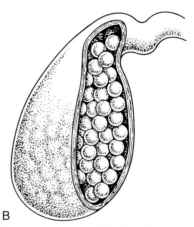

Figure 4–28. *A,* Numerous radiopaque calculi contained within a functioning gallbladder. The gallstones most likely contain a combination of elements. Calculi of this quantity and size are frequently referred to as gravel. *B,* Illustration of a gallbladder containing gravel-like calculi.

tion of the cystic duct. The concentration of calcium is directly proportional to the amount of obstruction (Fig. 4–28).

Treatment. Whatever the causative factor of cholecystitis, the usual premise is that if the inflammatory process cannot be controlled by diet, surgical removal of the gallbladder is required. This procedure is referred to as a cholecystectomy. After removing the gallbladder, the surgeon checks for further stones by making a direct injection of contrast media into the common bile duct. The surgeon's physical examination of the ducts is referred to as a common duct exploration. The subsequent injection of contrast media during radiographic exposure is referred to as a surgical or operative cholangiogram. The x-ray film of the bile ducts is processed and taken to a radiologist for immediate interpretation. The radiologist immediately reports to the surgeon about whether or not any stones remain. Many hospitals use a C-arm or portable fluoroscopy unit in surgery to facilitate immediate diagnosis. If the surgeon suspects additional stones that are not apparent at that time, he or she may insert a T-tube into the bile ducts. Additional x-ray films may be taken at a later date. The patient returns as an outpatient, and a T-tube cholangiogram is performed. The bile is first drained from the tubing. The radiologist then injects contrast media into the tubing. Care must be exercised not to inject air into the tubing, because air

can mimic the presence of stones. Once radiographs confirm that no stones are present, the tubing is removed, and the wound heals quickly.

A cholecystectomy usually follows the gallbladder examination within a matter of days. The patient may be in grave discomfort, and there is some suggestion that persistent cholecystitis predisposes to the development of carcinoma. Stones may eventually obstruct the ductal passageway, producing jaundice and perhaps an emergency condition. Under these circumstances, surgery poses a higher risk.

The Pancreas

Congenital Disorders

Cystic Fibrosis

General Information. Cystic fibrosis, also known as *mucoviscidosis,* is a generalized abnormality of the exocrine glands affecting multiple organs and systems to various degrees of severity. Cystic fibrosis is the leading fatal genetic disease of Caucasian children. About 50% of children affected with this chronic disorder die before the age of 16. With recent medical advances, the rate of survival is increasing, and some patients have survived to age 30.

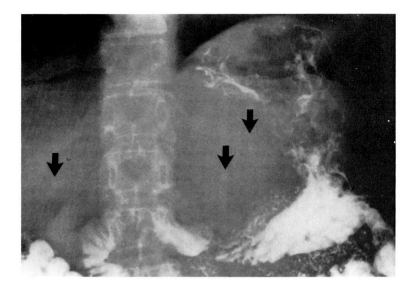

Figure 4–29. Calcifications noted in the midabdomen of a 64-year-old woman. The pancreas is significantly enlarged and appears to displace the stomach laterally. These findings are consistent with chronic pancreatitis.

Diagnosis. Elevated levels of sodium and chloride in sweat usually confirms the diagnosis of cystic fibrosis. This diagnostic procedure is called the *sweat test*, and it is performed in the clinical laboratory. The cystic fibrosis patient suffers from changes in the lungs, intestine, and pancreas. Intestinal distension and obstruction are not uncommon. Eventual obstruction of the pancreatic ducts ensues, resulting in insufficient quantities of trypsin, amylase, and lipase, preventing the absorption and conversion of fat and protein in the bowel. The result of this enzyme deficiency is extremely foul-smelling and fat-laden stools. Despite the abnormal changes occurring in the intestine and pancreas, the greatest threat from cystic fibrosis occurs when the bronchial air passageways of the lungs become plugged with mucus and when enzymatic necrosis of the pancreas and pancreatitis develop.

Treatment. There is no definitive cure for cystic fibrosis. The primary emphasis is treating the symptoms and effects of the disease while assisting the child in leading as normal a life as possible.

Inflammatory Disorders

Pancreatitis

General Information. Pancreatitis is usually a primary inflammation of the pancreas. It can occur in both acute and chronic forms. Pancreatitis is especially common in men who are alcoholics and in women with biliary disease. The mortality rate in alcoholics rises to about 60% when pancreatitis is associated with necrosis and hemorrhage.

Diagnosis. Increased levels of serum amylase and lipase are common with pancreatitis. The level of

serum calcium is elevated, and the white blood cell count is between 20,000 and 40,000. Plain films of the abdomen may reveal dilatation of the bowel or *calcifications* of the pancreas (Fig. 4–29). Pancreatitis is often associated with a left-sided pleural effusion. IVC can help differentiate acute cholecystitis from acute pancreatitis. However, CT and ultrasonography provide definitive means of imaging the pancreas (Fig. 4–30).

Treatment. The primary treatment of this disorder involves maintaining circulation and fluid volume, relieving pain, and decreasing pancreatic secretions. Shock is the most frequent cause of death in the early stages of acute pancreatitis; thus vigorous administration of intravenous fluids is essential.

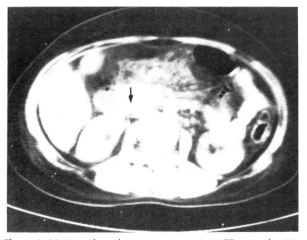

Figure 4–30. An enlarged pancreas, as seen on CT scan of a 46-year-old woman. This is consistent with pancreatitis.

Self-Assessment Quiz

For each of the following questions, select the one best response and circle the letter that precedes it.

1. Which of the following procedures can assess the degree of gallbladder function?
   a. cholecystography
   b. cholecystography and endoscopic retrograde cholangiopancreatography
   c. cholangiography and computed tomography
   d. endoscopic retrograde cholangiopancreatography and computed tomography

2. Gallstones that are usually nonopaque are composed of
   a. bilirubinate
   b. combined substances
   c. cholesterol
   d. calcium carbonate

3. Surgical removal of the gallbladder is called
   a. cholangiography
   b. cholecystogram
   c. cholecystectomy
   d. ERCP

4. Which method of cholangiography is primarily indicated to diagnose obstructive jaundice when no other method is possible?
   a. percutaneous transhepatic
   b. operative
   c. T-tube
   d. splenoportography

5. Which of the following imaging techniques is performed to determine the existence of portal hypertension and to differentiate between intra- and extrahepatic obstruction?
   a. cholecystography
   b. cholangiography
   c. hepatic angiography
   d. splenoportography

6. Which of the following imaging modalities can demonstrate both primary as well as metastatic tumors?
   a. cholecystography
   b. ERCP
   c. hepatic angiography
   d. splenoportography

7. Hepatobiliary abnormalities can be demonstrated using
   a. ultrasonography
   b. computed scanning
   c. nuclear liver scans
   d. ERCP
   e. all of the above

8. The most common acute inflammatory disorder of the hepatobiliary system is
   a. cholangitis
   b. pancreatitis
   c. viral hepatitis
   d. cirrhosis

9. The end stage of liver disease is termed
   a. hepatitis
   b. cholangitis
   c. cirrhosis
   d. obstruction

10. Cirrhosis is most often the result of
    a. acute alcoholism
    b. infection
    c. chronic alcoholism
    d. hepatitis

11. The most important waste product of red blood cell breakdown is
    a. bilirubin
    b. creatinine
    c. uric acid
    d. bile

12. The purpose of the cholecystogram is to determine the ability of the gallbladder to fill, concentrate bile, and empty.
    a. true
    b. false

13. Which of the following positions is employed to demonstrate layering or stratification of gallstones?
    a. PA
    b. LAO
    c. lateral decubitus
    d. RAO

14. Nonvisualization of the gallbladder may be due to
    a. cholelithiasis
    b. obstruction
    c. allergy to contrast media
    d. pancreatitis
    e. all of the above

15. The preferred method of imaging when obstructive jaundice is in evidence is
    a. intravenous cholangiography
    b. ERCP
    c. transhepatic cholangiography
    d. angiography

16. Which of the following imaging methods is safer to perform?
    a. transhepatic cholangiography
    b. ERCP

17. Which of the following are types of gallstones?
    a. bilirubinate
    b. cholesterol
    c. carbonate
    d. phosphate and carbonate
    e. bilirubinate, cholesterol, and carbonate

18. Which of the following disorders is also known as mucoviscidosis?
    a. cystic fibrosis
    b. hepatitis
    c. cirrhosis
    d. jaundice

19. The sweat test is used to diagnose
    a. cirrhosis
    b. cystic fibrosis
    c. obstructive jaundice
    d. hepatitis

20. Enzymatic necrosis is associated with
    a. cirrhosis
    b. hepatitis
    c. cholangitis
    d. pancreatitis

Study Questions

1. Describe the action of cholecystokinin in terms of gallbladder function.

2. List several reasons why intravenous cholangiography would be performed in place of oral cholecystography.

3. Explain why a common duct exploration would be performed following a cholecystectomy.

4. What are some of the long-term effects of chronic hepatitis and cirrhosis?

5. Which laboratory tests are performed in the presence of hepatobiliary disease?

6. What are the symptoms of acute hepatitis, chronic hepatitis, and cirrhosis?

7. What are combined and mixed gallstones?

Five

Genitourinary System

Related Terminology

agenesis
atrophic
azotemia
creatinine
ectopia
glomerulonephritis
hypoplasia
interstitial nephritis
megaloureter
nephrectomy
nephrocalcinosis
nephrolithotomy
nephrolithotripsy
nephrostomy
nephrotic syndrome
polycystic disease
pyelonephritis
reflux
urea nitrogen
uremia
ureterocele
uric acid

Objectives

Upon completion of Chapter 5, the reader will be able to

- List and describe the major congenital and inflammatory disorders of the urinary system.

- Explain the purposes of the intravenous urogram, retrograde pyelogram, and cystogram.

- Describe the advantages of specialized imaging of the urinary system, which includes angiography, computed tomography, percutaneous nephrostomy, and nuclear renal scans.

- List the important laboratory tests that are performed in conjunction with urinary disease.

- Identify urinary pathology on radiographic examinations.

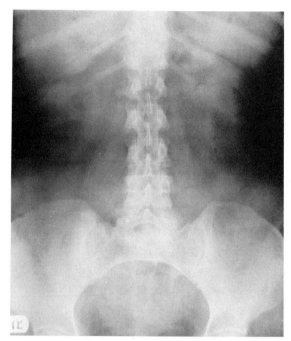

Figure 5–1. Abdominal scout film (kidney-ureter-bladder) that appears to be within normal limits.

Imaging the Urinary System

Diseases of the genitourinary system currently affect between eight and nine million Americans. These diseases vary from inconsequential to severe and life threatening. Because of the advances in diagnostic procedures and modes of treatment, people with urinary tract diseases are surviving much longer.

One of the primary purposes of the kidneys is to maintain homeostasis by filtering the blood. Waste products are sent to the kidneys for elimination. Certain products that are useful may be reabsorbed, and the wastes are eliminated. When the kidneys are not functioning properly, these wastes accumulate in excessive amounts, and the patient may be manifesting a level of kidney dysfunction. Radiographic and laboratory examinations play an important role in the diagnosis of most urological disorders, of which the majority are inflammatory. A most important aspect of many diagnostic radiographic procedures is the scout film (Fig. 5–1). The scout film is a plain film of the abdomen that includes the kidneys, ureters, and urinary bladder (KUB). It will demonstrate an outline of the kidneys—their size, shape, position, and location. Various types of abdominal calcifications may be identified. Calcifications may be signs of conditions such as developmental disorders, metastatic disease, or calculi. Occasionally we may determine the absence of a kidney shadow. This may be due to congenital agenesis, previous surgical removal, or possibly dysfunction. Retroperitoneal masses may

cause displacement of the kidneys and possibly nonvisualization of the psoas shadows. Conditions such as peritonitis and intraabdominal hemorrhage may also result in the absence of the psoas shadows. The excretory urogram or *intravenous pyelogram (IVP)* is a true measure of excretory function. The IVP demonstrates kidney filling, filtration, and excretion. It is the only diagnostic test that demonstrates the function of the kidneys, ureters, bladder, and urethra. The IVP demonstrates pathological conditions such as inflammation, calculi, obstruction, tumors, and cysts (Fig. 5–2).

The *hypertensive* or *timed* IVP is an excretory urogram designed to demonstrate differences in kidney function in smaller time intervals. Typically, the standard IVP uses venipuncture and injection of iodinated contrast medium over a 3-minute period, whereas the hypertensive or timed IVP necessitates a bolus injection of contrast medium in about 30 seconds. Radiographs are taken after about 30 seconds, after 1 minute, and then at 1-minute intervals for the first 5 minutes. Differences may be evident in comparing right and left kidney function (Fig. 5–3). On numerous occasions, renal artery stenosis is the reason for this visual difference, which may explain the reason for the patient's increased blood pressure. The radiographs following the 5-minute film are usually routine views of the kidneys, ureters, and urinary bladder. Another method of excretory urography is accomplished via a drip infusion of contrast medium into the venous system. This procedure often is used when kidneys are not functioning

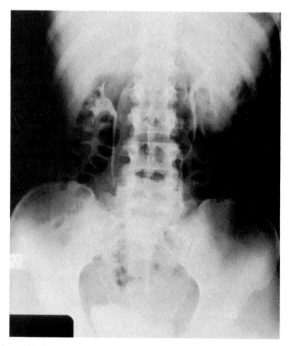

Figure 5–2. Intravenous pyelography, 15-minute film, essentially negative.

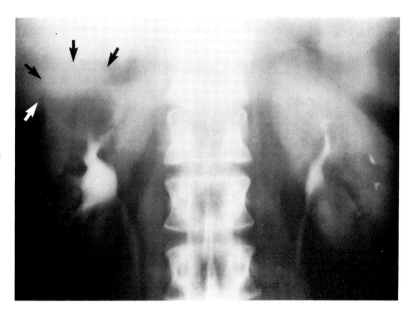

Figure 5–3. Intravenous pyelography revealing a 5-cm cyst of the right upper pole (arrows) in a 44-year-old man. There is no evidence of renovascular hypertension.

normally and their visualization is delayed. When tomograms are included (Fig. 5–4), a series of radiographic slices or cuts are taken at periodic intervals. Tomograms are useful when there are overlying bowel shadows that may obscure the renal outlines and parenchyma. After about 5 minutes, the kidneys begin to excrete, and it is then important to place the cassette so that the bladder is visualized. Following injection of contrast medium, the cassette may be placed crosswise to visualize the kidneys as they are filling. The patient is often placed in the upright anteroposterior (AP) position in order to demonstrate any change in position of the kidneys. Oblique views

in the upright position can distinguish the position of calcifications. The patient is usually asked to urinate first. A final film is then taken of the bladder after voiding. The position of calcifications in relation to the ureters may be determined.

Retrograde pyelography is a radiographic procedure usually performed in a specialized surgical urological suite. A catheter is passed into the ureters via the urethra and bladder. Contrast medium is then injected into the catheters. This procedure is referred to as *cystography* and *retrograde pyelography.* It primarily demonstrates the ureters and renal pelvis and is not a kidney function test. The contrast me-

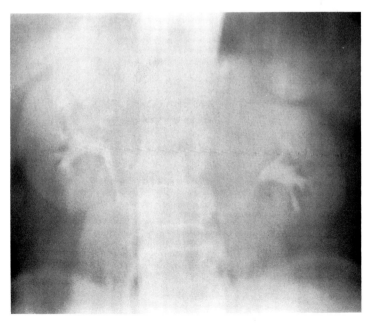

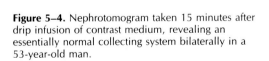

Figure 5–4. Nephrotomogram taken 15 minutes after drip infusion of contrast medium, revealing an essentially normal collecting system bilaterally in a 53-year-old man.

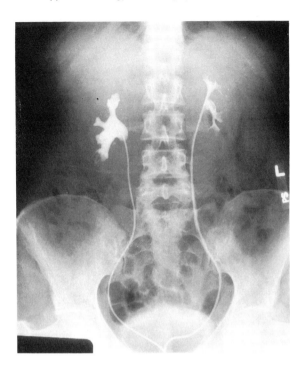

Figure 5–5. An essentially negative retrograde pyelogram of a 41-year-old woman.

dium is injected against the usual flow of urine and thus is described as retrograde (Fig. 5–5). In the event that an intravenous urogram and retrograde pyelogram are not possible, antegrade pyelography or percutaneous nephrostomy may be substituted. This procedure is especially useful with urinary tract obstruction. It is also useful in infants when cystoscopy is difficult or impossible (Fig. 5–6).

Renal angiography is a specialized imaging procedure that is usually carried out with the *Seldinger* catheterization technique via the femoral artery and is useful in distinguishing between a solid renal tumor and fluid-filled renal cyst. The catheter is introduced over a guide wire placed in the aorta. The catheter is selectively placed into the lumen of the affected renal artery, and contrast medium is injected into

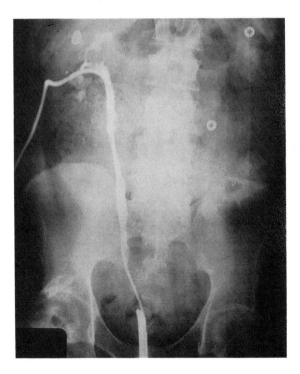

Figure 5–6. Percutaneous nephrostomy was performed in an attempt to remove calculi in this 47-year-old man with a history of renal and ureteral calculi.

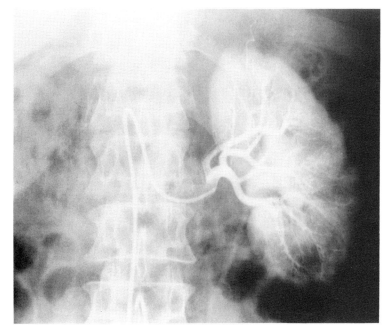

Figure 5–7. Selective renal arteriogram that proved to be essentially negative in a 60-year-old man.

the renal circulation. Using a rapid serial changer, radiographs are taken at a rate of 6 to 12 films per second. Numerous types of renal pathology are demonstrated with renal angiography (Fig. 5–7).

Cystography involves the passage of a retention catheter into the bladder. Contrast medium fills the bladder by the gravity method. Contrast medium is instilled into the bladder until the patient expresses discomfort. Radiographic and/or fluoroscopic filming may be performed during either nonvoiding or voiding. The retention catheter is first removed prior to voiding and filming. When filming takes place while the patient is voiding, the procedure is referred to as a voiding cystourethrogram (Fig. 5–8).

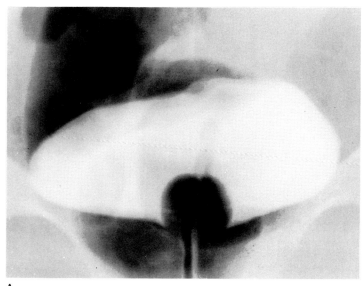

A

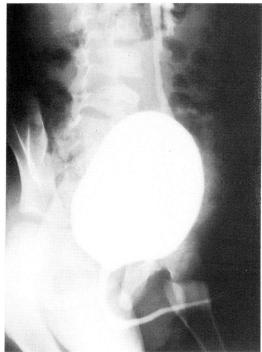

B

Figure 5–8. *A*, A normal-appearing cystogram of a woman. *B*, Left posterior oblique view revealing left ureteral reflux in a 6-year-old boy.

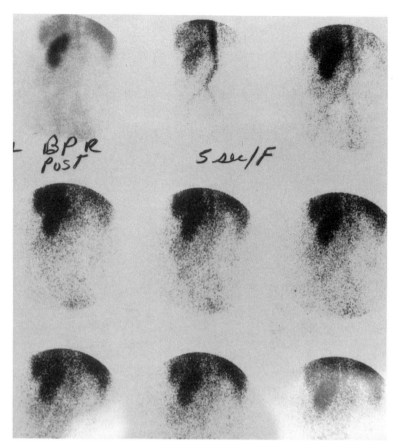

L BPR POST   5 sec/F

Figure 5–9. Renal scan and flow study revealing a normally functioning left kidney and a non-functioning right kidney in a 53-year-old woman.

Renal scans performed in nuclear medicine determine renal function by demonstrating the uptake of radioactive isotopes within the kidney (Fig. 5–9).

Renal biopsy is a process by which a specimen is obtained for histological diagnosis and determination of treatment. More recently, ultrasonography, computed tomography (CT), and magnetic resonance (MR) imaging have enhanced the diagnosis of urinary tract diseases (Fig. 5–10).

Important laboratory test results that can be correlated with the radiographic findings as well as with the patient's symptoms and signs include urinalysis, serum creatinine, uric acid, and blood urea nitrogen, as well as the complete blood count (CBC).

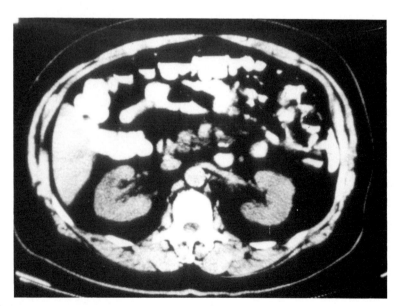

Figure 5–10. An essentially normal CT scan of the kidneys of a 65-year-old man.

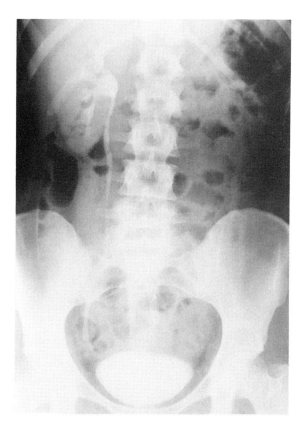

Figure 5–11. Congenital agenesis of the left kidney in a 27-year-old woman.

Kidneys

Congenital Disorders

Agenesis

General Information. Agenesis is congenital *absence* of an organ. Kidney agenesis is relatively uncommon. It is encountered in approximately 2 of every 1000 autopsies on fetuses and is most often associated with pulmonary hypoplasia. Unilateral agenesis is usually asymptomatic, is twice as common as bilateral agenesis, and is most common in males. This congenital condition includes absence of the ureters. As an isolated anomaly, it is usually compatible with life. When bilateral, it often is accompanied by many other anomalies and is usually incompatible with life.

Diagnosis. The patient's history may provide valuable information about the radiographic findings. A history of surgical nephrectomy is not uncommon, but an older adult may have forgotten to mention the previous surgery. It is possible on occasion for the patient not to have been aware of the surgical removal during infancy. If agenesis is present, no kidney shadow will be observed. This phenomenon should be detected on the scout KUB (Fig. 5–11).

Treatment. There is no treatment for this condition. It is most important to recognize the congenital

absence when it exists. Extreme care must be taken when the remaining kidney is afflicted with disease of any type.

Hypoplasia

General Information. True congenital renal hypoplasia is relatively uncommon. In most cases, it is found to be the result of other acquired diseases.

Diagnosis. Hypoplastic kidneys have atypically small vessels and a reduced number of calices and vary in size from barely perceptible to moderate size. The kidney never develops unless a ureter is present, and the kidney is a frequent site of infections. Most are unilateral. When an atrophic kidney is discovered later in life, it is difficult to determine whether it is a true congenital form or is an acquired form of hypoplasia (Fig. 5–12).

Treatment. As with agenesis, there is essentially no treatment for hypoplasia or atrophic kidneys. Infections of the normal kidney must be guarded against.

Polycystic Kidneys

General Information. Polycystic disease is considered to be the most important anomaly of the kidney.

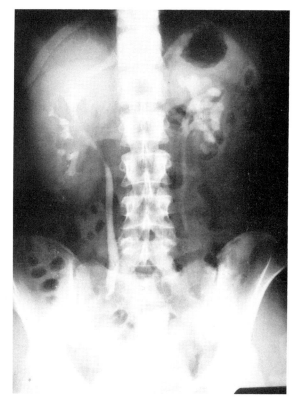

Figure 5–12. A small left kidney with a diffuse loss of cortical tissue and dilated unobstructed calculus of the lower pole of the left kidney collecting system in a 41-year-old woman. There is compensatory hypertrophy of the right kidney.

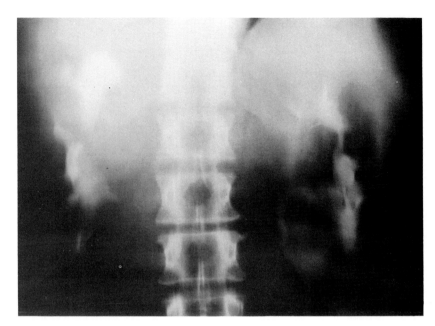

Figure 5–13. Drip infusion nephrotomogram revealing bilateral polycystic kidneys with dilated collecting systems in a 52-year-old man.

There are essentially three types of polycystic disease. Type I is produced by dilatation and hyperplasia of the collecting tubules of the kidney. Type I is bilateral and is usually fatal soon after birth. Type II is characterized by thick-walled cysts of different sizes, with fibroconnective tissue between the cysts. Type II can be unilateral or bilateral or can involve only a part of one kidney. When bilateral, it is incompatible with life and is only encountered in stillborn and newborn infants. Type III is most often bilateral and is found in adults. There is a mixture of normal and abnormal nephrons, and impaired renal function is characteristic. It is most common in the fifth or sixth decade of life. As the patient ages, the cysts enlarge, causing compression of the renal interstitium and resulting in ischemia. Death usually occurs from vascular complications and infection.

Diagnosis. IVP or retrograde pyelography reveals enlarged renal collecting systems, with elongation of the pelvis, calyceal flattening, and multiple cystic *indentations.* In neonates, the IVP reveals diminished excretion of contrast material. Tomograms reveal kidney enlargement and cystic lesions. The findings on urinalysis and the serum creatinine level are grossly abnormal (Fig. 5–13).

Treatment. As with most congenital kidney defects, polycystic disease has no treatment. It is most important to avoid infections and hypertension, which may affect the normal kidney.

Medullary Sponge Kidney

General Information. Medullary sponge kidney is a benign lesion consisting of parapelvic cysts, which may contain calculi. The exact cause is unknown, but it is thought to be related to polycystic disease. Although medullary sponge kidney may be found in both sexes and in all age-groups, it is found most frequently in men between the ages of 40 and 70. It is thought to occur in about 1 in every 5000 to 20,000 persons. Medullary sponge kidney bears no relationship to medullary cystic disease.

Diagnosis. Medullary sponge kidney is often an incidental finding in radiographic examinations of the urinary tract. The IVP is usually the major method of diagnosis. It will often show a characteristic *flower-like* appearance of the pyramidal cavities when filled with contrast media. Medullary sponge kidney must be differentiated from renal tuberculosis, tubular necrosis, tubular acidosis, and papillary necrosis (Fig. 5–14).

Treatment. Because renal calculi are a common complication, treatment may focus on the prevention of calculi. Calculi can be minimized by increasing fluid intake and by periodic examination of the patient's urine. This condition is usually quite manageable without surgery.

Horseshoe Kidneys

General Information. Horseshoe kidneys are a congenital deformity in which the lower poles of the kidneys are *fused.* Renal function is not usually impaired.

Diagnosis. The striking feature is the closeness of the lower poles to the spine. The kidneys are rotated so that their pelves point forward and the lower calyces point medially. On occasion, both lower poles lie on one side of the median sagittal plane. This is known as crossed renal ectopia. Horseshoe kidneys can be seen on plain posterior views (AP projection) of the abdomen, as well on the IVP (Fig. 5–15).

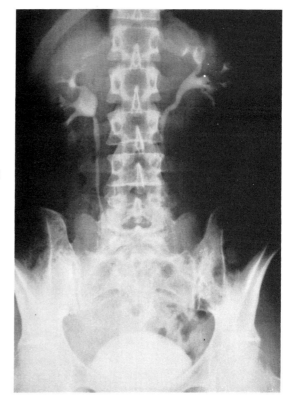

Figure 5–14. Intravenous pyelogram revealing a medullary sponge kidney bilaterally, with the presence of multiple small calculi. The collecting systems are otherwise normal in this 46-year-old woman.

Treatment. This congenital defect is usually an incidental finding and requires no treatment.

Duplication/Bifid Collecting Systems

General Information. Duplication of the renal collecting systems is one of the most frequent con-genital anomalies of the urinary tract. The only concerns are the complications of infection and obstruction. Otherwise, duplication is simply an incidental finding discovered by the radiologist.

Diagnosis. Duplication can be seen in many variations, as well as unilaterally or bilaterally on the excretory urogram (IVP). It is not uncommon for the

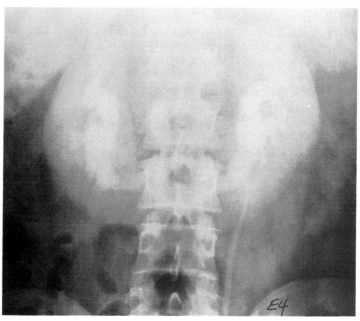

Figure 5–15. Congenital horseshoe kidneys that are fused at the lower poles in a 29-year-old man.

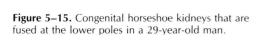

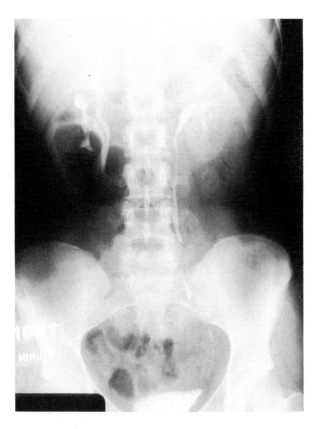

Figure 5–16. Double ureter–double renal pelvis in the right, with slight delay in emptying of the lower caliceal system. The left kidney, the ureter, and the bladder appear normal in this 27-year-old woman.

ureters to be bifid also. Kidneys with bifid collecting systems are as much as 2 cm longer than the normal opposite side (Fig. 5–16).

Treatment. No treatment is required for duplication. However, this variant may be of significance when infection or obstruction is present.

Renal Ectopia

General Information. During fetal development, the kidneys ascend within the abdomen. If this ascension is delayed or halted for any reason, an ectopic kidney results. These kidneys are usually found in the lower abdomen, in or near the pelvis. The ureter is extremely short and communicates directly with the urinary bladder.

Diagnosis. Ectopic kidneys are most often seen in IVP studies. Although most are found in the **pelvic** area, they can be found almost anywhere. Many variations are visible on x-ray studies. They may be bilaterally ectopic, or both kidneys can be found on one side of the midline or located together in the midline. For the most part, renal ectopia is an incidental finding and is of no consequence to the patient. The radiographer should consider ectopia when kidney shadows are absent. This consideration is more realistic than that of congenital agenesis. Careful examination should include the lower pelvic region. When the pelvic kidneys overlie bone, they may be a bit more difficult to visualize. The increased

density of the bladder region and the opaque visualization of the collecting system are easier to see because of the higher contrast. In many cases of pelvic kidneys, a lower abdominal mass may be palpable (Fig. 5–17).

Treatment. The presence of ectopic kidneys becomes significant in the presence of inflammatory or obstructive disease. Otherwise, ectopic kidney is simply an incidental finding.

Inflammatory Disorders

Glomerulonephritis

General Information. Glomerulonephritis is a kidney disorder that may develop in response to several different stimuli such as chemical agents, anoxia, ionizing radiation, and bacteria. Diseases of the glomeruli are usually separated into primary diseases and those that are secondary to systemic diseases. It is thought that the major cause of inflammation is immunological factors. In this regard, it is accepted that glomerulonephritis is a disorder that occurs secondary to inflammation. Many of these inflammatory responses are due to an allergic reaction or antigen-antibody response.

Diagnosis. In focal inflammation, some but not all of the glomeruli are affected. In segmental glomerulonephritis, only a portion of the glomerulus is affected. However, when the inflammation affects the

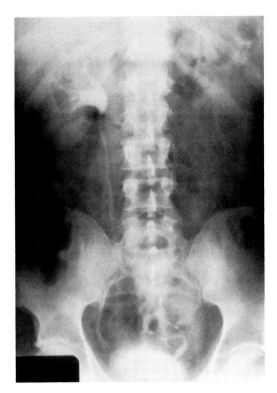

Figure 5–17. Left ectopic pelvic kidney in a 41-year-old man. Both kidneys appear normal otherwise.

majority of the glomerular system, diffuse glomerulonephritis is present. The more glomeruli that are affected, the worse the outlook for the patient. Patients with severe glomerular disease will usually develop the *nephrotic syndrome.* Both the acute and chronic forms of glomerulonephritis usually affect both kidneys. In the acute form, the kidneys appear slightly enlarged on the IVP radiographs. Laboratory tests provide the best chance for definitive diagnosis. Increased levels of creatinine and blood urea nitrogen indicate that the kidneys are failing. A renal biopsy can be used to confirm the diagnosis or assess renal tissue status.

Treatment. It is essential that the patient receive aggressive supportive care, including strict bed rest, fluid intake management, correction of electrolyte imbalances, and possibly dialysis. Antibiotic and diuretic therapy may be considered. The treatment is primarily directed toward minimizing the effects of the symptoms and preventing complications.

Pyelonephritis, Acute

General Information. Acute pyelonephritis, the most important inflammatory renal disease, is an acute inflammation of the kidney parenchyma and renal pelvis. This could be a hematogenous disorder, but most commonly the infectious agent is *Escherichia coli*, which usually enters the body in retrograde fashion via the urinary bladder and ureters. In females, bacteria have easy access into the bladder

because the urethra is relatively short. The possibility of this condition increases with insertion of instruments into the urethra. One prime example is the retention catheter, which is frequently inserted following surgery and in elderly persons. It is to be noted that diabetes mellitus is another frequent cause of acute pyelonephritis.

Diagnosis. Acute pyelonephritis presents symptoms of fever, malaise, pain at the costovertebral angle, dysuria, and urgency. Pus and bacteria are present in the urinalysis. The urine may also have a cloudy appearance and a fishy odor. A fever of 102°F or higher is not unusual and is accompanied by chills, flank pain, loss of appetite, and general fatigue. In addition to the urinalysis, a urine culture will be taken to identify the organism and help determine which antibiotic would be most effective in treatment. Radiographic studies of the kidneys are not too helpful at this point. The IVP is indicated when the patient does not respond to treatment and when complications such as obstruction may be present. In the presence of pyelonephritis there is little if any structural change of the kidney. The IVP is totally normal about 75% of the time. If any changes are noted, they usually involve renal enlargement, decreased density of collecting system contrast material, delayed calyceal appearance time, and dilatation of the collecting system.

Treatment. The treatment centers on identifying the antibiotic that will most effectively kill the offending bacteria (culture and sensitivity testing). An-

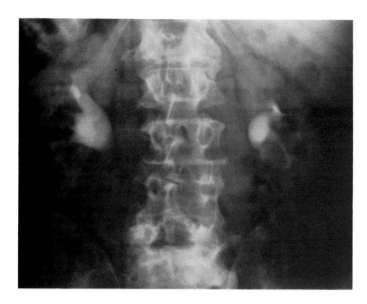

Figure 5–18. Smaller right kidney showing changes of chronic atrophic pyelonephritis with cortical scarring in a 72-year-old man.

algesics may be given for pain, and repeat urinalysis and cultures are performed periodically. In severe cases, complications such as vesicoureteral reflux, obstruction, abscess formation, and stones are not uncommon.

Pyelonephritis, Chronic Atrophic

General Information. A significant number of patients with chronic atrophic pyelonephritis had this disease since childhood. One or both kidneys may be affected, and vesicoureteral reflux is commonly associated. In afflicted children, this condition usually resolves as the bladder develops. Even when bilateral, this disease is more severe on one side.

Diagnosis. Patients having chronic pyelonephritis may have had a history of unexplained fever or bedwetting. Flank pain, anemia, proteinuria, an increased number of leukocytes in the urine, and hypertension are the major findings. Because of the long-term effects of the disease, the IVP demonstrates parenchymal atrophy. The pyramids are inflamed and atrophied, resulting in *clubbing* of the calyces. Radiographically, the kidney is asymmetrically small and scarred. The asymmetry is due to the uninvolved part of the kidney undergoing hypertrophy. This may even resemble a pseudotumor (Fig. 5–18).

Treatment. The primary treatment involves controlling the hypertension, eliminating the obstruction that is often found, and administering antimicrobial therapy.

Interstitial Nephritis

General Information. Interstitial nephritis is an exudative inflammatory disease of the tissue of the kidney. This infection may be localized or may involve all of the interstitium. Both acute and chronic forms are possible. The acute form is often found in association with other diseases such as diphtheria, scarlet fever, and Weil's disease. In chronic interstitial nephritis, there is an association with analgesics that contain phenacetin. Patients who ingest significant amounts of analgesics over a long period of time are often suffering from arthritic conditions or from migraine headaches.

Diagnosis. Chronic interstitial nephritis presents no overt symptoms at its onset, other than general malaise and increased levels of albumin in the urine. In the intermediate stage, edema occurs. Fluid is obvious in the face, legs, and arms. The final stage involves uremia, and by this time the damage to the kidneys is substantial and permanent. It is in this final stage when the kidneys begin to fail. Owing to kidney failure, injections of organic iodine (e.g., IVP) might be dangerous to the patient and thus are usually contraindicated.

Treatment. Control of interstitial nephritis is easiest in the early to intermittent stages. This is mostly accomplished by monitoring the blood and urine while maintaining a balanced diet. In the late stage, there is usually reduced kidney function. This is first apparent with the presence of azotemia, in which there is an accumulation of blood urea nitrogen and serum creatinine. Uremia is the final indicator of kidney failure, and the remaining treatment options are dialysis or transplant.

Vascular Disorders

Renal Artery Stenosis

General Information. Renal artery stenosis is a narrowing of the renal artery. This stenosis compromises the flow of oxygenated blood from the abdom-

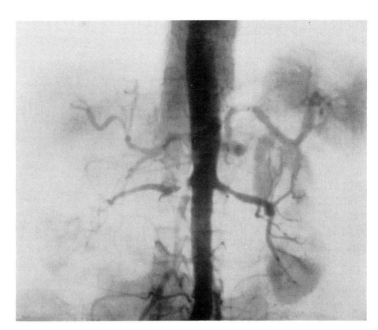

Figure 5–19. Stenosis of the right renal artery as revealed on a subtraction study from an abdominal flush aortogram in a 55-year-old man.

inal aorta to the kidney via the renal artery. As a result of this stenosis, the enzyme renin is released, causing vasoconstriction. This vasoconstriction results in an increased work load on the left ventricle, leading to elevation of blood pressure. Hypertensive heart disease is a form of hypertension that is not a disease of the heart. This form of hypertension is referred to as essential or idiopathic. It is a leading cause of hypertension.

Renal artery stenosis most often affects young adult women and is usually unilateral. The most frequent cause of this stenosis is fibromuscular dysplasia or hyperplasia. Atherosclerosis is the second most frequent cause. The stenosis is most often located at or near the origin of the renal artery. Hypertension in general is the most common serious chronic disease in the United States, affecting about half of the population over 60 years of age. Arterial hypertension is considered borderline when it reaches 140/90 mm Hg and is hypertensive when it reaches 165/95. Although the systolic pressure is a cause of concern, the high diastolic reading is considered dangerous. Approximately 5 to 10% of patients with high blood pressure are found to have renovascular stenosis. Renovascular hypertension is most common in persons under age 30 and over age 50.

Diagnosis. Although many methods of diagnostic imaging are possible, the renal arteriogram is the most definitive method of visualization and of evaluating renovascular stenosis. Renal angiography reveals the actual arterial stenosis or obstruction (Fig. 5–19). Other diagnostic studies include the renal flow scan performed in nuclear medicine. Rapid-sequence or timed IVP can detect abnormalities in renal blood flow. Often the IVP is essentially normal even in the presence of significant stenosis. A hypertensive or

timed IVP sequentially delineates comparative views of the collecting systems over short time intervals following a bolus injection of contrast medium. The timed IVP presents a delayed visualization of the affected collecting system. IVP can demonstrate renal artery stenosis about 20% of the time. In the 1960s, IVP was contraindicated when renal failure was suspected. In persons with decreased renal function, large amounts of contrast media are injected because the kidneys cannot concentrate well. The liver excretes the medium when the kidneys fail. However, extreme care must be exercised when the patient has elevated blood urea nitrogen. With limited kidney visualization, nephrotomograms can be taken via drip infusion over long periods of time. Angiography is the preferred method of demonstrating renal artery stenosis, however.

Treatment. Surgery is the treatment of choice for restoring adequate blood flow and for controlling hypertension. This may be accomplished by arterial bypass, endarterectomy, or angioplasty. Recently, the use of a balloon catheter to dilate the stenosed artery has been most successful. The advantage of the balloon catheter dilatation is that it can be performed as part of the angiographic procedure, eliminating the need for a more invasive surgical procedure. The patient is also maintained with antihypertensive drugs, diuretics, and a diet that restricts the intake of sodium.

Metabolic Disease

Nephrocalcinosis

General Information. Nephrocalcinosis is a condition characterized by numerous irregular deposits

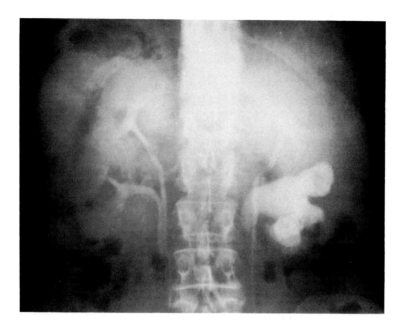

Figure 5–20. Huge staghorn calculus completely filling the markedly dilated lower collecting system on the left. There are bifid collecting systems bilaterally. The patient is a 56-year-old woman.

of calcium in the kidneys. Calcification within the kidney usually occurs as a result of one of many diseases such as hyperparathyroidism and other disturbances of calcium metabolism. It may also be associated with multiple myeloma or some metastatic cancers. Next to calculi formation, nephrocalcinosis is the most common calcification found in the kidney.

Diagnosis. Calcifications in the kidney may be observed on plain films of the abdomen or on an excretory urogram (IVP). In nephrocalcinosis, the calcium deposits are found throughout the kidney substance. These can be differentiated from renal calculi, which are found in the large collection passageways.

Treatment. The primary method of treatment is evaluation of the problem in terms of a specific metabolic origin. A high fluid intake is important, as is regulation of the patient's diet.

Renal Calculi

General Information. Fifty percent of persons with renal stones are found to have an abnormality of metabolism that accelerates stone formation. There are also underlying disorders that can promote the excretion of calcium. Afflicted persons may have a high intake of milk or vitamin D, together with hyperparathyroidism. Diseases such as gout and leukemia have been known to predispose to the formation of calculi. Urinary tract infections, which have the ability to alkalize the pH of urine, also predispose to the formation of stones. Calculi generally develop within the collecting system of the kidney and tend to migrate from the calyces to the renal pelvis. Renal

calculi occur mostly in men and at a rate of 1 of every 1000 persons. Afflicted men most often are between the ages of 30 and 50. Once stones occur, the chance for recurrence is extremely high. The southeastern United States, because of its hot and dry climate, is called the stone belt. Persons in this region have a more than average chance of stone formation due to both metabolic and infectious causes. Dehydration and obstruction are common occurrences. *Staghorn calculi* (Fig. 5–20) are common in bacterial infections. However, 90% of patients have multiple calculi that are 5 mm or smaller and that usually pass spontaneously. Calculi larger than 6 mm have less than a 20% chance of passage.

There are five distinct varieties of calculi. The stones vary in size, shape, contour, color, and consistency. *Calcium* stones are the most common and account for 50 to 75% of all stones. They may be pure or of mixed variety. They are often combined with *oxalate* or *phosphate*. Pure phosphate stones are usually massive and may form a cast of the entire renal pelvis and calyces. These massive phosphate stones are referred to as staghorn calculi. *Magnesium ammonium phosphate* stones are present in a pure or mixed form about 13% of the time. *Uric acid* stones account for about 10% of stones, and *cystine* stones account for about 3%. The type of stones formed is influenced by urine pH. For example, uric acid and cystine stones precipitate in acid urine. Phosphate calculi only precipitate in alkaline urine. Oxalate precipitates in urine that is either acid or alkaline.

Diagnosis. The two major complications of renal calculi are renal *colic* and urinary tract *obstruction.*

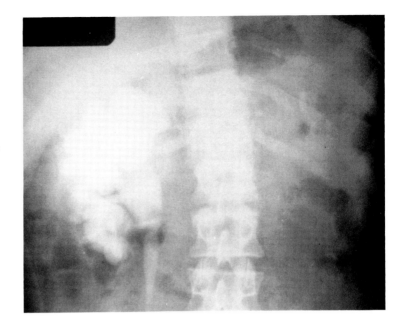

Figure 5–21. Enlarged right hydronephrotic kidney showing cortical thinning and extensive dilatation of the caliceal system in a 16-year-old male.

Renal colic is the severely intense pain due to either an obstructing stone or a stone making its way down the ureter. Obstruction by a stone causes pain that is constant and dull. In urinary tract obstruction, there is an abnormal dilatation of the renal pelvis, causing *hydronephrosis* (Fig. 5–21). When the stone is moving down the ureter, the pain is extremely sharp and severe, accompanied by nausea and vomiting. Chills, fever, and hematuria are also usually present. Most plain AP radiographs of the abdomen can reveal a calculus (Fig. 5–22). The urinary bladder often reveals calculi that have been passed. Intrave-

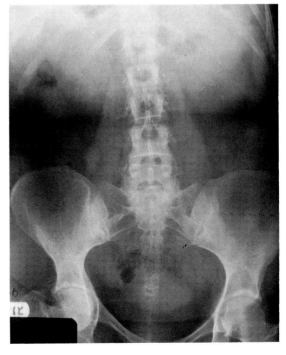

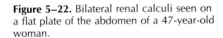

Figure 5–22. Bilateral renal calculi seen on a flat plate of the abdomen of a 47-year-old woman.

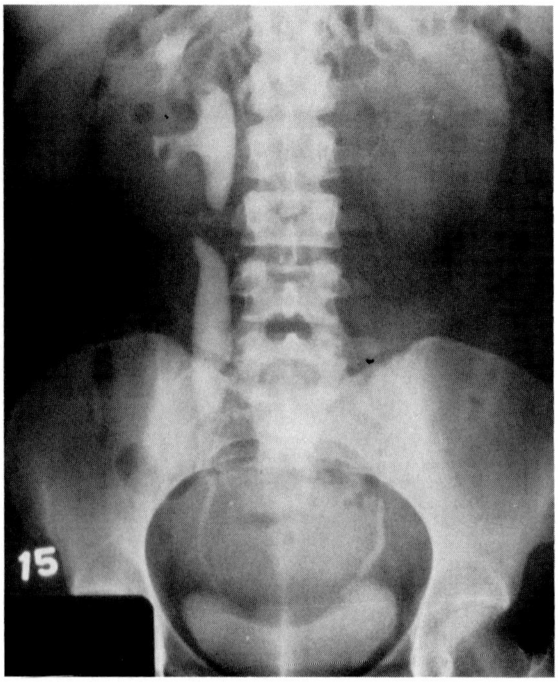

Figure 5–23. Intravenous pyelogram revealing the presence of a nonvisualizing but presumed ureteral stone at the level of the midureter, resulting in hydronephrosis of the right kidney and ureter. The patient is a 20-year-old woman.

Obstructive Disorders

Hydronephrosis

General Information. Hydronephrosis is a primary dilatation of the renal pelvis and calyces with urine. It can be the result of a congenital defect, ureteral tumor, stricture, blood clots, or inflammation, but most frequently is due to a calculus, usually in the ureter. The calculus may be located in the kidney itself, in the ureter, or at the ureteropelvic junction.

Diagnosis. Patients with hydronephrosis describe a recurring pain in the kidney region. The type of pain may vary from dull and nagging to sharp. The urine often contains pus and blood. Hydronephrosis is usually first seen on an excretory urogram (IVP) but is more definitive on a retrograde pyelogram (Fig. 5–24). In the event of an intrarenal obstruction, dilatation of the calyx proximal to the obstruction is usually seen (Fig. 5–25). Bilateral hydronephrosis most often is indicative of obstruction at the base of the urinary bladder or urethra (Fig. 5–26). Renal ultrasonography is another mode of diagnosis frequently employed for hydronephrosis.

Treatment. It is most important to maintain renal function. Depending on the causative factors and severity of obstruction, renal function may have been

nous urography confirms the diagnosis and reveals the size and location of calculi (Fig. 5–23). The abdomen films also aid in the differential diagnosis, including other possibilities such as calcified lymph nodes, gallstones, phleboliths, and fibroid tumors. Ultrasonography can detect obstructive changes, such as those in hydronephrosis. A urinalysis can help determine the type of calculi, based on the pH of the urine. A urine culture in the presence of a bacterial infection can assist in determining the medication of choice for treatment. The diagnosis must rule out appendicitis.

Treatment. Analgesics are indicated when the pain is most severe. When surgery is not contemplated, increased fluid intake is prescribed. All urine passed is strained for stone analysis. Calculi that are too large for normal pasage must be removed surgically. If the stone is in the ureter, it may be removed via cystoscope. A lodged stone may cause severe pain, stasis of urine producing infection, and even deterioration of renal function. The surgical removal of a kidney stone is referred to as nephrolithotomy. Most recently, a new procedure called nephrolithotripsy has been developed. The patient is submerged in water, and ultrasonic waves causing vibrations break up stones so that they can be passed through the urinary system. After the stone appears to have been passed, a follow-up IVP is taken.

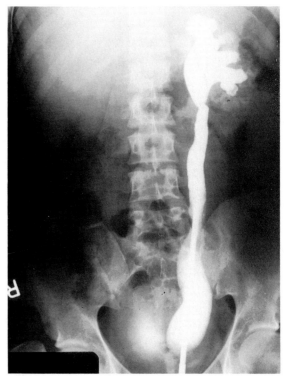

Figure 5–24. Marked dilatation of the upper collecting system with marked ureteral fullness, as seen on retrograde pyelogram of a 21-year-old man.

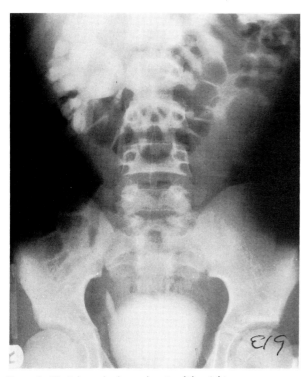

Figure 5–25. A huge hydronephrosis of the right upper collecting system due to an obstruction of the calyx proximal to the obstruction in a 12-year-old boy.

heart. The soft tissues of the body and bones are not affected by the pulsing sound wave, but the calculus shatters, just as glass is shattered by a sonic boom. The sandy remains are then flushed through the urinary system.

Nephrotic Syndrome

General Information. A syndrome is a collection or constellation of signs and symptoms, and the nephrotic syndrome is characterized by signs and symptoms of hypoproteinemia, proteinuria, hyperlipidemia, and edema. It is commonly associated with glomerulonephritis, diabetes, and many other less common diseases.

Diagnosis. About 75% of patients with the nephrotic syndrome have some form or effect of glomerulonephritis. The dominant feature is *edema* of the lower legs and ankles. The severity may vary from mild to severe. In severe cases, edema may lead to ascites and pleural effusion. Other signs such as lethargy, fatigue, anorexia, depression, and pallor are often evident. Complications such as malnutrition, infection, coagulation disorders, vascular occlusion, thrombosis, emboli, and atherosclerosis may develop. Consistently increased levels of protein in the urine strongly suggest the nephrotic syndrome.

compromised. Removal of calculi is of primary importance. Until recently, removal of calculi was only possible with surgery. In December, 1984, the U.S. Food and Drug Administration approved the general use of lithotripsy, a new treatment that destroys kidney stones with sonic shock waves, a procedure that could spare an estimated 80,000 people annually from painful and debilitating surgery. Lithotripsy is indicated for patients who have calculi that cannot be passed through the urinary system and must be removed through surgery. In a study of more than 800 patients, researchers at the Mayo Clinic removed renal and ureteral calculi using ultrasonic lithotripsy. A success rate of 95% was achieved with renal calculi, and 86% in removal of ureteral stones. This treatment results in reduced morbidity and a shortened hospital stay. Although this is considered a urological procedure, fluoroscopy is required for nephrostomy placement and manipulation of the catheter and guide wire. The success of the lithotripsy procedure depends on establishing good access for the nephroscope and creating a pathway that will allow direct visualization of the stone. With this treatment, the patient is strapped into a reclining chair and is lowered into a tub of water over the lithotripter. A probe nestles against the skin of the back and, during treatment, projects an intense sonic shock wave against the body, pulsing in time with the patient's

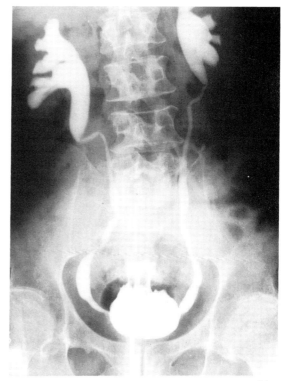

Figure 5–26. Bilateral vesicoureteral reflux in a 46-year-old man.

In most cases, when a patient exhibits renal failure, radiographic examinations such as an IVP may be dangerous to the patient. When they are performed, extreme care must be exercised. Contrast medium is usually introduced by drip infusion.

Treatment. Supportive treatment consists of a protein replacement with a nutritious diet, restricted sodium intake, diuretics for edema, and antibiotics for infection.

Chronic Renal Failure

General Information. Chronic renal failure is the end result of a gradual progressive loss of kidney function. Symptoms usually appear after loss of about 75% of the glomerular filtering apparatus, followed by deterioration of the renal parenchyma. Uremia toxins accumulate and produce potentially fatal physiological changes in all major organ systems. Chronic renal failure is usually the end stage of renal disease or the end result of many numerous diseases, including chronic glomerular disease. Other common causes are infections, congenital anomalies, vascular diseases, obstructive diseases, collagen diseases, toxic agents, and endocrine disorders.

Diagnosis. Major changes are noted in all body systems. Renal failure leads to hypertension, ventricular tachycardia or fibrillation, congestive heart failure, metabolic encephalopathy, convulsions, coma, anemia, clotting disorders, and arterial calcification. The blood urea nitrogen, serum creatinine, and serum potassium levels are greatly elevated. Diagnostic examinations used to determine the level of renal function include intravenous or excretory urography, nephrotomography, renal arteriography, and nuclear medicine renal scan. A kidney biopsy is used to differentiate the possible underlying causes of the renal failure. In renal failure, the kidneys cannot concentrate well, and large doses of contrast medium are used. Contrast medium is excreted by the liver when the kidneys fail. Tomography is used because the contrast within the renal pelvic structures is very poor and delayed films can be taken for many hours.

Treatment. Dialysis is the primary treatment, and it can control, eliminate, or decrease the manifestations of chronic renal failure. A proper diet is maintained, restricting the intake of sodium and potassium. Maintaining fluid balance is very important. Drugs such as diuretics help to excrete edema. Because chronic renal failure has many widespread clinical effects, its management must be coordinated.

Lower Urinary Tract

Congenital Disorders

Double (Bifid-Duplex) Ureters

General Information. The finding of congenital double or bifid ureters is usually of no clinical signif-

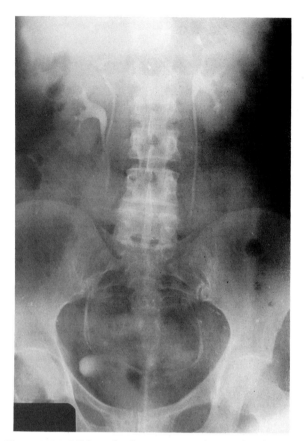

Figure 5–27. Bifid renal pelvis, ureters, and ureteral orifices, as seen on intravenous pyelogram of a 33-year-old woman. This is considered to be a normal variant.

icance. The ureters emerge separately from one or two collecting systems and may unite at some point or individually join the urinary bladder. When two individual collecting systems are present, the upper system is usually dysplastic.

Diagnosis. Double ureters can be seen on the emptying phase of the IVP or intravenous urogram, usually after the 5-minute film (Fig. 5–27). They can also be observed if they are filled with contrast medium during a retrograde pyelogram. Double ureters are often associated with ureterocele.

Treatment. No treatment is required for this condition.

Primary Obstructive Megaloureter

General Information. Primary obstructive megaloureter is associated with pelviureteral obstruction. Congenital megaloureter is more common in males than in females and can occur bilaterally.

Diagnosis. The IVP usually reveals **dilatation** and **hypertrophy** of most of the ureter, and there is a short terminal segment of normal caliber that does not permit reflux. Although the pathogenesis of this anomaly is unknown, the abnormality is thought to be associated with the narrow segment (Fig. 5–28).

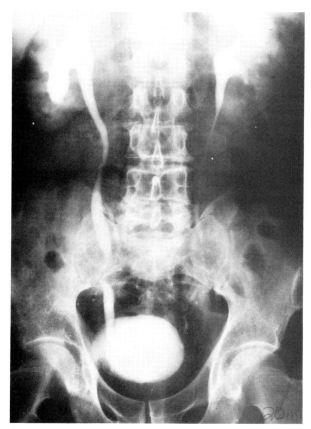

Figure 5–28. A primary obstructive megaloureter and hydronephrosis on the right as a result of a ureterocele at the pelviureter junction, as seen on intravenous pyelography in a 63-year-old man.

Treatment. Correction of this condition involves the removal of the obstruction. This is first attempted through retrograde pyelography. When this fails to correct the condition, surgery is the only recourse. Prevention of infection is an important part of this treatment. Antibiotic therapy is sometimes started prior to retrograde pyelography.

Ureterocele

General Information. A ureterocele is a dilated terminal segment or ureter within the bladder wall, usually unilaterally. It occurs mostly in girls and in cases of ureteral duplication.

Diagnosis. Ureterocele is most likely caused by congenital *stenosis* of the ureterovesical junction. As the terminal ureteral segment enlarges, it invaginates into the bladder and may cause urinary tract infection. When the ureterocele appears without ureteral duplication, it is usually asymptomatic and is not discovered until adulthood. When the ureterocele is associated with ureteral duplication, there is almost always substantial obstruction, producing a megaloureter with hydronephrosis. This condition is usually demonstrated on an intravenous urogram (Fig. 5–29).

Treatment. A ureterocele is usually surgically removed. This allows for an increased diameter of the ureterovesical junction and the increased flow of urine into the bladder, thereby reducing pressure and eliminating the hydronephrosis.

Vesicoureteral Reflux

General Information. Vesicoureteral reflux occurs when urine from the bladder flows backward into the ureters in retrograde fashion. This may be myogenic, because the prevention of reflux depends on the integrity of the ureterovesical junction and the compression of the submucosal portion of the ureter against the underlying muscles. Reflux may also occur as a response to inflammation, especially in the bladder. Infection frequently accompanies this condition and may lead to either acute or chronic pye-

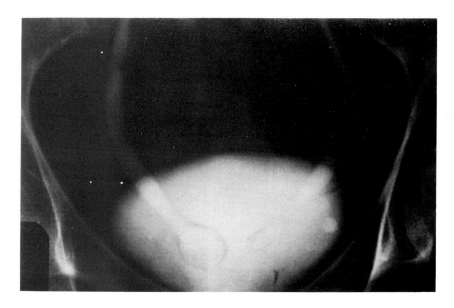

Figure 5–29. Bilateral ureterocele, as seen on the intravenous pyelogram of a 61-year-old woman.

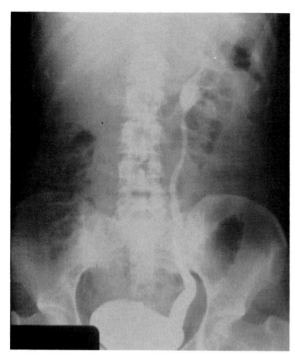

Figure 5–30. Vesicoureteral reflux on the left side of a voiding cystogram in a 30-year-old woman.

lonephritis. This condition is most common in infant boys and in girls between the ages of 3 and 7 years.

Diagnosis. Vesicoureteral reflux first manifests itself as a urinary tract infection. The patient experiences frequent, urgent, burning urination. The urine is especially foul smelling and may contain blood. The specific symptoms depend on whether the upper or lower kidney tract is involved. In children, the condition may not be diagnosed until puberty or even adulthood, when signs indicating renal impairment develop. These symptoms may include anemia, hypertension, and lethargy. Following the discovery of hematuria and foul-smelling urine, a hard mass can be palpated over the pelvic region. This mass represents a hard, thickened bladder. A midstream catch of urine reveals an extremely high number of bacterial colonies. The blood urea nitrogen and serum creatinine levels may be elevated. Radiographically, the IVP may reveal a dilated distal ureter and possibly hydronephrosis. Voiding cystourethrography may identify and determine the degree of *reflux* (Fig. 5–30). Fluoroscopic spot views are usually taken before, during, and after voiding. When necessary, nuclear medicine renal scans and bladder ultrasonography may be employed to demonstrate reflux.

Treatment. The primary goal of treatment is to prevent further damage to the urinary tract while trying to correct the initial problem. Because many patients are in the mid to late stages of the disease when diagnosed, it is necessary to prevent renal dysfunction. Significant damage can be done by long-term pyelonephritis. In reflux caused by a neurogenic bladder or infection, antimicrobial therapy is most effective. Despite the fact that reflux usually diminishes once the infection is eradicated, 80% of young females with vesicoureteral reflux will have recurring urinary tract infections within a year. With recurrent infection, medical treatment could be required for a long while, along with follow-up cystography and intravenous urography.

Inflammatory Disorders

Cystitis

General Information. Cystitis is almost always caused by bacterial organisms. If not treated quickly and effectively, pyelonephritis is the usual result. Bacteria enter the body through the urethra. Poor personal hygiene, catheterization, or a fistulous tract may precipitate infection. Stasis within the bladder enables the bacteria to remain, rather than be washed away.

Diagnosis. The classic sign of cystitis is a burning pain (dysuria) on urination, with hematuria. There is often a forced urgency and frequency of urination. Cystitis can be both acute as well as chronic. Chronic disease is usually the result of a persistent acute disease or underlying renal diseases. Fluoroscopic spot views while voiding during cystourethrography identify the infection, with the demonstration of ureteral reflux. When there is chronic inflammation, the smooth bladder contour is replaced by irregular bladder *trabeculae* (Fig. 5–31). The cystogram also helps rule out other structural abnormalities such as bladder or urethral strictures (producing obstruction), diverticula, and neoplasms.

Treatment. The usual treatment for cystitis includes antibiotics, forced fluids, and bed rest. Surgical dilatation via cystoscopy may be indicated when urethral stricture is in evidence.

Bladder Diverticula

General Information. Bladder diverticula may develop as a result of inflammation, chronic obstruction to the bladder outflow, or congenital defect. Because of urinary stasis, calculi as well as tumors may arise within the diverticulum. Most diverticula occur in middle age, with 95% in men.

Diagnosis. Diverticula are best demonstrated during a voiding cystogram and on the IVP film after voiding, when the bladder contracts. In about one-third of cases, two or more diverticula are present. Most are small, but they may expand into a larger mass (Fig. 5–32).

Treatment. Treatment usually consists of attempting to relieve the symptoms of the condition. This will ultimately remove the source of infection, and urinary excretion should return to normal. Although the diverticulum may not totally disappear, its size can be minimized. The usual course of treatment includes forcing fluids and administering antibiotics.

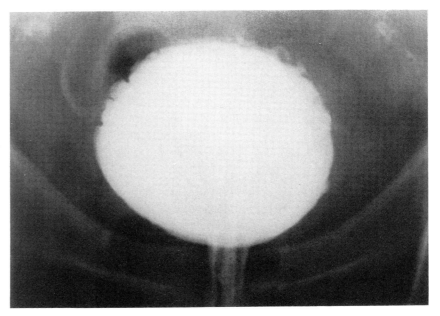

Figure 5–31. Mild bladder trabeculae, as seen on the cystogram of an 80-year-old man.

Vesicovaginal Fistula

General Information. In the lower urinary tract, the most common fistulous communication is between the bladder and vagina. It is not uncommon for a fistulous communication to develop between the bladder and the bowel and skin, most often because of inflammation, pelvic neoplasm, or radiation therapy. Carcinomas of the colon and cervix are the most common lesions that produce vesicovaginal fistulas. Crohn's disease and diverticulitis are the inflammatory conditions that produce fistulous tracts involving the bladder. Radiation-induced inflammation and necrosis are complications of radiation treatments for cervical cancer and are known to produce fistulous tracts.

Diagnosis. Vesicovaginal fistulas can be demonstrated with cystography. Fluoroscopic spots are taken by the radiologist with the patient in the supine and posterior oblique positions.

Treatment. Most fistulous communications of this type are corrected surgically.

Prostatic Hypertrophy

General Information. Prostatic hypertrophy is a benign condition that the majority of males suffer sometime after the 50th year of life. Practically all men over age 50 have some enlargement of the prostate gland. The cause of this condition seems to

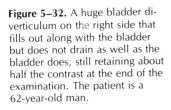

Figure 5–32. A huge bladder diverticulum on the right side that fills out along with the bladder but does not drain as well as the bladder does, still retaining about half the contrast at the end of the examination. The patient is a 62-year-old man.

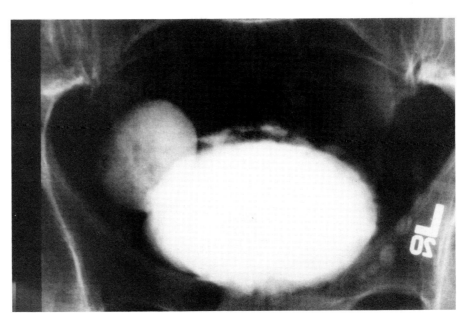

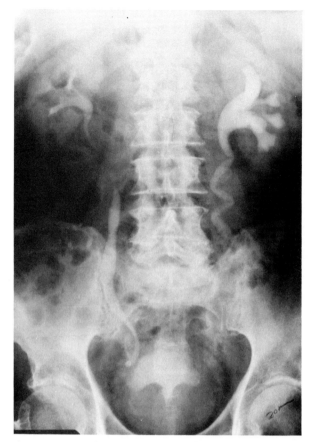

Figure 5–33. A filling defect at the bladder base, consistent with a markedly enlarged prostate gland causing a marked degree of bladder outlet obstruction in an 84-year-old man.

be a decrease in the production of androgenic hormones.

Diagnosis. The prostate gland is examined via the rectum. The physician is able to feel the entire surface of the gland. The greatest amount of hypertrophy is anterior with this benign condition. If the swelling is on the posterior surface of the gland, a nodule is often palpable. This nodule often signifies carcinoma of the prostate gland.

The earliest symptoms include reduced caliber and force of the urine stream, difficulty in initiating urination, and the feeling of pressure remaining in the bladder. As the gland enlarges, the patient urinates less but always feels the urge to urinate. The pressure of the distended bladder increases, and low back pain is present. As the level of urinary stasis increases, infections become more prevalent. As the condition worsens, the accumulation of nitrogenous wastes in the blood increases, indicating renal dysfunction, and the level of nitrogenous ammoniated wastes increases. This often results in central nervous system depression, stupor, and finally coma.

The excretory urogram often indicates tract obstruction, stone formation, and possibly tumors. The bladder filled with contrast medium often reveals the extent of prostatic hypertrophy. The lesion appears as a *filling defect* (Fig. 5–33).

Treatment. Initially, the treatment is conservative. Prostatic massages, sitz baths, and catheterization offer only temporary relief. Because of the potential complications as this condition worsens, surgery is the only means of relieving the discomforts associated with acute urinary retention. Transurethral resection is the procedure of choice. Excess tissue is removed with a rectoscope with a wire loop and electric current. Other surgical options include removal of the prostate gland.

Self-Assessment Quiz

For each of the following questions, select the one best response and circle the letter that precedes it.

1. Which of the following is routinely performed in the presence of hypertension?
   a. retrograde urogram
   b. cystogram
   c. timed IVP
   d. nephrogram

2. Which of the following is a true kidney function test?
   a. IVP
   b. cystogram
   c. retrograde pyelogram
   d. nephrostomy

3. The Seldinger technique is used with
   a. nephrotomography
   b. IVP
   c. retrograde pyelography
   d. renal angiography

4. A retention catheter is used in conjunction with
   a. IVP
   b. cystography
   c. retrograde pyelography
   d. nephrostomy

5. Which of the following is the most important laboratory test when evaluating the urinary system?
   a. creatinine
   b. urinalysis
   c. BUN
   d. bilirubin

6. Results of which of the following tests will be abnormal in persons with renal dysfunction?
   a. BUN and creatinine
   b. uric acid
   c. BUN and bilirubin
   d. bilirubin

7. The term *agenesis* usually refers to congenital
   a. absence
   b. enlargement
   c. duplication
   d. cyst formation

8. An underdeveloped kidney may be described as
   a. cyst-like
   b. metastatic
   c. atrophic
   d. hypertrophic

9. Fusion of the lower poles of the kidneys produces a particular configuration referred to as
   a. polycystic kidneys
   b. bifid kidneys
   c. horseshoe kidneys
   d. sponge kidney

10. Duplication or bifid collecting systems is a congenital disorder and is considered as an incidental finding on an IVP by the radiologist.
    a. true
    b. false

11. The term *ectopia* refers to
    a. duplication
    b. cyst formation
    c. displacement or malposition
    d. a size decrease

12. A kidney condition that occurs secondary to inflammation and is due to immunological factors is
    a. pyelonephritis
    b. cystitis
    c. glomerulonephritis
    d. nephrolithiasis

13. The most important and serious kidney disorder is
    a. acute pyelonephritis
    b. nephritis
    c. glomerulonephritis
    d. cystitis

14. The large majority of urinary tract infections are caused by
    a. bacteria
    b. a virus

15. Ingestion of large amounts of analgesics can cause
    a. renal ectopia
    b. pyelonephritis
    c. interstitial nephritis
    d. nephrocalcinosis

16. The kidney releases renin in the presence of
    a. diabetes
    b. cystic disease
    c. cancer
    d. renal artery stenosis

17. Renal artery stenosis is often the cause of idiopathic
    a. diabetes
    b. hypertension
    c. hypotension
    d. fibrillation

18. Delayed filling of the kidneys may be demonstrated by
    a. nephrotomography
    b. cystography
    c. retrograde urography
    d. CT scanning

19. Which of the following is an error in metabolism?
    a. renal ectopia
    b. cystic disease
    c. nephrocalcinosis
    d. agenesis

20. The terms *oxalate, phosphate, uric acid,* and *cystine* refer to types of
    a. stones
    b. cysts
    c. tumors
    d. urine

21. Overdistension of the renal pelvis due to an obstructing calculus is termed
    a. nephrocalcinosis
    b. calculosis
    c. hydronephrosis
    d. hydrocele

22. The terms *hypoproteinemia, proteinuria, hyperlipidemia,* and *edema* are usually included together when discussing
    a. renal agenesis
    b. nephritis
    c. renal angiography
    d. nephrotic syndrome

23. A dilated terminal segment of ureter located within the bladder wall is known as
    a. hydrocele
    b. ureterocele
    c. megaloureter
    d. stenosis

24. The backward flow of urine into the ureters in retrograde fashion describes
    a. achalasia
    b. ectopia
    c. uremia
    d. reflux

25. A transurethral resection is a surgical procedure used in the treatment of
    a. bladder cancer
    b. prostatitis
    c. prostatic hypertrophy
    d. obstruction

Study Questions

1. Which laboratory tests would tend to yield abnormal results when urinary tract infections are present?

2. What is nephrolithotripsy and how is it used?

3. Describe each type of kidney stone.

4. What may be seen on a microscopic examination of a urine specimen of a patient with a urinary tract infection?

5. What are some of the complications of nephrolithiasis?

6. Describe the process of renal dialysis.

7. Under what circumstances is a renal transplant considered?

Six

Osseous System and Joints

Related Terminology

achondroplasia
acromegaly
ankylosing spondylitis
aseptic necrosis
Brodie's abscess
bursitis
equinovarus
gout
kyphosis
Kienböck's disease
Köhler's disease
Legg-Calvé-Perthes disease
Marfan's syndrome
Osgood-Schlatter disease
osteogenesis imperfecta
osteomalacia
osteomyelitis
osteopetrosis
osteoporosis
Paget's disease
rheumatoid arthritis
rickets
Scheuermann's disease
Schmorl's nodes
scoliosis
spondylolisthesis
spondylolysis
spondylosis
Still's disease
tendinitis

Objectives

Upon completion of Chapter 6, the reader will be able to

- List the most common disorders of the osseous system and joints.

- Identify the major radiographic features of the most common disorders of the osseous system and joints.

- Describe the various imaging modalities used in demonstrating the osseous system and joints.

- List several methods of treatment used for the osseous system and joints.

- Describe the major complications that often accompany many bone and joint disorders.

Imaging the Osseous System and Joints

Radiography of the osseous system and joints often involves a certain amount of decision making by the radiographer. Initially, the radiographer must observe the physical characteristics of each patient and establish what level of communication will be necessary. The requisition states the nature of the request and the patient's vital statistics. In addition, the requisition should include the patient's history. Unfortunately, the extent of a patient's recorded history will vary with the individual and the situation.

The radiographer should double-check that the patient is the one who is listed on the requisition. In addition, it can be useful to verify the patient's history. The emergency room is often busy, and a history may be incomplete, incorrect, or even absent. It is important to establish whether or not an injury has taken place and, if so, how and when the accident occurred. If there is no injury, consider the patient's age, the specific description of what the patient is experiencing in terms of type and location of pain, and to what extent function of the part is impaired.

When no injury is apparent, the patient's age and the location of the pain are important. The radiographer should be aware of the importance of demonstrating the soft tissues as well as the bony structures. Many types of bone reactions are possible, and the radiographic technique factors should be adjusted to reveal as much anatomy as possible. It is advantageous to discern as many shades of gray as possible in the adjacent structures.

Although it is understood that the radiographer is not supposed to establish a diagnosis based on radiographs, it is generally accepted that the radiographer should be able to correlate the patient's history with the radiographic findings. The more knowledgeable the radiographer, the better he or she will be able to produce the most diagnostic radiograph.

It is the radiographer's responsibility to be sure that the radiographs are properly labeled in terms of right and left markers and patient identification. Once processed, the radiograph should be completely scanned to assure that all pertinent anatomy has been properly demonstrated anatomically as well as photographically. When making x-ray films of bones and joints, it is essential that at least two views be obtained at right angles to each other. In addition, when long bones are involved, both the proximal and distal joints must be identified. The radiographer is responsible for conducting procedures that will minimize radiation exposure to the patient.

In addition to plain films, other means of imaging are common. These methods include tomography, computed tomography (CT), and radionuclide bone scanning. Tomography is most useful in demonstrating bones that are of mixed shape. For example, routine radiography of the bony orbit, sacrum, or sternum often do not reveal the structures to best advantage. CT is better able to distinguish bony elements and soft tissue planes. Some bones and joints simply are inadequately demonstrated radiographically. This is especially true of the hip, which often has irregular fractures that may be missed on plain films. Radionuclide bone scans are most useful in demonstrating areas of metastasis, fracture, or infection.

Bone lesions can be categorized in two groups: those in which there is a loss of density of the bony matrix and those in which there is an increase of bone. The term *osteolytic* is used in denoting a loss of bone or referring to bone destruction. The term *osteoblastic* refers to the formation of additional bone or forming bone.

Some conditions that may be classed as osteolytic include osteoporosis, which is an overall loss of bone density with thinning of the cortex, and osteomalacia, which is a generalized softening of bone. Within osteolytic bone, we may also observe a change of the trabecular pattern such as in hyperparathyroidism. Various forms of growth disturbances present osteoblastic or osteolytic bone changes. These conditions will be discussed in Chapter 8.

The periosteum, as well as the inner bony trabeculae, is also subject to changes. Periosteal reactions may reflect an early stage in the life of many abnormalities. In the early stages, periosteal reactions are often difficult to differentiate. The cortex of bone is similarly affected, and the patient's age, sex, symptoms, and history are of great importance. Specific types of lesions are common in certain locations of the body. Again, it is important to emphasize the capabilities of the radiographer, who is increasingly aware of the various types of lesions and the best ways to demonstrate them radiographically. Thus, certain judgments are necessary regarding radiographic exposure and positioning. Based on a patient's complaints and history, an alert radiographer may suspect the possibility of a particular lesion. Early and accurate detection of a lesion by a radiologist may be enhanced by the capabilities of the radiographer.

Congenital Disorders

Congenital Clubfoot

General Information. Congenital clubfoot is referred to as the *talipes equinovarus* deformity. This condition is considered to be the most common congenital disorder of the lower extremities and is two times more common in males than in females. It

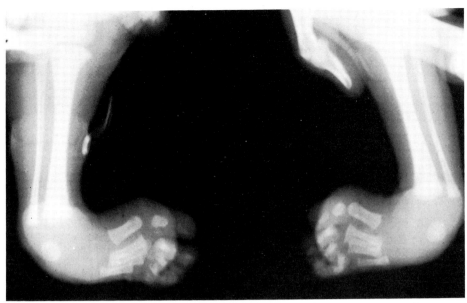

Figure 6–1. Bilateral equinovarus deformity of the feet, commonly known as congenital clubfeet, in a neonate.

may be associated with other abnormalities such as myelomeningocele and spina bifida and may be caused by a combination of genetic and environmental factors. If one sibling is affected with this condition, there is a 1 in 15 chance that other siblings will be similarly affected. Afflicted parents have a 1 in 10 chance that their offspring will have the same condition. From the environmental point of view and in the absence of family history, it is thought that the defect is formed during the 9th and 10th weeks of embryonic life (period of foot development).

Diagnosis. The foot turns *downward* (equino) and *inward* (varus), and the front of the foot curls toward the heel. The talus is shortened, and the calcaneus is shortened and flattened. A shortening of the achilles tendon produces the club-like appearance of the foot (Fig. 6–1). This condition also involves muscle abnormalities, and there may be a variation in the length and insertions of muscle. This condition can vary in severity and must be distinguished from a condition known as metatarsus adductus or the pigeon-toed deformity. In metatarsus adductus, there is a characteristic superimposition of the talus and calcaneus.

Treatment. Congenital clubfoot is corrected in three stages: (1) In forefoot adduction, the foot is uncurled away from the heel. (2) Varus deformity correction involves the turning of the foot so that the sole faces outward (eversion). (3) Equinus is corrected by casting the foot with the toes pointed upward in dorsiflexion. This correction may be accomplished in several stages of manipulation and casting over a 5-to 6-week period followed by remanipulation, recasting, and so on. When treatment is begun early, the usual correction time will not exceed 3 to 4 months. A resistant deformity may require surgical correction. When surgery is performed, complete correction is seldom achieved. After the condition is corrected, the patient must follow a strenuous exercise program, use night splints, and wear orthopedic shoes when walking.

Congenital Hip Dysplasia

General Information. Hip dysplasia is the most common congenital hip disorder. It is actually a malformation of the *acetabulum* rather than of the femoral head, which is displaced in relation to the acetabulum. This condition is much more common in firstborn females (83%) and is 10 times more common in breech fetal presentations. Although the exact cause is unknown, it has been postulated that certain hormones that relax the maternal ligaments in preparation for labor may also cause laxity of the infant's ligaments around the capsule of the hip joint.

Diagnosis. The earliest diagnosis usually takes place during a routine examination by a pediatrician. Extra folds of gluteal tissue when the infant is placed in both the supine and prone positions are among the earliest signs. When the infant is prone, the buttock fold is higher on the affected side. When supine, abduction is restricted. Radiographically, the hips are viewed in the anteroposterior (AP) position

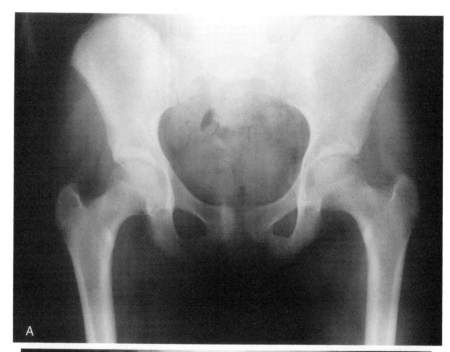

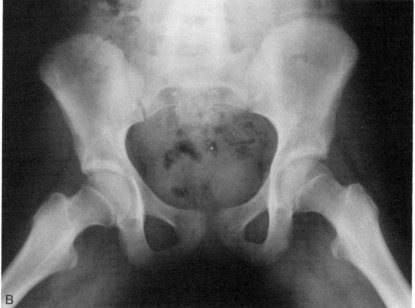

Figure 6–2. *(A)* Internal and *(B)* external rotational views of both hips, which were within normal limits, in a 12-year-old girl.

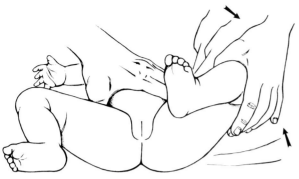

Figure 6–3. Ortolani's sign.

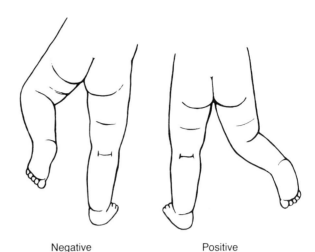

Negative   Positive

Figure 6–4. Trendelenburg's sign.

with complete extension and with the legs abducted 45 degrees in full internal rotation (Fig. 6–2). In addition to the abnormal buttock folds, two other signs are positive for dysplasia. (1) To demonstrate **Ortolani's sign,** the infant is placed in the supine position, with the hips flexed in abduction and then adducted while the femur is pressed. This will dislocate the hip. A characteristic *clicking* sound is heard when the femoral head moves over the acetabular ring. Subluxation is more common between birth and the age of 1 month. Dislocation is more common after age 1 month (Fig. 6–3). (2) To demonstrate **Trendelenburg's** sign, the infant is placed on the affected side and the opposite knee is lifted. The pelvis drops on the normal side because of the weak abductor muscles on the affected side. If the child stands and the opposite knee is lifted, the pelvis remains horizontal. With Trendelenburg's sign, the

pelvis will reveal the location of the femoral head and a shallow acetabulum (Fig. 6–4). In general, the earlier the treatment the better the prognosis.

Some of the late signs of this disorder include a unique pattern of walking that resembles a **duck waddle** and that is indicative of bilateral hip dysplasia. This is most common after the age of 2. Joint degeneration typically occurs after the age of 2. There are three forms of severity: (1) In unstable hip dysplasia, the position of the hip is normal but the hip can be dislocated with the least effort. (2) In subluxation, the femoral head rides on the edge of the acetabulum. (3) In complete dislocation, the femoral head is totally outside the acetabulum (Fig. 6–5).

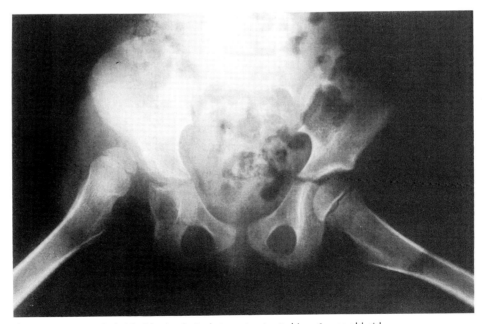

Figure 6–5. Congenital right hip dysplasia that went untreated in a 6-year-old girl.

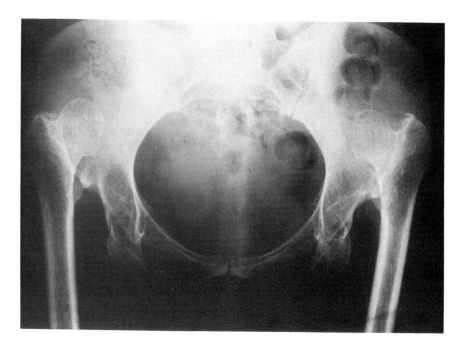

Figure 6–6. Bilateral congenital hip dysplasia that went untreated in a 45-year-old woman.

Treatment. The treatment of congenital hip dysplasia varies depending on whether the condition is discovered early or late. When it is discovered before the infant is 3 months of age, gentle manipulation and reduction are followed by immobilization with splints, braces, or a plaster cast for 2 to 3 months, followed by 1 month with night splints or braces. The treatment of choice in a child from the ages of 3 months to 2 years is bilateral skin traction. If the infant is walking, skeletal traction or closed reduction is followed by application of a spica cast for 4 to 6 months. If that is not successful, open reduction is performed followed by application of a spica cast for 6 months. If a child is older than 5 years, restoration is rare (Fig. 6–6).

Achondroplasia

General Information. Achondroplasia is the most frequent cause of *dwarfism* and is a result of defective ossification of the growth plate, where there is inadequate proliferation and calcification of endochondral tissue. In 99% of cases, this condition occurs as a result of spontaneous mutation. Characteristically evident are the short arms and legs but a normal-size head and trunk and almost a total vertebral lordosis. Although the size of the head is normal, the forehead is markedly rounded or bossed. The nose is sunken (saddlenose), and there is prominence of both the upper and lower jaws (prognathism), especially the mandible. The foramen magnum is atypically small, and the cranial base is usually flat (platybasia), with upward displacement of the upper cervical vertebrae and bony impingement on the brain stem. This is referred to as the basilar impression. A trident or three-fingered hand and varus deformities of the knees are often present. The intelligence of an achondroplastic dwarf is not usually impaired.

Diagnosis. Radiographically, the skull reveals a thin growth plate and a heavy cylinder of compact or cortical bone. There is characteristic *trumpeting* of the shafts and *widening* of the proximal and distal ends (Fig. 6–7).

Treatment. As in other congenital and inherited disorders, treatment is not usually required. However, because most congenital defects are multiple, it is possible that other associated conditions may produce complications in the early and middle adult years.

Osteogenesis Imperfecta

General Information. Osteogenesis imperfecta is referred to as the *brittle bone* disease. The skeleton is extremely fragile and will fracture on the least amount of impact or stress. This condition is a defect of osteoblastic activity and abnormal collagen synthe-

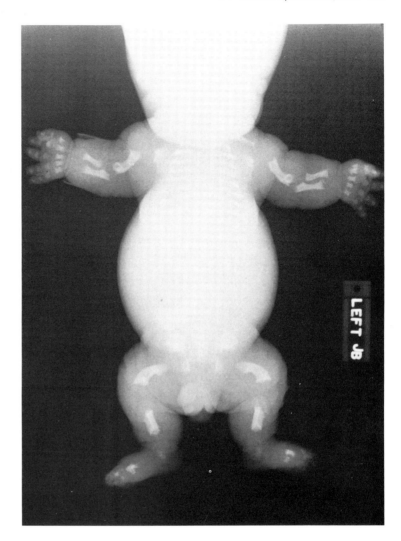

Figure 6–7. Postmortem radiograph of a thanatophoric dwarf.

sis. Osteogenesis imperfecta is characterized by numerous signs, which include but may not be limited to bulging of the temporal region, a triangle-shaped head and face with prominent eyes, blue sclera, and protruding ears. One-third of patients suffer deafness between the ages of 30 and 40 years. Also present are subcutaneous skin hemorrhages, which are both large and small (petechiae and ecchymoses). Later, the patient may develop aortic valve incompetency and bluish-gray discolored teeth. The tooth discoloration is due to a lack of dentin, and affected teeth are more prone to caries and fracture easily. Muscle atrophy is apparent, and there is hypermobility of the joints owing to the laxity of the ligaments around the joint capsule.

Osteogenesis imperfecta presents two forms, one that is congenital and the other that is delayed. The congenital form is the most serious and is an autosomal recessive disorder in which fractures are present at birth. This form is usually fatal within a few days to a few weeks. Osteogenesis imperfecta *tarda* is the most common and least severe form and is an autosomal dominant disorder. The newborn infant appears normal at birth but has recurring fractures during the first year of life.

Diagnosis. The cardinal sign of osteogenesis imperfecta is *fracture,* which occurs with the least trauma. X-ray films usually reveal the existence of old healing fractures with abundant callus formation along with the fresh fracture. Many fractures of the extremities become apparent during the first year of life and are usually painless. When the child is brought to the emergency room for treatment, the hospital personnel may suspect child abuse. Most fractures are of the greenstick variety. The incidence of fractures decreases after puberty. The repeated fractures account for the stunted growth, especially when the epiphyseal plate is involved. Skull x-ray

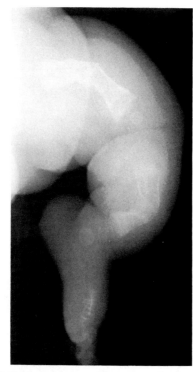

Figure 6–8. Thickened bones with numerous healing fractures and deficit demineralization compatible with congenital osteogenesis imperfecta, in a 1-day-old boy.

films reveal wide sutures, with irregular bone islands of the occipital region, usually referred to as wormian bones (Figs. 6–8 and 6–9).

Treatment. There is essentially no treatment for this disorder other than the treatment of specific fractures and their effects and complications. It is important to give the patient strong psychological support and to encourage ambulation. Obviously, the patient must avoid strenuous activity and contact sports. Parents must be taught how to recognize and splint fractures until medical care can be received. Nutrition counseling will ensure proper nourishment.

Marfan's Syndrome

General Information. Marfan's syndrome or arachnodactyly is a rare, inherited, degenerative, and generalized disease of connective tissue. Affected are the ocular, skeletal, and cardiovascular systems. Males and females are afflicted with equal frequency. Death, when it occurs, is usually from cardiovascular complications. Marfan's syndrome is an autosomal dominant disease in which 85% of reported cases presented with a family history. The remaining 15% are the result of a mutation that most often occurs with advanced paternal age. In practically all reported cases, the clinical effects are not apparent at birth. President Abraham Lincoln suffered from Marfan's

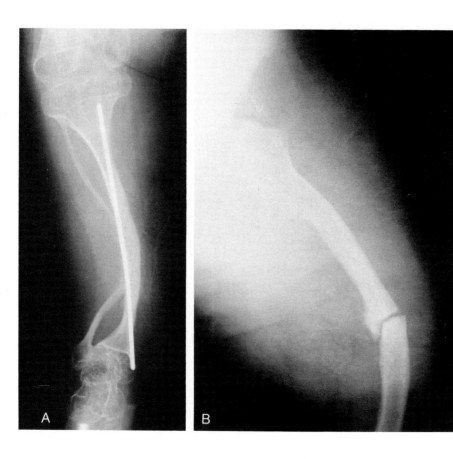

Figure 6–9. *A,* An intermedullary rod inserted into the right tibia of an 18-year-old male. This is compatible with osteogenesis imperfecta tarda. *B,* An old ununited fracture of the left femur in the same patient. The femur is quite distorted in position. Callus formation is minimal.

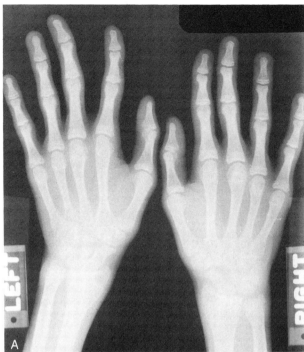

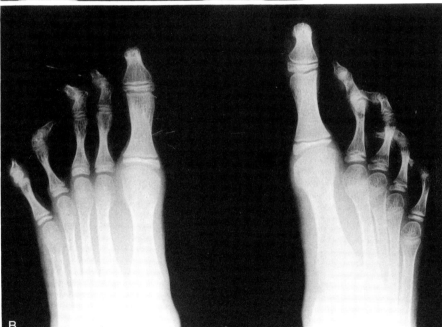

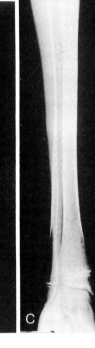

Figure 6–10. Abnormally long, slender, and tubular metacarpals *(A)*, phalanges *(B)*, and lower leg *(C)* in a man. These findings are consistent with Marfan's syndrome.

syndrome, as did Flo Hyman, a U.S. volleyball player who distinguished herself at the 1984 Olympics and who later collapsed and died during a volleyball game in Europe.

Diagnosis. The long bones are *slender, tubular,* and unusually *long.* The fingers are characteristically long and slender and are sometimes referred to as spider fingers (Fig. 6–10).

The patient's arm span exceeds the patient's height. The individual is taller than average for the family. The upper half of the body is shorter than average, whereas the lower half is longer than average. In addition, there is a marked weakness of the ligaments, tendons, and joint capsules. Joints are hyperextensible, and dislocation is frequent. There is excessive growth of the ribs, and anomalies such as pectus excavatum and pigeon breast are common. A most important sign is eye lens displacement. This occurs in about 75% of reported cases. There is also a quivering of the iris with eye movement, myopia, and retinal detachment. Glaucoma occurs in some cases. Another unique finding is the relative absence of subcutaneous body fat.

This condition includes many serious complications such as weakness of the aortic media. This weakness usually involves the ascending aorta and results in aortic regurgitation due to valvular insufficiency. Rupture of the aorta is always a possibility. Because of this complication, pregnancy is discouraged. Other complications include inguinal hernia, cystic lung disease, recurring spontaneous pneumothorax, and severe scoliosis. Because this is a hereditary disorder, the diagnosis may be suspected when a close family relative is afflicted. The skeletal and ocular defects, in addition to family history, usually confirm the diagnosis.

Treatment. There is essentially no treatment for Marfan's syndrome. The treatment is primarily palliative, in that an attempt is made to control the effects of the complications that can accompany this disorder. Treatments may include surgical repair of the vascular and ocular defects and administration of steroids and hormones to induce puberty. The drugs stop the early advancement of bone growth. Sudden death most often occurs during the greatest periods of bone growth and during physical exercise. Death is usually the result of aortic rupture. Genetic counseling would discourage pregnancy because of the possibility of aortic rupture and because of the increased probability that offspring might be similarly afflicted.

Osteopetrosis

General Information. Osteopetrosis is a congenital condition having many eponyms, including Albers-Schönberg disease, osteosclerosis, marble bones, chalk bones, and ivory bones. This condition results from a failure of resorption of cartilaginous intercellular substance. The growth plate does not mature, and bone retardation and brittleness result.

Osteopetrosis is an inherited disorder that can be dominant or recessive. The dominant form, resulting from a gene of a single parent, is usually benign, and patients usually enjoy a normal life span. The recessive form results from the genes of both parents, is usually malignant, and is mostly present in children. The recessive form is usually fatal before the age of 20.

Diagnosis. Osteopetrosis is characterized by thickening and increased density of atypically soft bone. It is considered to be the exact opposite of osteoporosis, in which there is a decrease in bone density.

Radiographically, osteopetrosis presents a *chalky white* or opaque appearance with a loss of distinction between the bony cortex and trabeculae. Because of the increased thickening and widening of the cortex, there is a reduction in size and loss of distinction of the medullary cavity. The ends of the long bones appear club shaped, and there are alternating areas of radiolucency and radiopacity, depending on the stage of the disease. This unique condition is radiographically apparent in the vertebrae, pelvis, and cranial base, as well as in the long bones (Fig. 6–11).

The most frequent complication of osteopetrosis is fracture. Other complications include osteomyelitis, anemia, osteosclerotic marrow, otosclerosis, cataracts, abnormal teeth, and hepatosplenomegaly. In the late stage of the disease, pressure is created on the cranial nerves, causing optic atrophy, deafness, and facial palsy.

Treatment. There is no definitive treatment for osteopetrosis, other than palliative measures. The emphasis is placed on controlling the effects of the complications.

Metabolic Disorders

Osteoporosis

General Information. Osteoporosis is a condition characterized by a loss of bone density or rarefaction of bone. This condition may also be described as a reduction in the amount of calcified bone mass per unit volume of skeletal tissue, resulting in porous and brittle bone.

Although there are many causes of osteoporosis, we can categorize them into two groups: primary and secondary. Primary or idiopathic osteoporosis is further identified according to the age of onset. Included in this group are juvenile, postmenopausal, and senile forms. Secondary causes include Cushing's syndrome, steroid therapy, osteogenesis imperfecta, disuse atrophy, rheumatoid arthritis, diabetes mellitus, prolonged heparin administration, sickle cell anemia, multiple myeloma, and scurvy. A radiological diagnosis of osteoporosis is usually made only after other diseases have been ruled out.

Juvenile osteoporosis afflicts younger people, and in this particular case the cause is usually idiopathic rather than metabolic.

Postmenopausal osteoporosis is related to a lack of estrogen, which is necessary to stimulate production of new osteoblasts. This is considered to be a metabolic disorder.

Senile osteoporosis is by far the most common type. It affects elderly persons and leaves the bones very susceptible to fracture.

Diagnosis. Radiographically, osteoporosis may be

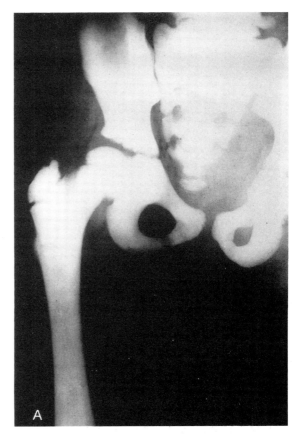

Figure 6–11. Bones of the pelvis, hip, femur *(A)*, ribs, and thoracic spine *(B)* showing a chalky-white appearance in a girl. The medullary canal of the long bones is indistinguishable. These findings are compatible with osteopetrosis.

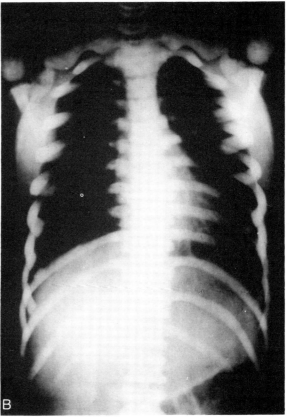

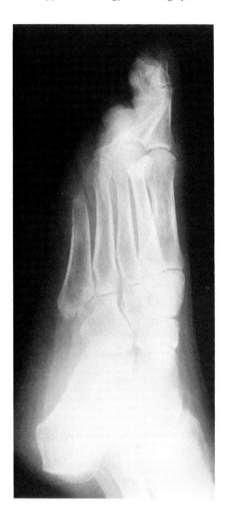

Figure 6–12. Moderate osteoporosis of the foot in a 57-year-old woman. Noted is the previous amputation of the fifth phalanx and head of the fifth metatarsal.

noted best in the distal extremities, joints (Fig. 6–12), pelvis (Fig. 6–13), flat bones of the skull (Fig. 6–14), and vertebral column, especially in the lateral view of the dorsolumbar spine. In addition to the decreased bone density, there is widening of the disk space, obvious calcification of the cartilaginous rim surrounding the vertebral body, and perhaps a partial collapse centrally of one or more vertebral bodies. A

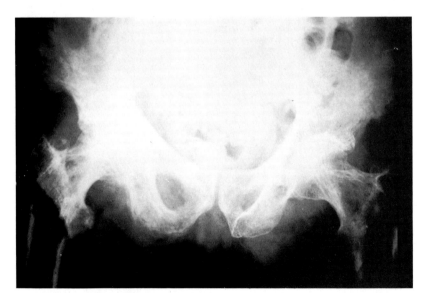

Figure 6–13. Severe osteoporosis and osteoarthritis of the pelvis, hips, and proximal femurs in an 82-year-old man.

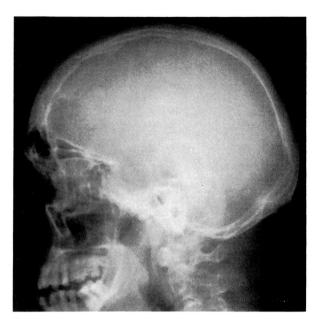

Figure 6–14. Osteoporosis of the skull, most prominently in the flat bones, in a man.

collapse is actually a compression fracture, which results in the vertebral bodies appearing *wedge shaped* or biconcave (Fig. 6–15). The long bones reveal an extremely thin cortex. For all types of osteoporosis, a decrease in radiographic exposure is warranted. For postmenopausal women, the milliampere seconds (mAs) should be decreased by about 15%. For senile osteoporosis, a decrease in mAs of about 25% is required. The major complication involves spontaneous fractures of the proximal femur and thoracic and lumbar spine. Osteoporosis is the leading cause of intertrochanteric hip fracture in the elderly. These fractures occur with the least bit of trauma and are often referred to as *pathological* or trophic fractures.

Treatment. The treatment of osteoporosis is essentially based on the symptoms presented. Fracture prevention and pain control are the major emphasis of treatment. The patient is encouraged to take part in simple exercise, whether in physical therapy or at home and outdoors. Fractures must of course be treated according to their severity. Hip fractures almost always require an open-reduction surgical

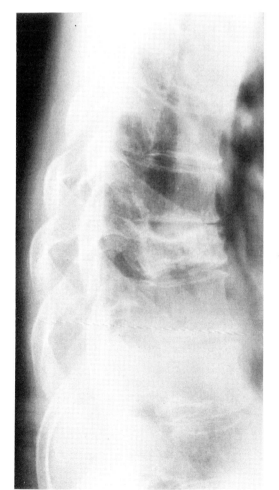

Figure 6–15. Osteoporotic compression and collapse, with the lower lumbar vertebrae appearing biconcave or wedge-shaped, in a 75-year-old woman.

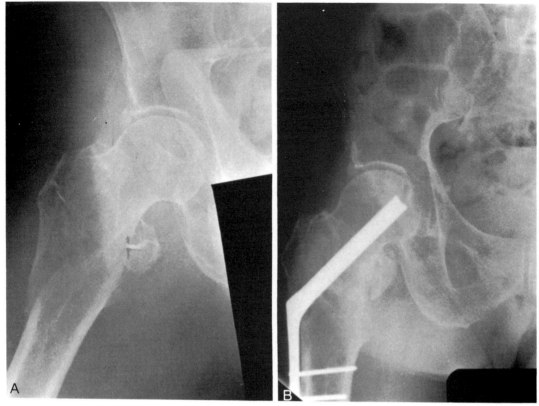

Figure 6–16. *A,* Intertrochanteric fracture of the left femur, with the fractured fragments in excellent alignment and position, in an 87-year-old man. *B,* Open reduction of the left hip with a Jewett nail situated in the head and neck of the femur to immobilize the fracture.

procedure in which metallic fixation devices immobilize the fracture (Fig. 6–16). When osteoporosis is too advanced for metallic pinning or nailing, a complete artificial joint replacement is provided. This involves surgical removal of the entire proximal remur and the insertion of a total hip replacement (Fig. 6–17).

Hormonal Disorders

Hyperparathyroidism

General Information. Hyperparathyroidism is a disease characterized by overactivity of one or more of the four parathyroid glands. This results in excess secretion of parathyroid hormone (PTH), promoting bone resorption and leading to hypercalcemia and hypophosphatemia. This condition usually occurs between the ages of 30 and 50 but has been known to afflict the very young and the elderly. Women are affected two to three times more often than men.

Diagnosis. Radiographs usually reveal *diffuse demineralization* of bones, outer compact bone absorption, and subperiosteal erosion of the radial aspect of the middle fingers. A high concentration of serum PTH on radioimmunoassay, together with hypercalcemia, confirms the diagnosis.

Treatment. Treatment of this condition depends on the exact cause of the disease. Surgical removal of one or more of the parathyroid glands or one of several types of dietary therapy is the usual method of treatment.

Acromegaly

General Information. Acromegaly is a chronic and progressive condition that results from hypersecretion of growth hormone from the pituitary gland. This condition is rare and usually occurs in adults following epiphyseal closure. Overproduction of growth hormone in children before the onset of puberty is referred to as gigantism. Increased growth of long bones and exaggerated height are the major characteristics of gigantism. In adults, long bone growth ceases at puberty, thus deformity of the bones of the face, jaw, hands, and feet are those that are most apparent.

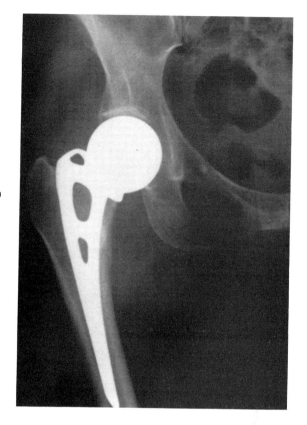

Figure 6–17. An Austin Moore prosthesis surgically implanted in a 71-year-old woman who sustained a fractured hip that could not be repaired with conventional pinning because of advanced osteoporosis.

Diagnosis. The overproduction of growth hormone is most often the result of a pituitary adenoma. In addition to the prominence of the hands, feet, and facial features, a characteristic **ballooning** of the sella turcica may be seen on lateral skull radiographs.

When diagnosed early, a double line, a sloping sellar floor, appears as a result of the asymmetric enlargement of the pituitary fossa (Fig. 6–18). Hand radiographs reveal prominent tufts on the terminal phalanges, with widening of the metacarpophalangeal

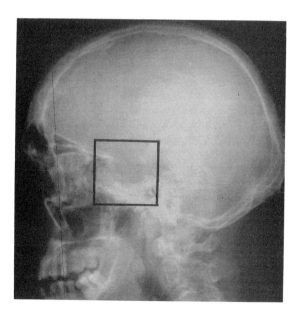

Figure 6–18. Significant enlargement of the sella turcica, as seen on a right lateral view of the skull of a 58-year-old man. This finding is consistent with acromegaly.

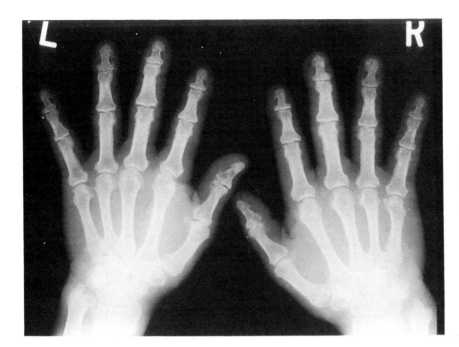

Figure 6–19. Extraordinarily large man's hands, revealing prominent tufts of the terminal phalanges with widening of the metacarpophalangeal joint spaces.

spaces due to overgrowth of articular cartilage (Fig. 6–19).

Treatment. The treatment of acromegaly centers on surgical removal of the tumor. Pituitary tumors are often deep seated and difficult to remove. Radiation therapy is almost always used, whether for palliative purposes or to initiate a cure.

Nutritional Disorders

General Information. A deficiency of vitamin D can result in rickets or osteomalacia, conditions in which there is a lack of calcium in the body tissues with decreased mineralization of osteoid. Rickets occurs before the unification of the diaphysis and epiphyses, whereas osteomalacia occurs after epiphyseal closure. There are three primary causes: (1) Dietary deficiency of vitamin D or lack of exposure to sunlight, (2) impaired absorption of calcium or vitamin D, and (3) renal disease, in which the condition develops despite normal amounts of vitamin D.

Diagnosis. Rickets, the *juvenile* form of osteomalacia, is most profound where the greatest activity of growth is taking place. For that reason, radiographs of the knees, wrists, and ankles of affected persons usually show widening and irregular mineralization of the metaphyses, which have a frayed appearance. There is usually decreased bone density accompanied by bone softening, which results in *bowing* deformity often accompanied by greenstick fractures (Fig. 6–20).

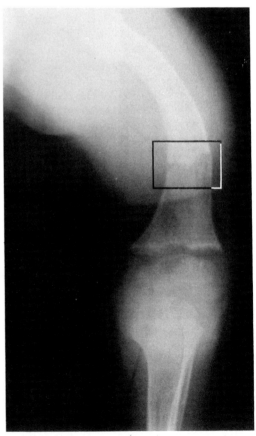

Figure 6–20. Pathological or trophic fracture of the distal one-third of the left femur of a 2½-year-old boy, with considerable bowing of the proximal and middle one-third, which is compatible with rickets.

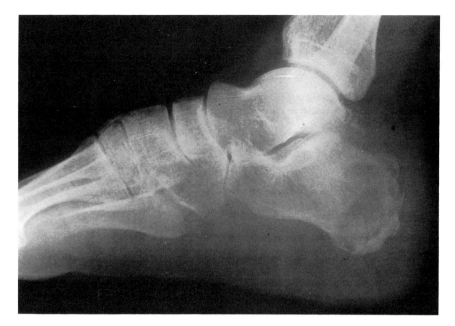

Figure 6–21. A periosteal reactive formation and loss of cortical margins about the calcaneus. This is consistent with osteomyelitis.

Treatment. The treatment of vitamin D deficiency disorders primarily involves the administration of massive doses of vitamin D or cod-liver oil. Patients are encouraged to eat foods that are high in vitamin D.

Inflammatory Disorders

Osteomyelitis

General Information. Osteomyelitis is a bone infection that may be acute or chronic. It most commonly results from *hematogenous* spread of bacteria from a distant location. It may arise as an invasion of bone from adjacent septic arthritis, as the result of penetrating trauma, as a complication of fractures, as a postoperative complication, or as a usual result of certain diseases, such as sickle cell anemia and the late stage of diabetes. Drug addicts are also susceptible.

Osteomyelitis is usually a localized infection, but it can spread through the bone from the periosteum, cortex, and marrow. This can result in bone destruction and joint stiffening, and the limbs may be shortened if the growth center is destroyed.

Three types of osteomyelitis are identified. (1) Pyogenic osteomyelitis typically affects children and adolescents, especially boys, and usually involves the femur, tibia, humerus, and radius. Although the causative organism is not always apparent, it is usually presumed to be *Staphylococcus aureus*. (2) Chronic osteomyelitis is the continuation of the acute condition that has not been properly treated. Recurrences are common at intervals of months or years. (3) Tuberculous osteomyelitis is a hematogenous form affecting both children and adults. The initial site of this form is usually not apparent. However, involvement of the vertebral column is usually apparent, with destruction and collapse of the vertebral bodies. Other joints such as the hips, knees, ankles, and hands may be affected.

Diagnosis. In the acute stage, the patient may complain of localized pain in the affected extremity. A portion of the bone may feel warm to the touch and appear red. An increase in the body temperature may be apparent. The onset may be sudden, with the patient complaining of chills, fever, and acute pain.

The initial radiographic sign of osteomyelitis is soft tissue swelling with loss of the fat planes. In about 10 days, there is a visual loss of the cortical margins, and a *periosteal reaction* may be observed (Fig. 6–21). This reaction is rapidly followed by patchy destruction of cancellous bone and formation of a new wall or periosteum to offset the reactive process. The visible reactive process involves an abscess containing a pool of pus, which consists of dead cells, bacteria, and intracellular fluid and is referred to as *sequestrum*, which is a Latin term that means "to seclude." Once the infection becomes chronic and walled off, two areas become clinically significant. When an abscess is found in the distal ends of long bones, especially the tibia, the lesion is known as *Brodie's abscess.* Typically, Brodie's abscess presents a lucent appearance with clear-cut margins in the metaphysis adjacent to the epiphyseal plate or with a small tail

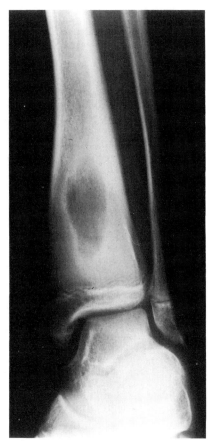

Figure 6–22. A Brodie's abscess on the distal tibia of a 16-year-old.

running down to the plate itself (Fig. 6–22). In addition to radiography, bone scanning is most useful because technetium polyphosphonate can reveal the infection within 48 hours of the onset. A gallium scan is useful in distinguishing between cellulitis and osteomyelitis (Fig. 6–23).

When considering the patient's age and history, the radiographer should pay particular attention to the complaint of pain in the absence of trauma or previous history of trauma. In the absence of trauma, diseases of bone are common among all age-groups. The radiographer should also consider adjusting the exposure factors to maximize the visualization of soft tissue as well as bone. A 15% reduction in mAs enhances the visualization of soft tissue and adjacent structures. A specimen is removed from the abscess via needle aspiration. The specimen is then cultured in the bacteriological section of the clinical laboratory. The culture can usually identify the bacterial organism and determine the proper course of treatment.

Treatment. The treatment of osteomyelitis involves the administration of antibiotics and surgical debridement. After the organism is identified, futher cultures indicate both sensitivity and resistance of

the organism to several different antibiotics. Without identification of the organism, the administration of antibiotics at best is arbitrary. The wound is debrided, and new bone cells may be implanted. The iliac crest is often a source of red bone marrow for bone implant.

Acute Arthritis

General Information. Acute arthritis is a suppurative and septic form of arthritis. The offending organisms may be staphylococci, streptococci, or gonococci. This condition is characterized by a sudden onset of pain when the organism invades a joint space, resulting in loss of joint motion and accompanied by joint stiffness, tenderness, and increased temperature of the affected area. Of the offending organisms, staphylococci are the most common and are usually spread through the bloodstream. This infection usually spreads from a primary site to a joint and is consistent with a concurrent bacterial infection.

Primary infections of the upper respiratory and genitourinary tracts often precipitate acute arthritis.

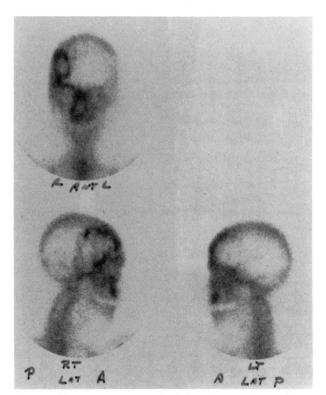

Figure 6–23. A postoperative infection study of a 35-year-old man. The gallium scan was negative for osteomyelitis. Increased uptake is seen to have the configuration of a craniotomy site, with the normal uptake in the margins of the craniotomy site, where reactive bone change would normally produce increased uptake of the radioisotope.

This secondary infection is also caused by other long-term illnesses, such as malignancy, renal failure, diabetes, cirrhosis, alcoholism, drug addiction, tuberculosis, fungal diseases, and syphilis. Infection can also result from nonsterile technique in joint injections. A similar condition may be caused by a virus as part of an autoimmune reaction. When a virus is present, this condition is referred to as Reiter's syndrome.

Diagnosis. Diagnosis is made through needle aspiration and culture of the debris. Radiographs taken 1 to 2 weeks after the onset usually reveal distension of the affected joint capsules and narrowing of the joint space (Fig. 6–24).

Treatment. Treatment involves the administration of large doses of antibiotics.

Rheumatoid Arthritis

General Information. Rheumatoid arthritis is referred to as an immunopathological joint disease and is a chronic, systemic, inflammatory collagen disease. It attacks the peripheral joints and surrounding muscles, tendons, ligaments, and blood vessels. It usually requires lifelong treatment and results in total disability in 10% of affected individuals. Most of the time the course of the disease is intermittent, and normal activities are permitted.

Rheumatoid arthritis affects females three times more often than males. It may affect any age-group. The juvenile form is most severe and is referred to as *Still's disease.* Women between the ages of 20 and 60 have the highest incidence, with the peak onset period being between the ages of 35 and 45 years.

At any one time, approximately 6.5 million Americans are affected with rheumatoid arthritis. Although the exact cause is unknown, it is thought to be the result of genetic defects that impair the autoimmune system.

Some of the frequent causes include stress, trauma, menopause, childbirth, surgery, endocrine imbalance, nutritional and metabolic factors, occupation, and psychosocial factors.

Rheumatoid arthritis usually develops in four stages: (1) synovitis, involving inflammation of the synovial membrane; (2) pannus, the formation of thickened layers of granulation tissue, which involves cartilage and eventually destroys the joint capsule and bone; (3) fibrous ankylosis, in which scar formation occludes the joint space and at which stage the bone atrophies and the joint becomes misaligned and deformed; and (4) ankylosis, a final stage involving calcification and a bent, deformed, and fused joint.

Diagnosis. The joints primarily affected are the proximal interphalangeal and metacarpophalangeal joints. The effect may be unilateral or bilateral. Stiffness and pain are apparent after periods of inac-

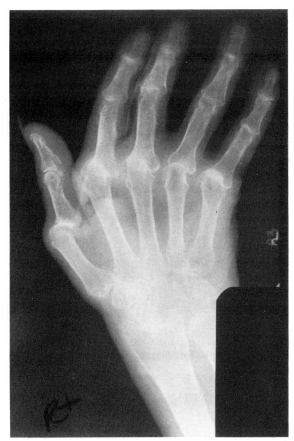

Figure 6–24. Extensive severe changes of rheumatoid arthritis involving all the joints of the right hand and wrist, including volar subluxations at the metacarpophalangeal joints and volar subluxation of the carpus with respect to the radius. The patient is a 64-year-old woman.

tivity or on rising in the morning. In the later stages of the disease, pain and stiffness may be noted in the wrists, knees, elbows, and ankles. Pain is usually experienced even when at rest. Joint function is usually diminished. Later, the interphalangeal and metacarpophalangeal joints swell dorsally. There is volar (palmar) subluxation and stretching of tendons, which may pull fingers to the ulnar side. There is a gradual apearance of rheumatoid nodules on the elbows. In the advanced stages of rheumatoid arthritis, severe changes involving the affected bones and joints are in evidence, especially in the hands. Loss of cartilage and joint spaces is most common, as is periarticular bone erosion and joint subluxation. Swelling is usually evident around the affected interphalangeal joints (Fig. 6–24).

A blood test referred to as the rheumatoid antibody (RA) latex fixation test demonstrates the level of antibodies in the serum. This is known as the rheumatoid (R) factor. The R factor is an immunoglobulin antibody directed against one's own immune system

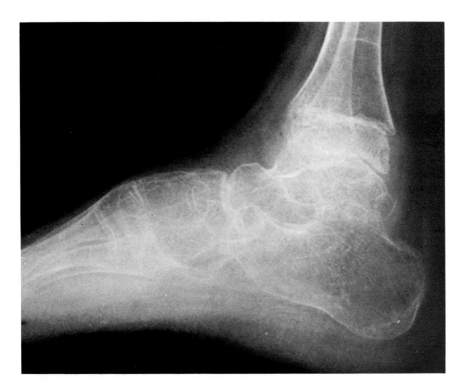

Figure 6–25. Juvenile arthritis of the foot and ankle in a 10-year-old girl.

and is usually elevated in persons with collagen diseases. Of all patients with symptoms of rheumatoid arthritis, 75 to 80% have elevated levels of the R factor.

The sedimentation rate indicates the rate at which erythrocytes settle out of unclotted blood in an hour's time. This test is based on the principle that an inflammatory process causes an alteration in blood proteins, resulting in aggregation or clumping of red blood cells, making them heavier and more likely to fall rapidly when placed in a special vertical test tube. In persons with rheumatoid arthritis, the sedimentation rate is increased, indicating the presence of an inflammatory process.

Treatment. The treatment of rheumatoid arthritis depends on the severity of the condition. Ordinarily, analgesics are taken for pain. Steroids are administered to decrease inflammation. Patients are encouraged to use the affected areas as much as possible.

Juvenile Rheumatoid Arthritis

General Information. Juvenile rheumatoid arthritis is also called *Still's disease* or acute febrile arthritis. It affects mostly girls under the age of 16 and is marked by remissions, exacerbations or increases in severity, and chronic synovitis. It can occur as early as the sixth week of infancy, but rarely before the sixth month. The peak period of onset is between the ages of 1 and 3 and 8 and 12 years.

Juvenile arthritis is considered to be the major rheumatic disease. The word *rheumatic* describes a variety of disorders characterized by inflammation, degeneration, or metabolic derangement of connective tissue structures, especially bones and joints. As many as 250,000 persons (mostly females) in the United States are affected at one time.

Diagnosis. Juvenile rheumatoid arthritis is characterized by lymph node enlargement, splenomegaly, swelling, edematous and painful joints, limited movement, anemia, leukocytosis, and a spiking fever. The systemic effects are often worse than the joint symptoms. In diagnosis, two forms of this disease must be distinguished: polyarticular and pauciarticular juvenile arthritis. The *polyarticular* form exclusively affects females and presents two subtypes according to serotype. Serotype refers to the type of microorganism determined by its constituent antigens. The seronegative type is the most common and least severe form of juvenile arthritis. Ninety percent of reported cases usually are seronegative. This form affects four or more joints, including the hands, wrists, knees, ankles, elbows, and feet. Involvement of the hands occurs first and most frequently. The other area affected is the axial skeleton, most commonly the cervical spine, hips, and shoulders. Patients have a low-grade fever, noticeable developmental retardation, and subcutaneous nodules on the elbows and heels. The seropositive type occurs in 10% of affected individuals and is the most severe form of the two subtypes. It becomes apparent in late childhood and is a destructive form of juvenile arthritis that mimics the adult form. It has an extremely poor prognosis (Fig. 6–25).

The *pauciarticular* form of juvenile rheumatoid arthritis affects both male and female children and adolescents. When it affects females, only a few of the larger proximal joints are involved, mostly the knees. It usually affects no more than four joints. In children between the ages of 4 and six, the elbows and ankles are usually affected. When it occurs in males, the condition is usually more severe, and the hips and knees are among the most affected joints. Early in the course of illness, an afflicted boy will suffer from Achilles tendinitis, and much later he will develop ankylosing spondylitis and sacroiliitis. In general, not all forms of juvenile rheumatoid arthritis are demonstrable radiographically in the early stages of the disease. Later, erosion of cartilage and bone is evident.

A similar form of Still's disease referred to as *Felty's syndrome* is found in adults. This presents all the same signs and symptoms as juvenile rheumatoid arthritis.

Treatment. Although there is no known cure, steroid and analgesic therapy is usually indicated.

Ankylosing Spondylitis

General Information. Ankylosing spondylitis is an unusual form of rheumatoid arthritis that affects males in the third decade of life. It is commonly referred to as *Marie-Strümpell* disease or *bamboo spine.* Ankylosing spondylitis primarily affects the vertebrae and sacroiliac joints. It may also affect the intervertebral and costovertebral ligaments. It presents cardiovascular complications such as aortic valve insufficiency. A unique finding is inflammation of the sites of insertion of ligaments and tendons into bone. The course of this disorder is slow and insidious. Pain originates in the lower lumbar spine. It is not uncommon for the patient to complain of low back pain and stiffness on rising in the morning. This discomfort usually abates with exercise.

Diagnosis. Ankylosis of the spine is considered to be a separate entity from rheumatoid arthritis, since rheumatoid arthritis occurs mostly in females. This form may not involve the peripheral extremities. It is also unique because of the later cardiovascular changes. Ankylosis first takes place in the lumbar spine. It then migrates to the thoracic spine and finally the cervical spine. Radiographs reveal *sacroiliitis* with ossification and eventually complete sacroiliac obliteration. Osteoporosis of the vertebral bodies occurs, with obliteration of the anterior concavity so that the vertebral bodies appear *square* rather than cylindrical. Calcification of the anulus fibrosus gives the spine its *bamboo* appearance (Figs. 6–26 and 6–27).

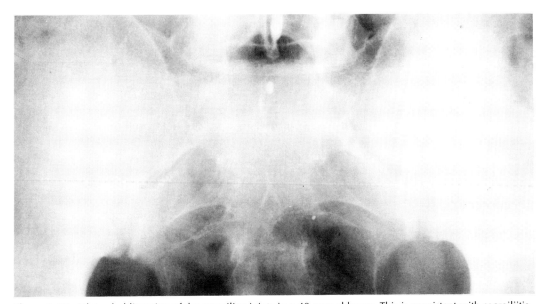

Figure 6–26. Bilateral obliteration of the sacroiliac joints in a 40-year-old man. This is consistent with sacroiliitis secondary to ankylosing spondylitis.

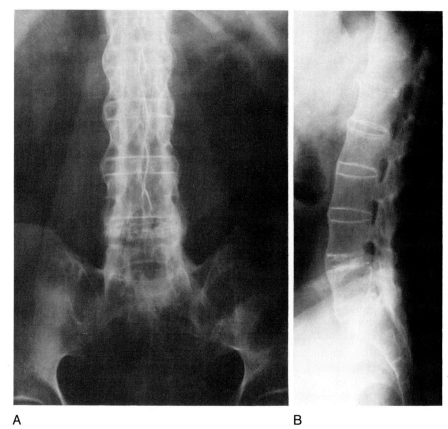

A   B

Figure 6–27. *(A)* Anteroposterior and *(B)* lateral views of the lumbar spine revealing ankylosing spondylitis. There is fusion of the total spine in this 48-year-old man.

In addition to the cardiovascular defects, complications involving the ocular, respiratory, and gastrointestinal systems are evident.

Treatment. The primary treatment consists of analgesics and steroids. There is a significant mortality due to the complications previously described. In the most severe cases and in the later stage of the disease, suicide is not uncommon.

Bursitis

General Information. Bursitis is an inflammatory condition involving one or more of the bursae. The bursae are lubricated with small amounts of synovial fluid, which facilitates the motion of muscles and tendons over a bony prominence. Inflammation most often occurs in the subdeltoid region of the shoulder, but can be found in the olecranon, trochanteric, calcaneal, or prepatellar bursae.

Bursitis occurs in middle age and results from recurring trauma that stresses or puts pressure on a joint. An inflammatory joint disease associated with rheumatoid arthritis or gout is another cause. This condition is highly related to an individual's particular

activities. For example, a baseball pitcher may injure the shoulder, a football player may injure the knee, and a tennis player may injure the elbow. Injuries are also frequent in individuals who intermittently participate in these sports and who overextend themselves without warming up properly or overexert themselves and become fatigued. Often the joint was used beyond its normal limits, or perhaps the person was not adequately trained for that type of activity. A person who jogs for 2 miles without first training or gradually building up the distance can suffer severe muscle cramps or may even strain a muscle. The shoulder joint can suffer similar trauma. In baseball, a pitcher frequently tries to make the ball move erratically, such as to rise, sink, curve, and so on. This type of action results in forced rotation of the rotator cuff and can cause soreness or, even worse, a torn rotator cuff. Baseball injuries involving the shoulder and elbow are most common for this reason. In some cases, calcium deposits develop in the bursae, further worsening the condition.

Diagnosis. This condition may be diagnosed on the basis of the presenting signs and symptoms, which involve the collection of fluid in the bursa causing irritation, inflammation, and sudden or gradual pain

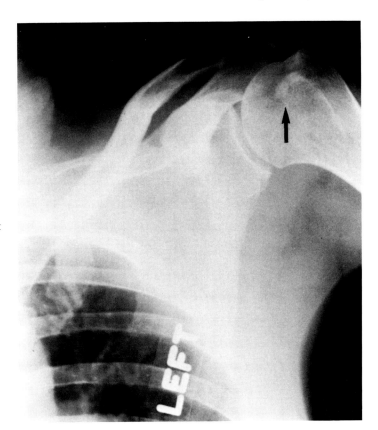

Figure 6–28. A soft tissue calcification over the head of the humerus, consistent with calcific bursitis, in a 34-year-old man.

with limited movement. Involvement of the subdeltoid region impairs the most simple shoulder movements. Housemaid's knee is a form of bursitis resulting from the activities of climbing stairs and washing floors. When there is inflammation of the hips, it is virtually impossible to cross the legs over each other. Usually there is localized pain and inflammation, with a history of unusual strain or injury occurring 2 to 3 days prior to the onset of pain. The patient may often first recognize this condition on waking or by about the fourth day after the injury. The patient usually attributes the pain to sleeping on the arm, but after consideration will usually remember some incident or activity that could explain the cause. Bursitis is radiographically significant only when deposits of *calcium* are present in the subdeltoid region of the shoulder (Fig. 6–28).

Treatment. The treatment for bursitis is initially conservative. Immobilizing or resting the joint is the first approach. The application of a sling forces the individual not to use the arm. Mild analgesics such as aspirin or acetaminophen are used to combat pain. If pain persists, a local injection into the joint is made with a combination of lidocaine and a steroid such as prednisone. Orally administered steroids can damage the stomach lining, so patients are encouraged to take them with milk rather than water. Warm moist heat is often used for temporary relief.

Tendinitis

General Information. Tendinitis is a painful inflammation of the tendons and their muscle attachments to bone. The shoulder and elbow tendons are commonly damaged in the same way as in bursitis. The achilles tendon and hamstring muscle are very common sites of tendinitis. Trauma and athletic activities are two of the most common causes. The patient usually complains of restricted shoulder movement (especially abduction) and local pain, which is most severe at night and often interferes with sleep. With shoulder involvement, pain extends from the acromion to the deltoid muscle insertion. Fluid accumulates and causes swelling.

Diagnosis. Calcific tendinitis involves calcium deposits in the tendon, causing proximal weakness. Calcium may erode into adjacent bursae, creating calcific bursitis. Radiographs reveal bony *fragments,* osteophyte sclerosis, or calcium deposits. Arthrograms usually fail to show cartilaginous disruption

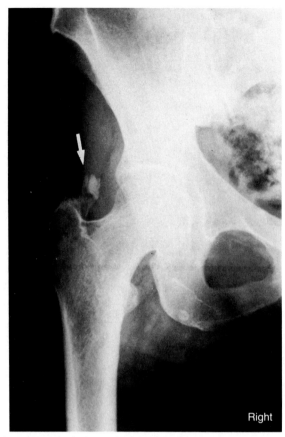

Right

Figure 6–29. Calcific tendinitis of the right hip just above the greater trochanter in a 55-year-old woman.

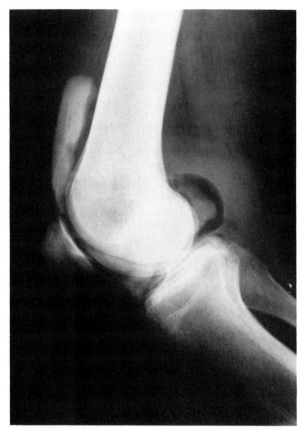

Figure 6–30. Double-contrast arthrogram and lateral view of the knee of a 28-year-old man. The examination results were negative.

(Figs. 6–29, 6–30, and 6–31). Diagnosis of tendinitis must rule out other causes of shoulder pain, such as myocardial infarct, cervical spondylosis, and tendon rupture.

Treatment. Unlike bursitis, tendinitis is aggravated by heat. Cold packs are usually more comfortable and bring relief. All other bone and joint conditions except tendinitis usually respond to heat application. Analgesics and steroids are administered orally. This condition usually abates with rest and immobilization.

Degenerative Disorders

Gout

General Information. The name *gout* is derived from the latin word *gutta*, meaning drop. At one time, a poison was thought to drop into weakened joints. Gout is a metabolic disease marked by the presence of urate deposits (salt of uric acid) in the blood serum. It causes painfully arthritic joints. The feet, especially the metatarsophalangeal joint of the great toe, are primarily afflicted.

There are two types of gout, primary and secondary. The most common form is primary gout, which affects men over 30 years of age and postmenopausal women. Scondary gout occurs mainly in the elderly and is often associated with other diseases such as polycythemia, leukemia, and multiple myeloma. Gout may also result from drug therapy, especially diuretics, which interfere with the excretion of uric acid. Gouty arthritis often follows an intermittent course and frequently leaves patients totally free of symptoms for years between attacks. It can lead to chronic disability or incapacitation, but the prognosis is good with early treatment. The exact cause of this condition is unknown. It is thought to be linked to a genetic defect in purine (amino acid metabolism) in the DNA, causing overproduction of uric acid (hyperuricemia), retention of uric acid, or both. The increased concentration of uric acid leads to urate deposits called tophi in synovial joints or tissues, causing local necrosis or fibrosis.

Gout develops in four stages: (1) In the asymptomatic stage, the serum urate levels are elevated but produce no symptoms. (2) In the acute state there may be hypertension or nephrolithiasis, with severe back pain. The first acute attack strikes suddenly and

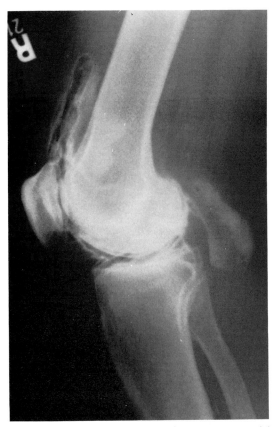

Figure 6–31. Baker's cyst in the popliteal space posterior of the knee, as seen on double-contrast arthrogram. This man had sustained a previous knee injury.

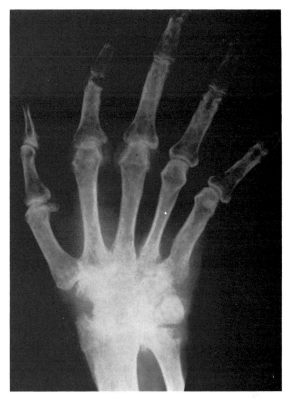

Figure 6–32. Urate deposits in the metacarpal and distal interphalangeal joints, with an outward displacement of the overhanging bone margins, in a 74-year-old man. These findings are consistent with gout.

peaks quickly. It affects only a few joints but is extremely painful. The affected joints appear hot, tender, inflamed, dusky red, or cyanotic. Initially, there is inflammation of the first metatarsophalangeal joint (podagra), progressing to the instep, ankle, heel, knee, or wrist joint. The symptoms may include low-grade fever, followed by mild acute attacks that subside quickly but tend to recur at regular intervals. The attacks may persist for days or weeks. (3) There is a symptom-free interval between gout attacks. The second attack begins within 6 months to 2 years of the initial attack and in some cases may be delayed for several years. The delayed attacks are more common in those who have gone untreated. (4) Polyarticular gout develops in the final unremitting stage. This stage is characterized by the formation of tophi in cartilaginous and synovial membranes, tendons, and soft tissues. Pain is persistent.

Diagnosis. In the chronic stage, tophi form in the helix of the ear above the lobe. This is the classic sign of the fourth stage of gout. Urate deposits form in the fingers, hands, knees, ulnar sides of the forearms, and achilles tendons. The skin over the tophus may ulcerate and emit a chalky white exudate or pus. The fourth stage then progresses to a point

where the joint degenerates and eventually becomes permanently deformed and the patient is disabled. The kidneys may also become involved during the fourth stage, leading to tubular damage and renal dysfunction. Radiographically, bone changes are most visible during the chronic stage. Clearly defined punched-out areas of bone *lysis* (decomposition or destruction) are visible. The erosion in the late stage is similar to that in other types of arthritis, but only gout manifests outward displacement of the overhanging margins from the bone contour (Fig. 6–32). RA latex fixation blood tests will distinguish gout from rheumatoid arthritis, as results are negative in gout.

Treatment. The treatment for gout involves reducing uric acid levels; bed rest; analgesics; heat or cold applications; administration of colchicine (an alkaloid), which prevents acute attacks and may be injected intravenously or intramuscularly or directly into a joint; and aspiration of the joint. Reducing levels of uric acid is most important. This may be accomplished by the administration of allopurinol, which inhibits uric acid production. This drug is to be used cautiously when associated renal problems are present. Uricosuric agents are used to promote

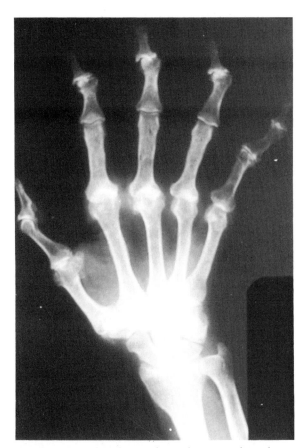

Figure 6–33. A marked degree of joint disease involving the distal interphalangeal joints and metacarpophalangeal joints of several fingers can be seen in this 77-year-old woman. There is a joint space calcification at the third metacarpophalangeal joint of the right hand. There is subluxation of several metacarpophalangeal joints. These findings are consistent with degenerative joint disease or senile osteoarthritis.

uric acid excretion. Patients with gout must avoid purine-rich foods, especially meat, fowl, and fish such as sardines and anchovies. They must avoid alcohol, especially beer and wine, which raise urate levels. Daily intake of at least 2 liters of fluid helps prevent the formation of stones. Weight reduction is suggested for obese patients.

Osteoarthritis

General Information. Osteoarthritis is also referred to as senile arthritis, arthritis deformans, and hypertrophic arthritis. It is the most common form of arthritis, usually affecting persons older than 40. About 50% of cases occur after the age of 50. Osteoarthritis occurs equally often in both sexes.

Rather than a primary inflammation, osteoarthritis is essentially a degenerative condition of the articular (hyaline) cartilage, with reactive and hypertrophic changes in underlying bone (formation of new bone at the joint margins), referred to as *lipping.* This

results from a breakdown of chondrocytes, most often in the hips and knees. The course of the disease worsens with advancing age. There are two types of osteoarthritis: (1) Primary osteoarthritis is an age-related process due to genetic predisposition. (2) Secondary osteoarthritis is usually due to other primary sources such as trauma, infection, stress, and disorders of metabolism. In addition, important environmental factors are related to types of activities, employment, and personal habits. Football and basketball players, workers who operate pneumatic drills, and parachutists are at increased risk. Osteoarthritis may develop as a postoperative complication and is found more frequently in grossly obese individuals.

Diagnosis. The symptoms of osteoarthritis include joint pain, which is the foremost symptom, especially following exercise or long periods of weight bearing, and is relieved by rest. Joint stiffness is at its greatest on rising in the morning. The joint aches respond to changes in the weather, especially humidity and barometric pressure. There is a characteristic grating of the joint during motion (crepitus) and a limited range of motion of the joint itself. Often there is associated fluid in the joint space. The severity of all effects vary with the patients' age and overall condition. Other considerations such as poor posture, obesity, and occupational stress play an important role in the progression of this condition. There are also changes in the bones themselves. The distal interphalangeal joints form small pea-shaped nodules called ***Heberden's nodes.*** The proximal interphalangeal joints form small pea-shaped nodules referrred to as ***Bouchard's nodes.*** When the interphalangeal joints are affected, there is accompanying joint narrowing and derangement. Osteoarthritis of the interphalangeal joints is considered irreversible. The distal

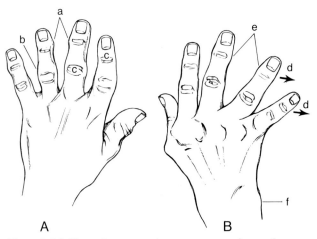

Figure 6–34. Illustration comparing two common forms of arthritis. *A,* Osteoarthritis reveals the following: a = Heberden's nodes; b = Bouchard's nodes; c = joint narrowing and derangement. *B,* Rheumatoid arthritis demonstrates the following: d = volar subluxation; e = swelling at the interphalangeal joints; f = swelling of the wrist.

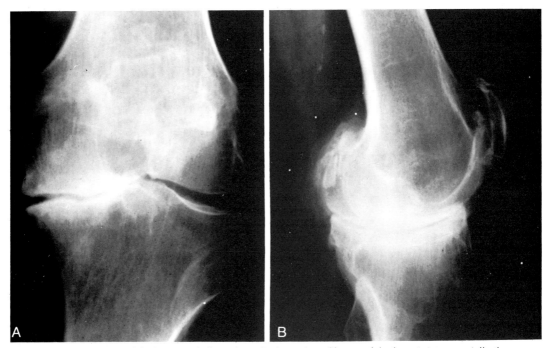

Figure 6–35. Narrowing of the knee medially with marked spurring of bones of the knee joint, especially the anterior and posterior lower femur and superior aspect of the patella, on standing anteroposterior *(A)* and lateral *(B)* knee study. The patient is an 85-year-old man.

joints are affected first, followed by the proximal joints. Both Heberden's and Bouchard's nodes become red, swollen, and tender, with numbness and loss of manual dexterity (Figs. 6–33 and 6–34).

Radiographs usually reveal narrowing of the joint space or margins, cyst-like bony deposits in joints and margins, joint deformity, and bone growths on weight-bearing joints such as the hips, knees, and vertebrae (Fig. 6–35). These periosteal growths form on the joint margins and are specifically evident in the vertebrae. This is called lipping or spondylitis deformans (Fig. 6–36). This condition may lead to

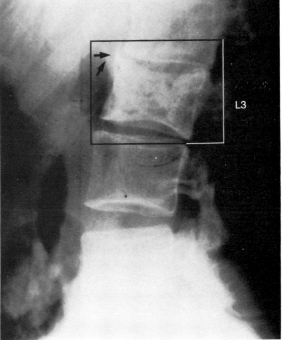

Figure 6–36. Osteoporotic demineralization and wedging of the body of L3, with anterior osteoarthritic lipping, in a 63-year-old woman.

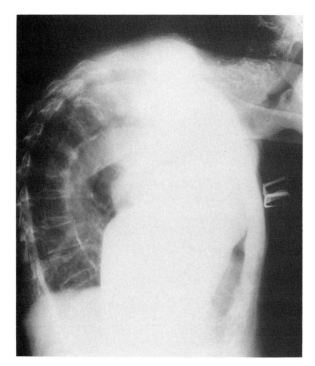

Figure 6–37. Extreme dorsal kyphosis, often referred to as humpback deformity, in a 77-year-old woman.

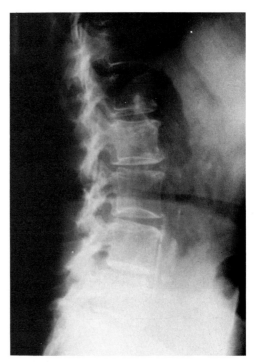

Figure 6–38. Hypertrophic spondylosis of T-12 and all five lumbar vertebrae in a 65-year-old woman. There is abdominal atherosclerotic disease with calcification of the aorta.

kyphosis, extreme rigidity (poker back), and osteophytic outgrowths on nerve roots (Fig. 6–37). There may be associated breaking down of the vertebra (*spondylosis*), along with degenerative changes. In the spine, the apophyseal joints are most affected (Fig. 6–38).

Treatment. The treatment of osteoarthritis is mainly palliative. Analgesics are administered for pain, and steroids are given to reduce inflammation. In more severe cases, this medication is given parenterally (by injection) rather than by mouth. Steroids can delay nodular development. A reduction in stress can be achieved by frequent periods of rest between weight-bearing exercise or by the use of a cane or walker. Moist heat and a paraffin dip for the hands will temporarily relieve the pain and lessen joint stiffness. In the more serious cases and when the patient's condition permits, surgery may be in-

dicated. Operative procedures include the following: (1) Arthroplasty is a partial to total joint replacement with a prosthesis. This operation is commonly used on the hips and knees. (2) An arthrodesis is a surgical fusion, as with a laminectomy. (3) An osteoplasty is used to scrape deteriorated bone away from the joint space. (4) An osteotomy is performed to change bony alignment to relieve stress. This is accomplished by excising or cutting out a wedge of bone.

Idiopathic Disorders

Paget's Disease

General Information. Paget's disease, or *osteitis deformans* as it is also known, is a common bone disorder that affects 3 to 4% of the population over

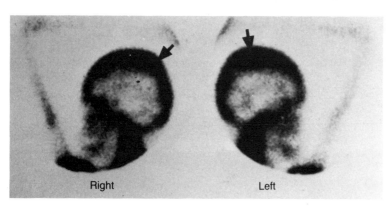

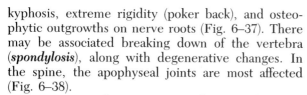

Figure 6–39. Gallium scan revealing an increased uptake of isotope throughout the skull, secondary to Paget's disease, in a 73-year-old woman.

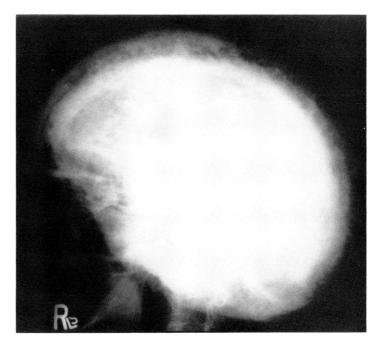

Figure 6–40. Lateral view of the skull revealing increased thickening of the calvarium and presenting a cotton-wool appearance, which is typical of Paget's disease, in a 75-year-old woman.

40 years of age, or approximately 2.5 million people. This disease is characterized by bone deformity, especially of the long bones of the lower limbs, the pelvis, the lumbar vertebrae, and the skull. Paget's disease usually follows a two-stage process: (1) The bone is first hyperemic and soft, and bowing occurs. (2) In the secondary phase, the bone becomes increasingly hard and brittle. As a result of the brittleness, fractures may occur. The fractures are often of the stress type and are undisplaced. Paget's disease is also associated with malignant neoplasm such as osteogenic sarcoma.

Diagnosis. Radiographs usually reveal increased bone expansion and density. Because radionuclide bone scans are more sensitive than x-rays, Paget's lesions are identified by increased radioisotope concentrations in the areas of active disease (Figs. 6–39, 6–40, and 6–41).

Treatment. Primary treatment includes drug therapy, which decreases the resorption of bone.

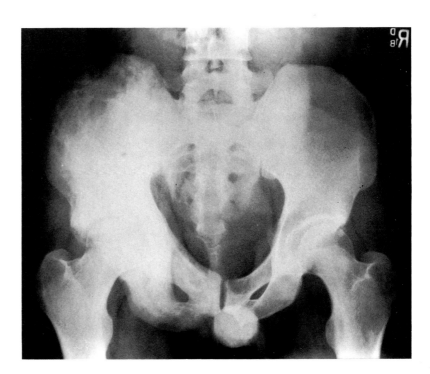

Figure 6–41. Extensive Paget's disease involving the pelvis, hip joints, and proximal femurs in a 46-year-old woman.

Aseptic/Avascular Necrosis

General Information. Aseptic/avascular necrosis is necrosis without the presence of infection or inflammation. There are two types: (1) The first type is the result of an interruption of the circulation, such as occurs at the site of a fracture. (2) The second type, idiopathic aseptic necrosis, occurs for no apparent reason in the epiphyses of growing children. Idiopathic aseptic necrosis may be due in part to heredity and is usually found to be bilateral. Several forms of idiopathic necrosis are known. These include Legg-Calvé-Perthes disease, involving the hip joint; Osgood-Schlatter disease, of the tibial tubercule; Köhler's disease, of the tarsal scaphoid; and Kienböck's disease, of the carpal lunate.

Legg-Calvé-Perthes Disease

General Information. Legg-Calvé-Perthes disease is also called coxa plana and *osteochondritis deformans.* It is ischemic necrosis leading to the flattening of the head of the femur caused by vascular interruption, resulting in osteochondritis of its epiphysis. The disease tends to occur in families and is usually unilateral, but it can be found in both femoral heads. This condition largely affects boys between the ages of 4 and 10. Typically, this condition is unilateral in males and bilateral in females. Legg-Calvé-Perthes disease usually runs its course in 3 to 4 years. It may lead to joint problems later in life. This disease occurs in four stages: (1) In the initial 1 to 3 weeks, there is a spontaneous vascular interruption causing ischemic necrosis of the femoral head. (2) In the second stage, a new blood supply causes bone resorption and deposition of new osteoblasts. A deformity may appear as a result of pressure on the weakened area. This stage occurs between 6 months and 1 year from the onset of the disease. (3) About 2 to 3 years after the initial onset of disease, new bone replaces necrotic bone. (4) Finally, healing is completed, and the femoral head is restructured and just about equal to the unaffected side.

Diagnosis. Legg-Calvé-Perthes disease is usually first noticed when the patient exhibits a persistent limp when walking. The limp becomes more severe as the pain increases. Initially there is a mild hip and knee pain that is aggravated by activity and relieved by rest. This usually occurs during the second stage of the disease. As this condition progresses, there is muscle spasm, atrophy of the muscles in the upper thigh, slight shortening of the leg, and severely restricted abduction and rotation of the hip.

The diagnosis is made in combination with a physical examination and the patient's clinical history. Radiographs usually reveal **misalignment** of the acetabulum and a **flattened** femoral head. The radiographer should consider the possibility of aseptic necrosis when there is pain without a history of trauma and limping is observed. Before making the exposure, the radiographer should shield the patient's reproductive structures with lead and should take care to assure that the examination is completed with the minimum number of exposures. Radiographs of the hips are taken in abduction and adduction and are repeated every 3 to 4 months to record progress of the disease. Because acute arthritis may cause similar signs and symptoms at its onset, aspiration and culture of synovial fluid are performed. Bacteria are present in the fluid if the condition is acute arthritis (Fig. 6–42).

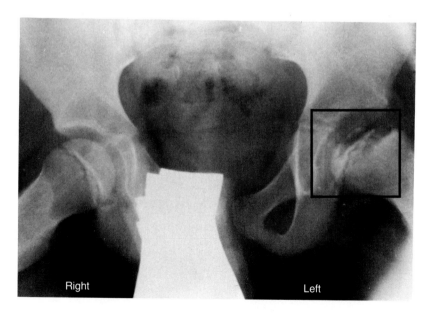

Figure 6–42. Evidence of fragmentation of the ossification center for the head of the left femur in an 8-year-old boy. This radiograph was taken about 1 year after the initial diagnosis of Legg-Calvé-Perthes disease.

Treatment. The treatment for Legg-Calvé-Perthes disease is quite conservative, since the healing in most cases will occur spontaneously as the disease runs its course. Protection for the femoral head is most important. The activities have to be monitored to assure minimizing stress to the femoral head. When muscle spasm is severe, bed rest is indicated and traction may be considered. In some cases, night braces are worn while sleeping. Plaster casts can be applied with the hip in abduction, and a weight-bearing brace can be worn, again with the hip in abduction when the patient ambulates.

Occasionally, the damage to the femoral head is severe in the early stages. In this event, surgical procedures are used to minimize permanent damage. Osteotomy and subtrochanteric derotation provide maximum confinement of the epiphysis within the acetabulum to allow return of the femoral head to its normal shape and full range of motion. Following this procedure, a *spica cast* is applied for about 2 months.

Osgood-Schlatter Disease

General Information. Like Legg-Calvé-Perthes disease, Osgood-Schlatter disease is one of several forms of *osteochondritis dissecans,* which means dissected or separated. This condition is characterized as a painful, incomplete separation, avulsion, or strain of the epiphysis of the tibial tubercle (tuberosity) from the proximal anterior tibial shaft. Osgood-Schlatter disease is more common in adolescent males between the ages of 10 and 15 years and is frequently bilateral. In severe cases, there may be permanent enlargement of the tubercle.

Although Osgood-Schlatter disease is often present without any traumatic history, it most frequently results from some form of trauma before the epiphysis

has completely fused to the tibia. The most common cause is repeated knee flexion against a tight quadriceps muscle, such as occurs when riding a bicycle. There is also a locally deficient blood supply. Genetic factors are thought to play a part, since parents who had this disease frequently have offspring who develop a similar condition. Usually, the first symptom is pain. Because of the age-group involved and the ongoing activities in which adolescents participate, the pain is often dismissed as an insignificant complaint. The parents assume that the patient simply received a minor injury that is typical of that age, and are not overly concerned. It is only after the patient continues to complain of the pain and insists that no injury took place that the parent takes the child to the family doctor. At this point, the pain is best described as an ache that does not abate with rest. The pain and tenderness below the patella worsen with any activity that causes forcible contraction of the patellar tendon. Localized swelling is present, with warmth of the part and tenderness to the touch.

Diagnosis. On examination, the physician forces the tibia into internal rotation while slowly extending the patient's knee from 90 degrees of flexion. About 30 degrees of flexion produces pain that subsides with external rotation of the tibia. Radiographs of the knee may show normal findings or epiphyseal *separation* and soft tissue swelling for up to 6 months following onset. The radiographs may eventually reveal *fragmentation* of the tibial tubercle. The radiographer reduces the overall film density about 15 to 20% in order to demonstrate the adjacent soft tissues as well as the presence of fragmentation of the nonossified tubercle (Fig. 6–43).

Treatment. After the initial diagnosis, the knee is immobilized for 6 to 8 weeks. This immobilization can be provided by reinforced elastic knee supports,

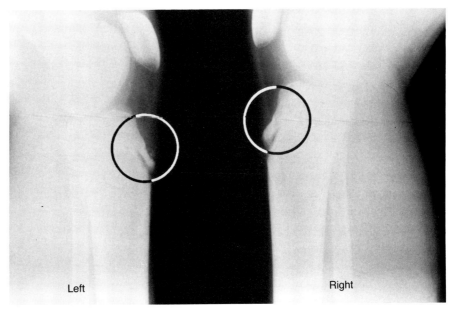

Figure 6–43. Evidence of fragmentation of the tibial tubercle epiphysis on the left knee, with soft tissue swelling over the area, in a 7-year-old girl. No changes of this type were noted on the right knee.

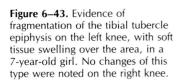

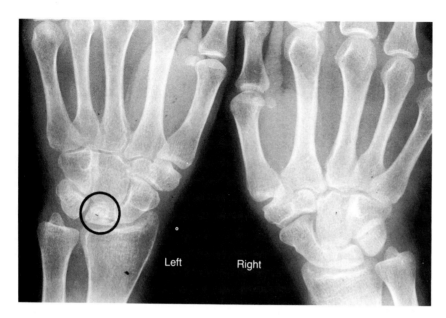

Figure 6–44. Evidence of fragmentation, with increased density of the left carpal lunate. This is compatible with Kienböck's disease or lunatomalacia. The diseased lunate was removed surgically. The right side appears normal in this 26-year-old man.

plaster cast application, or various types of splints. This immobilization allows for the revascularization and reossification of the tubercle and minimizes the stress or pulling of the quadriceps muscle. Bed rest, restricted activity, and cortisone injections all are methods of treatment. Although the treatment is conservative, it is usually successful. In severe cases, surgical removal or fixation of the tibial tubercle is necessary.

Köhler's Disease

General Information. Köhler's disease is best described as aseptic necrosis or osteochondritis of the **tarsal scaphoid.** It may also be referred to as tarsal scaphoiditis. This disease of unknown cause usually has a history of sudden onset at about the age of 5 years. Aching in the region of the instep and limping are the main features. There is some tenderness in the area of the scaphoid. Many patients with Köhler's disease present a history of trauma.

Diagnosis. Köhler's disease may be demonstrated on routine dorsoplantar and oblique radiographic positions of the foot. Radiographs of the foot reveal increased density and fragmentation. Its radiographic appearance is somewhat similar to Kienböck's disease of the lunate bone of the wrist.

Treatment. The primary treatment is quite conservative, and the emphasis is placed on resuming the blood supply to the affected area. A plaster cast is applied to immobilize the foot and restore the blood supply. The cast is left in place for usually 6 to 8 weeks. Complete spontaneous recovery may take place after this treatment. If the necrosis continues despite treatment, the tarsal scaphoid is surgically removed. The patella is another bone that may be affected by this disorder, but far less commonly.

Kienböck's Disease

General Information. Kienböck's disease is a form of osteochondritis affecting the carpal **lunate.** It is also referred to as **lunatomalacia** because of the generalized softening of the lunate bone of the wrist joint. It is primarily a disease of young men, who present with complaints of a stiff and aching wrist. This slowly progressive osteochondrosis is a result of aseptic necrosis. Like the other forms of aseptic necrosis, the cause is unknown, but it is often related to trauma such as a sprain of the wrist.

Diagnosis. Routine AP, oblique, and lateral views usually reveal a possibly **fragmented** lunate bone of increased density (Fig. 6–44).

Treatment. The treatment of Kienböck's disease involves immobilization of the wrist by a plaster cast for several months. If there is no significant improvement in healing, surgical removal of the lunate usually takes place.

Fibrous Dysplasia

General Information. Fibrous dysplasia is a condition that is neither a congenital disorder nor a neoplasm. It may affect one or more bones but typically involves a disturbance of **cancellous** bone. It is thought that the condition results from disorganization of the tissue differentiation and modeling of the diaphyses. The shafts are often thickened and painful.

Diagnosis. Radiographs usually reveal well-defined zones of **rarefaction** surrounded by narrow rims of sclerotic bone. Irregular ossification and cystic areas are characteristic. The severity of the bone deformity varies (Fig. 6–45).

Treatment. Although there is basically no treatment for fibrous dysplasia, the condition generally is not life threatening. The major complication is pathological fractures, which usually heal without incident. If the lesion is local, it can be treated by curettage or resection. If the condition involves several bones, treatment is discouraged because the lesion ceases growth after puberty.

Disorders of the Vertebral Column

Scheuermann's Disease

General Information. Scheuermann's disease was first cited in the early 1900s as the precipitating cause of an increase in the normal kyphosis of the thoracic spine. It is particularly a disease of adolescents and is sometimes referred to as adolescent kyphosis. Clinically, patients appear to have an increase in the kyphotic curve and usually stand with their shoulders dropping forward.

Diagnosis. Radiographically, the upper and lower ends of the vertebral bodies show some lack of

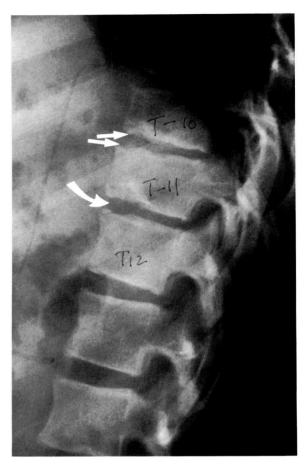

Figure 6–46. Scheuermann's disease of T10–12 and vertebral centra with end-plate irregularity in a 13-year-old girl.

organization and fragmentation of the epiphyseal areas of ossification (Fig. 6–46).

Treatment. Treatment usually consists mainly of exercises designed to strengthen the back and the use of a full-length back support or brace to be worn during daytime hours. The patient is to avoid movement in which vigorous spinal flexion is involved. This condition usually resolves when growth of the vertebral bodies is complete. If treatment is initiated early, the deformity can be limited.

Scoliosis

General Information. Scoliosis is typically thought of as a lateral curvature of the spine, but most scoliotic spines also usually present a rotary deformity, usually referred to as rotoscoliosis. In rotoscoliosis, the vertebral bodies are rotated toward the convex side of the curve and may produce a rib cage deformity. Scoliosis may be found in the thoracic, lumbar, or thoracolumbar regions of the spine. Dextroscoliosis is characterized by a curve with a convexity to the right and is usually a thoracic curvature. Levoscoliosis is a curvature with convexity to the left and is more

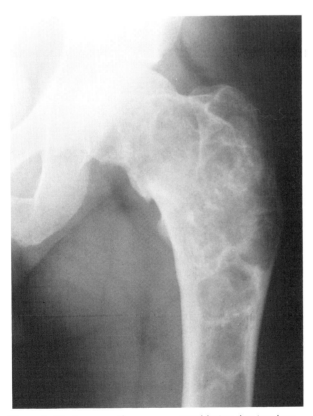

Figure 6–45. An expansile, many-septated lesion that involves the left femoral neck and proximal left femoral shaft in a 36-year-old man. There is a secondary valgus deformity in the proximal femur, and there are linear horizontal lucencies medially beneath the greater trochanter. These lucencies apparently represent stress fractures. All these findings are consistent with fibrous dysplasia.

common in the lumbar region. Thoracolumbar scoliosis usually consists of both dextro- and levoscoliosis. Scoliosis may be associated with kyphosis and lordosis.

Scoliosis is classed into two primary groups, functional and structural. Functional scoliosis is often the result of poor posture or discrepancies in leg length. Structural scoliosis may be further classified into four subcategories: (1) Osteopathic scoliosis is the form that includes congenital anomalies and deformities that are a result of trauma or disease. (2) Neuropathic scoliosis includes deformities that are the result of muscle imbalance caused by neurological lesions such as those in poliomyelitis and cerebral palsy. (3) Myopathic scoliosis consists of primary disorders of muscles. (4) Idiopathic scoliosis is the most common form of structural scoliosis. It is congenital but has no clear inheritance pattern. This form appears most commonly with a previously straight vertebral column and is most active during the growth years. The age of onset is most significant in idiopathic scoliosis. Infantile idiopathic scoliosis usually becomes evident within the first 3 years of life. Juvenile idiopathic scoliosis afflicts the age-group between 4 and 9 years. In adolescents, the curve appears after the age of 10 and before skeletal maturity is attained. The clinical assessment of adolescents with scoliosis is most difficult, and many patients suffer a rapidly worsening condition. This is especially true of females, who often have a severe convexity to the right.

Diagnosis. In most functional and structural forms of scoliosis, the curvature first develops in the thoracic spine, with convexity to the right. In addition, compensatory curves of the cervical and lumbar segments with convexity to the left are often present. As the spine becomes convex laterally, the compensatory or S curves develop to preserve body balance, and these mark the deformity. The symptoms of scoliosis are often not apparent until the deformity is well established. Thoracic curvatures are the most common form and usually result in distortion of the chest, with the ribs on the convex side appearing more prominent posteriorly. This deformity is most apparent when the patient bends forward. Thoracolumbar and lumbar curves often shift the upper body to one side relative to the pelvis when the curve is not associated with a compensatory curve in the thoracic region. This effect appears to make the iliac crest more prominent on one side.

Radiographically, there are two common methods of demonstrating and determining the degree of severity. Ferguson in 1939 reported a method of distinguishing a deforming curve from a compensatory curve. The patient is radiographed erect using 14 × 17-inch cassettes, either in the seated or standing AP or posteroanterior (PA) position. The midsagittal plane is centered, and the arms are down at the sides. The bottom of the cassette should include about 1 inch of the iliac crests. For the second radiograph, the side affected with the convexity is elevated at least 4 inches and is supported. The central ray is directed horizontally to the midpoint of the film. The second common method consists of four projections of the thoracolumbar spine. These posi-

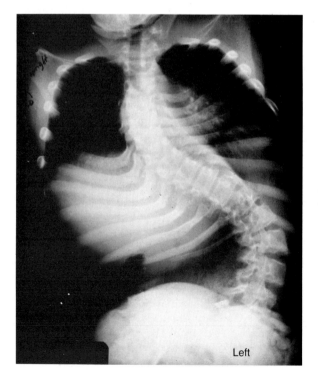

Figure 6–47. Congenital spina bifida with dextroscoliosis of 65 degrees extending from T-2 through T-9 and levoscoliosis of 125 degrees from T-10 to L-5 in a 12-year-old boy.

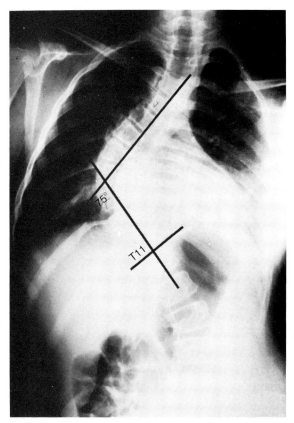

Figure 6–48. Marked scoliosis of the dorsal spine, with convexity to the right, in an 11-year-old girl. The center of the curve is at the level of T-8. The angle from the upper margin of T-4 to the lower margin of T-11 measures 75 degrees.

One such device, the Milwaukee brace, is a corset that is well supported by the pelvis and has a framework that extends upward to a head support. The chin rests on a padded support, which relieves the pressure of the head on the spine. The degree of curvature during the period of rapid growth may be minimized with this brace. A procedure referred to as *spinal fusion* is the typical procedure used with the most severe cases. In this procedure, the articular cartilage and underlying cortical bone are removed posteriorly and bone grafts are placed in these spaces. Postoperatively, the spine is held in the position of maximum correction by a plaster cast or internal fixation plates or rods. When deformities include protrusion of various bones such as the scapula, the protruding parts of these bones may be surgically removed for cosmetic purposes. In a recently developed technique, the ribs on the convex side of the curve are surgically fused or bound with tape. The results of this new treatment have proved favorable.

Kyphosis

General Information. Kyphosis is a continuation or exaggeration of the normal kyphotic curve resulting from increased anterior convexity of the thoracic

tions include standing erect AP, supine, and supine right and left bending or flexion. As before, 1 inch of the iliac crests is included and a central ray is directed to the film midpoint. On the AP radiographs, a line is drawn along the superior surface of the upper vertebra of the curve and a second line along the inferior border of the lower vertebra of the curve. Where the lines meet, the angle between them is measured. This procedure is described as the ***Lippman-Cobb*** method of measurement. The degree of curvature is then described. Methods of radiation protection other than shielding the thyroid gland and optimum collimation may compromise the examination (Figs. 6–47, 6–48, and 6–49).

Treatment. When the degree of curvature is severe, the patient's height is affected. Curves greater than 30 degrees may interfere with pulmonary efficiency. Gross curvatures may disrupt the spinal canal and lead to tension on the spinal cord, possibly resulting in paraparesis or paraplegia. Once detected, scoliosis must be periodically observed radiographically. Although the treatment is typically conservative, surgery is indicated in the more severe cases. The conservative treatment includes participating in exercises and wearing special braces and supports.

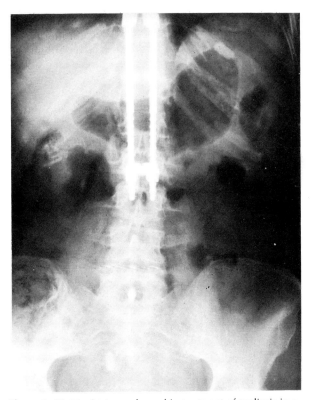

Figure 6–49. Harrington rods used in treatment of scoliosis in a woman. The rods are placed just above and below the site of surgery.

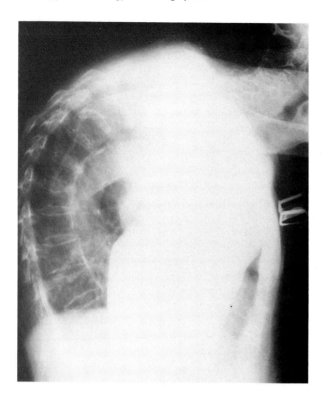

Figure 6–50. Extreme dorsal kyphosis in a 77-year-old man.

spine. This condition most frequently is referred to as the *hunchback* deformity and has also been called roundback and humpback. Kyphosis may be the result of an acquired disease (vertebral tuberculosis, spondylitis, poliomyelitis, Paget's disease), an injury, or a congenital disorder. This deformity can also result when trauma to the thoracic spine is not treated or is inadequately treated. Older adults who are affected may show associated age-related degenerative and inflammatory diseases. Back pain and an increased lack of mobility are associated with kyphosis.

Diagnosis. Physical examination provides a presumed diagnosis, which can be supported by x-rays. AP and lateral recumbent radiographs typically reveal vertebral wedging and Schmorl's nodes. Schmorl's nodes are bone defects in the upper or lower margin of the vertebral body into which the nucleus pulposus of the intervertebral disk herniates (Figs. 6–50 and 6–51).

Treatment. Typically, this condition is in the advanced stages when diagnosed. Treatment depends on the amount of pain and loss of mobility. Because this condition is mostly age related, the treatment is usually conservative. Corrective surgery includes posterior spinal fusion with insertion of Harrington rods, iliac bone grafting, and plaster immobilization. The surgical approach is considered as a treatment for adolescent kyphosis, referred to as *Scheuermann's disease,* which may result from growth retardation of a vascular disturbance affecting the vertebral epiphysis.

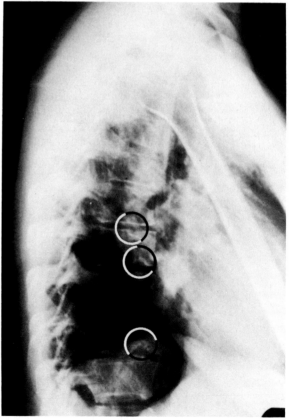

Figure 6–51. Multiple Schmorl's nodes in the dorsal spine of a 24-year-old woman.

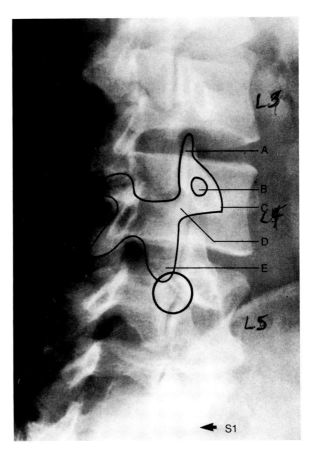

Figure 6–52. A defect in the pars articularis (corresponding to the collar in a Scottie dog) at the L4–5 level, consistent with spondylolysis. There is narrowing of the L4–5 disk space. The patient is a 24-year-old man. A (ear) = superior articular process; B (eye) = pedicle; C (nose) = transverse process; D (collar) = pars interarticularis; E (leg) = inferior articular process.

Spondylolysis

General Information. Spondylolysis is a condition in which there is a loss of bony continuity of the neural arch of a vertebra. This condition may or may not be symptomatic and usually does not result in any neurological deficit, but it is a common cause of low back pain. The gap or loss of continuity usually occurs at the junction of the lamina when the vertebra is viewed from above or between the superior and inferior articular processes (pars articularis or apophyseal joints) when viewed from the side. Spondylolysis most commonly afflicts the fourth and fifth lumbar vertebrae.

Diagnosis. This defect is most commonly visualized with the patient lying in the recumbent lateral and oblique positions on the radiographic table. This condition and both articular processs are most advantageously visualized when both right and left posterior oblique positions are filmed for comparison. While in the supine position, the patient is adjusted into a 45-degree angle of rotation, with the spine centered to the middle long axis of the table. A 45-degree foam pillow assures the correct position and provides stability and comfort for the patient. In this position, the outline of the lamina, the superior and inferior articular processes, and the transverse process resembles the appearance of a small Scottish terrier. This is called the **Scottie dog sign,** and the pars interarticularis corresponds to the neck of the dog. The defect appears as a collar on the dog (Fig. 6–52).

Treatment. Treatment of spondylolysis is usually quite conservative. The use of specialized back supports usually corrects the problem. There is little danger of the vertebra further giving way; however, recheck x-rays are advisable.

Spondylolisthesis

General Information. Spondylolisthesis is the *forward* movement of one vertebra on another as a result of fracture of the neural arch, separation into two parts as a result of spondylolysis, and gross osteoarthritis. This condition is most common in the fifth lumbar vertebra, in which there is a forward shift of L-5 on the sacrum. It is less often seen at L-4.

Diagnosis. Spondylolisthesis most often is demonstrated on a coned-down lateral view of the **L5–S1** junction. This view also reveals the L4–L5 junction

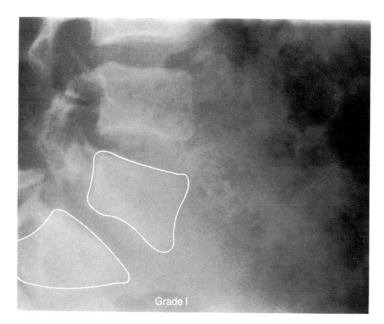

Figure 6–53. Grade I spondylolisthesis of L5–S1, which is secondary to a large defect of the pars articularis at this level, in a 13-year-old boy.

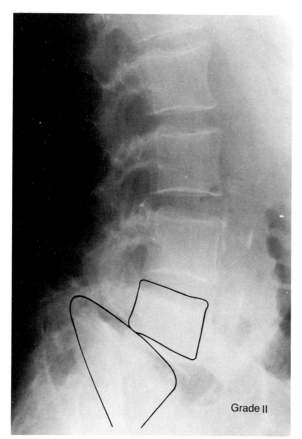

Figure 6–54. Anterior displacement of L5–S1, a grade II spondylolisthesis, with marked narrowing at this level, in a 52-year-old man. Calcification of the lower aorta is noted.

in the event of joint involvement at that level. Spondylolisthesis may be graded on a scale of 1 to 3 according to the degree of displacement (Figs. 6–53, 6–54, and 6–55).

Treatment. The severity of displacement decides the course of treatment. Treatment ranges from simply wearing a back support to spinal fusion, which is more serious but usually uncommon.

Trauma

General Information. Traumatic injury of the osseous system and joints primarily involves the bones and soft tissues. Sprains, strains, fractures, and disloctions are the most common forms of injury. Injuries such as abrasions and lacerations do not usually require x-rays and thus will not be discussed in this chapter.

Fractures are by far the most frequent affliction of bone. Trauma and disease are the two primary mechanisms for fracture. The sites of fracture vary with sex and age. Traumatic fractures are most common in males between the ages of 20 and 40 years and mostly involve the extremities. Fractures in children most often involve the clavicle and humerus. Elderly persons, especially women, are prone to fractures of the femoral neck and spine as a result of osteoporosis and osteoporotic compression.

The ability of a fracture to heal properly is related to the severity of the fracture as well as to the overall health and condition of the patient. Callus formation is an indication of healing and is more rapid in the

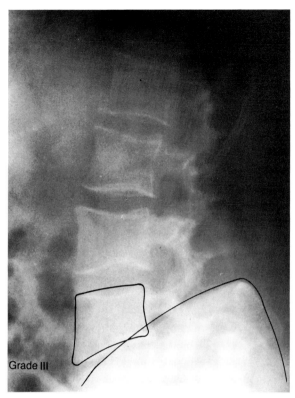

Figure 6–55. Anterior displacement of L5–S1, a grade III spondylolisthesis, in a 47-year-old man.

young and much slower in the elderly. Many age-related diseases such as arteriosclerosis and osteoarthritis often impair and limit the healing process. After injury, the area surrounding the fracture is remodeled with new osteoblasts from the fracture margins and is eventually formed into mature bone. Through this process, the bone usually returns to normal and the original structure and function are restored. However, the process of remodeling is inhibited in the elderly, in whom complete healing is not always possible. Demineralization of bone produces osteoporosis and generalized weakness and softening of bone. Joint replacement is sometimes necessary because porotic bone cannot contain a metallic fixation device, which either breaks or moves out of the desired location. In the elderly, joint replacement is common in weight-bearing joints such as the hips and knees.

Despite great advances in orthopedics, fractures are not without complications. Lack of bony union implies that healing will take place by fibrous union. The patient seldom recovers full use of an extremity when the healing of a fracture takes place with fibrous or secondary union. Perhaps the worst complication of fracture is infection. Open or compound fractures often are complicated by infection, especially when

the trauma drives dirt or cinders deep into the wound. Some of the consequences of infection include osteomyelitis, nonunion, and eventual deformity. Fractures that are comminuted and displaced are difficult to stabilize and slow to heal. If a fracture interrupts a joint, mobility is affected. Patients of advanced age often succumb from the effects of the trauma, fracture, and infection. Elderly patients must be stabilized before surgical correction can be initiated. The elderly often go into shock as a primary effect of the traumatic injury or as a result of secondary causes. Shock is often fatal to elderly patients who are injured. Posttraumatic and surgical complications such as fat or pulmonary emboli and pneumonia are especially common in the elderly when they remain bedridden and are unable to ambulate.

Fractures

General Information. As stated previously, fractures are the most frequent affliction of bone. Fractures and dislocations are almost always associated with soft tissue injury and may be life threatening because of injury to major arteries and nerves. Fractured fragments can also cause secondary injury to the thoracic, abdominal, and pelvic viscera.

Fracture is defined as any disruption in the continuity of bone or, simply, the breaking of a part. A fracture line is present when the cortex is penetrated. A fracture can also be described as the result of any force that tends to change the state of uniform motion of the body or body part. The type of fracture present is often indicative of the type of external force applied. This external violence may be either *direct* or *indirect.* When the trauma is direct, the fracture is at the site of impact. When the trauma is indirect, the intensity may be deflected and subsequent fracture may occur in a distant location. The importance of carefully taking the patient's history cannot be overemphasized. How a fracture occurred bears a direct correlation with the type of fracture to expect. Because pathological fractures occur in the presence of disease and with the least amount of stress, the patient's prior medical history is most important. Patients with terminal cancer are often bedridden and are unable to come to the radiology department for their x-rays. Mobile x-rays of the chest, abdomen, and extremities are frequently ordered for these patients. It is essential that the radiographer stop at the nurses' station and verify all important patient information. If the patient has cancer and is bedridden, the radiographer must request assistance from nursing personnel in order to avoid injury to the patient. Because a pathological fracture can occur with the least amount of stress, it is imperative that all of the patient's body parts be supported when being moved onto a cassette.

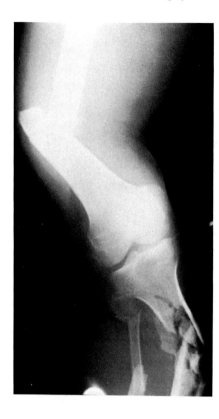

Figure 6–56. Compound fracture of the distal one-third of the right femur, with severe lateral displacement and a multiple comminuted fracture of the proximal one-third of the lower leg. This 25-year-old man was injured in a motorcycle accident.

Classification of Fractures

The primary classifications of fracture are **open** and **closed.** An open or **compound** fracture is one in which the fractured bone pierces the skin and is exposed to the external environment. Open fractures usually occur as a result of extreme violence or trauma such as motorcycle accidents (Fig. 6–56). A closed fracture is one that does not produce an open wound. In the past, closed fractures were referred to as **simple**

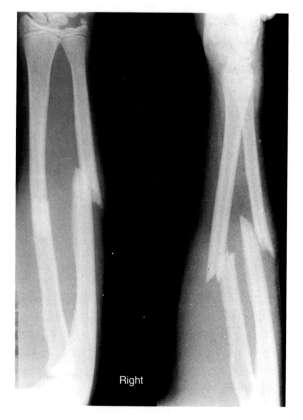

Figure 6–57. Closed oblique fracture of the middle third of the ulna, with 1 cm overriding of the fragments. Transverse fracture, middle third of the radius, with moderate ventral angulation of the fragments and slight overriding of the fragments. Note that both proximal and distal joints are incompletely visualized. Both ends of a long bone must appear on the radiograph. The patient was 14 years old.

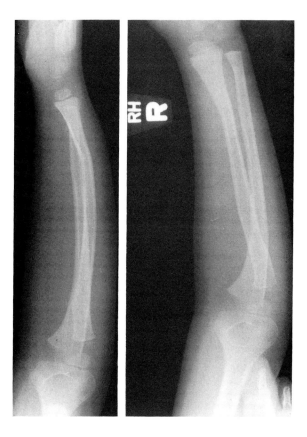

Figure 6–58. Incomplete fracture, greenstick, of the distal one-third of the radius, with ventral angulation. This 16-month-old patient's hand is incorrectly pronated for the anteroposterior projection. The hand is always to be supinated.

fractures. Because many closed fractures are severe and involve considerable trauma, that term appears to be quite inappropriate (Fig. 6–57).

An *incomplete* fracture extends only partially through the bone. These fractures are typically referred to as *greenstick* fractures and are common in children, whose bones are soft and pliable and absorb the force of the injury. This absorption of force also explains the mechanics of a fracture in a child who falls on the outstretched hands while running. The force is distributed through the upper extremities and often results in a fracture of the surgical neck of the humerus or, most commonly, the clavicle. If the direction of force is equally distributed, both clavicles may be fractured. Because this applied stress is indirect, the fracture occurs at a location distant from the impact. The fracture in this event is usually found in the middle third of the clavicle. The clavicle forms a joint with the acromion process of the scapula and with the manubrium of the sternum. Thus, the middle third is the point of least resistance and is most commonly the site of fracture (Fig. 6–58). A complete fracture is one that extends through the entire cross section of bone. The complete fracture is the most common fracture type, and it affects all age-groups. Numerous types of complete fractures are possible, and many are related to the traumatic intensity and the position of the body part (Fig. 6–59).

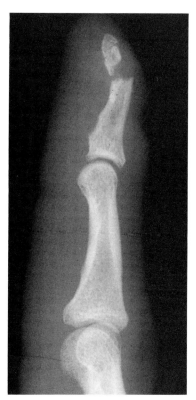

Figure 6–59. Complete transverse fracture, distal phalanx of the left index finger, as seen on the lateral view in a 32-year-old man.

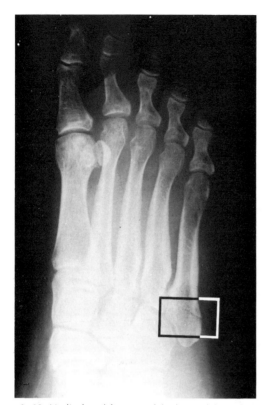

Figure 6–60. Undisplaced fracture of the base of the right fifth metatarsal in a 32-year-old woman.

Fractures can also be described in terms of alignment. A *nondisplaced* fracture is one in which the bone ends or fragments remain in reasonable alignment. Nondisplaced fractures are immobilized with a plaster cast or splint and do not require any manipulation or reduction (Fig. 6–60). A *displaced* fracture is one in which the force of injury causes bone end to be knocked out of alignment. Before the bone can be placed in a plaster cast, the fractured sections have to be placed in reasonable apposition or alignment with each other so that proper healing can occur with minimal deformity. The fracture must be manipulated or reduced so that it may heal properly. Once a fracture is in normal alignment, it is expected to heal without incident. When healing is complete, the bone resumes its prior structure and function. The more displaced the fracture, the more delayed the healing. In *closed reduction,* the orthopedist skillfully manipulates the bone ends or fragments until alignment is achieved. An attendant in the cast room often is asked to assist the physician by applying stress to an extremity during manipulation. If proper alignment cannot be attained, such as with unstable fractures of long bones, the proper alignment will be achieved through a surgical procedure referred to as *open reduction.* An incision is made, and the fractured fragment is maintained in direct contact with adjacent bone by means of metallic devices such as screws, nails, pins, plates, and

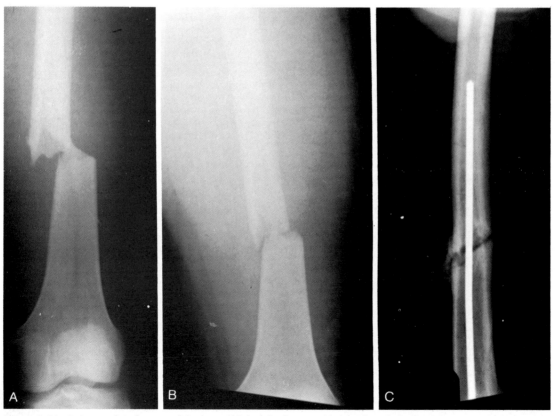

Figure 6–61. *A,* A complete fracture of the lower third of the femur, with 22% lateral displacement, in a 20-year-old man. *B,* After closed reduction. *C,* Postoperative film reveals the presence of an intramedullary rod situated above and below the fracture site, placing the femur in reasonable alignment.

rods. A plaster cast is then applied to further immobilize the extremity. Depending on the type and severity of fracture, the cast may be applied only to the injured joint, in which case it is referred to as a short arm cast or short leg cast. When further immobilization is necessary, both proximal and distal joints are immobilized. This is referred to as a long leg or arm cast. The metallic fixation devices may be removed after healing is complete or may be left in place permanently. The radiographer must be present for both closed and open reduction of fractures. In surgery, the radiographer controls the operation of a portable fluoroscopic unit that is often referred to as a C-arm (Fig. 6–61).

Types of Fractures

Transverse

Transverse fractures are complete fractures that are at right angles to the long axis of the bone. The fracture site occurs at the point of impact (Fig. 6–62).

Fissure

A fissure fracture is a type of incomplete fracture that extends from the surface into but not all the way through a long bone (Fig. 6–63).

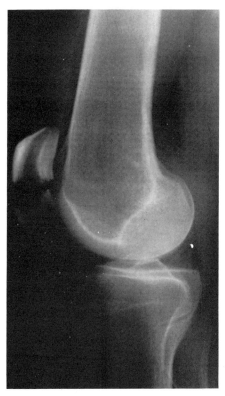

Figure 6–62. Complete transverse fracture of the patella, with considerable separation of the major fragments, in a 52-year-old man. The lower one-half of the patella was surgically removed.

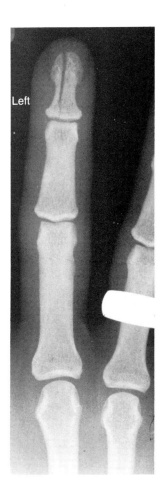

Figure 6–63. Fissure or cleft fracture of the distal phalanx of the left middle finger in a 47-year-old woman.

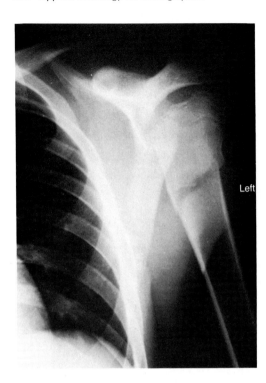

Figure 6–64. Oblique fracture of the surgical neck of the left humerus in a 13-year-old boy.

Oblique

In an oblique fracture, the axis of the fracture is neither parallel nor perpendicular to the bone. The length and angle of the fracture depend on the rotational stress (Fig. 6–64).

Spiral

In a spiral fracture, the bone appears to be twisted apart (Fig. 6–65). This is very common in the humerus, femur, and especially the tibia of skiers.

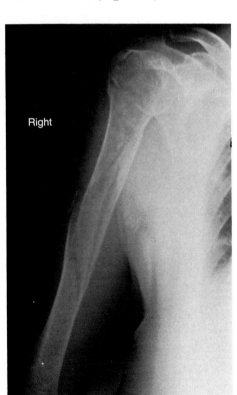

Figure 6–65. Long spiral fracture of the shaft, with mild posterior displacement and angulation of the major distal fragment, in a 90-year-old woman. There is also a comminuted fracture of the humeral neck.

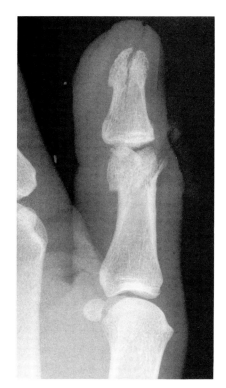

Figure 6–66. Longitudinal fracture, distal phalanx of the thumb (L).

Longitudinal

A longitudinal fracture is a lengthwise break in a bone (Fig. 6–66).

Impacted

In an impacted fracture, one bone fragment is driven into another. This injury is very common in the shoulder, where the proximal humerus is driven into the humeral head (Fig. 6–67).

Torus

A torus fracture is a type of impacted fracture that is especially common in the distal radius of children, where a bulging of the periosteum of the distal radius

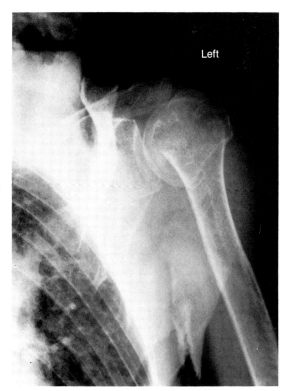

Figure 6–67. Impacted fracture of the surgical neck of the left humerus in an 89-year-old woman. Diffuse bone demineralization is also present.

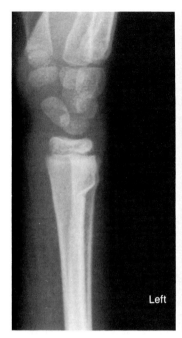

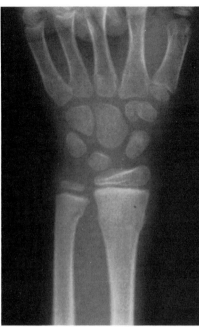

Figure 6–68. Torus-type greenstick fracture of the distal radius and ulna in an 8-year-old girl.

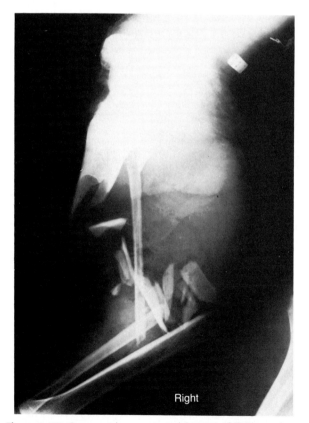

Figure 6–69. Compound, comminuted fracture of the lower leg and transverse fracture of the femur. This 21-year-old man was struck by a forklift.

can be seen. It is particularly likely to occur when a child falls on the outstretched hand. It can also be seen in the distal femur of a child who has jumped from a height such as from a tree (Fig. 6–68).

Comminuted

In a comminuted fracture, the bone is separated into two or more and often numerous fragments. It is especially common as result of severe vehicular accidents, gunshot wounds, and crush injuries (Fig. 6–69).

Double

Fracture of a bone in two distinct places is a double fracture. This is common in the upper and lower proximal extremities as a result of severe trauma (Fig. 6–70).

Salter

Salter types of fractures are five distinct variations of epiphyseal plate fractures in which there is trauma with hemorrhage into the growth plate, resulting in retardation or cessation of growth. When occurring in the lower limb, a Salter fracture may result in a significant shortening of the limb and a permanent limp (Fig. 6–71).

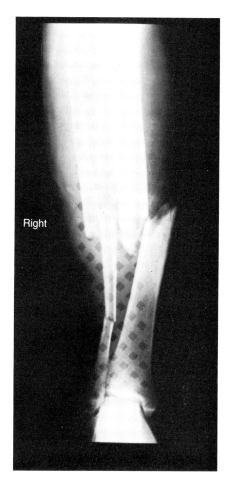

Figure 6–70. Double fracture of the right fibula and complete transverse fracture of the right tibia, with medial angulation of the distal fibula, in a 44-year-old man.

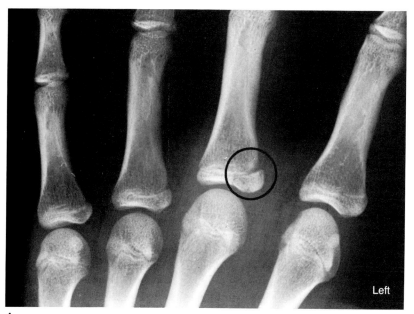

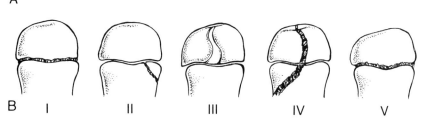

Figure 6–71. *A,* Nondisplaced Salter type III fracture of the epiphysis of the proximal phalanx of the left third digit in a 14-year-old. *B,* The five types of Salter fractures.

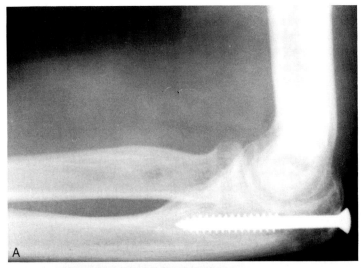

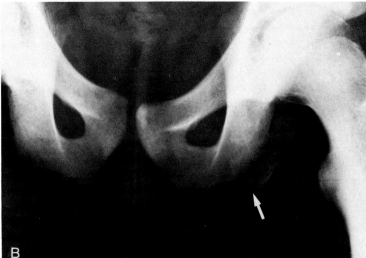

Figure 6–72. Avulsion fracture of the left ischial ramus. The patient is a 20-year-old male gymnast who suffered the injury while doing the splits during floor exercises.

Avulsion

Avulsion fractures occur at sites of muscle origin and are seen in both adults and children. One of the more common types of avulsion fractures involves the olecranon process in an adult. The olecranon is completely separated from the ulna as the triceps contracts (see Fig. 6–72A). Avulsion fractures are common in athletes, especially baseball players and gymnasts. These two sports involve stretching while running. Avulsion fractures of the ischial tuberosity are very common (Fig. 6–72B).

Stress/Fatigue

Stress or fatigue fractures are especially common in the second, third, and fourth midmetatarsals in track athletes, especially sprinters, who are required to attain maximum speed in a few steps after starting from a standing stop position. Joggers and ballet dancers often suffer stress fractures in the distal tibia. Stress fractures are encountered in soldiers who have to march excessive distances, thus the name fatigue or march fractures. If a soldier or hiker carries a heavy backpack for long distances, stress fractures may be noted in the surgical neck of the humerus. Ordinarily the patient will not be able to cite any traumatic event. The radiographer in this case may ask the patient what types of activities he or she has recently been engaged in. Callus formation can be seen 3 to 6 weeks after the first symptoms. A bone scan within 48 hours of the incident reveals a fracture (Fig. 6–73).

Pathological/Spontaneous

Any disease process involving bone usually leads to an inherent weakness of that bone, ultimately producing a spontaneous fracture or one that occurs

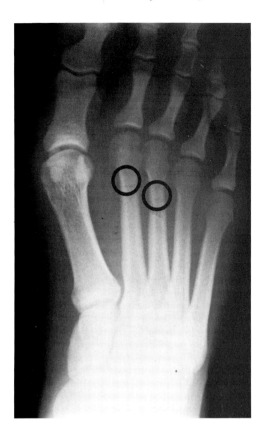

Figure 6–73. Stress fracture of the distal thirds of the second and third metatarsals in a 20-year-old man.

with the least bit of stress. Primary bone cysts and tumors, osteolytic bone metastases, age-related osteoporosis and bone degeneration, and nutritional disorders are common precipitants. The most common cause of pathological fractures is metastatic cancer, particularly from primary carcinoma of the breast in women and from the lung in men (Fig. 6–74).

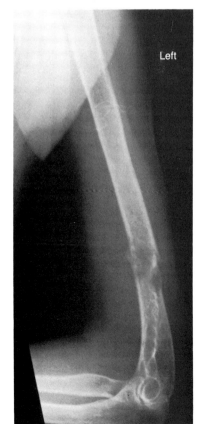

Figure 6–74. Pathological fracture of the left humerus just below the midshaft in a 79-year-old woman.

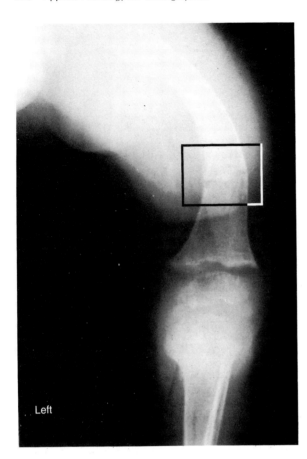

Figure 6–75. Pathological trophic fracture of the distal one-third of the left femur, secondary to rickets, in a 1½-year-old boy.

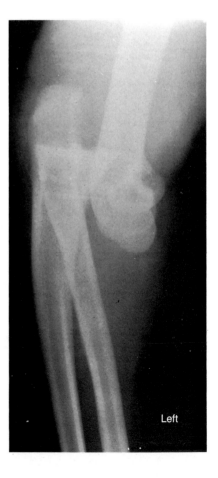

Figure 6–76. Dislocation of the elbow joint and fracture of the radial head in a 49-year-old man.

Trophic

Trophic fractures are pathological fractures that occur specifically as a result of nutritional disorders such as rickets and osteomalacia (Fig. 6–75).

Fracture-Dislocation

Fracture-dislocation is a fracture of a proximal or distal segment of bone near a joint that also dislocated as a result of its position at the time of impact (Fig. 6–76).

Common Fractures

Bennett's Fracture

Bennett's fracture is a fracture of the base of the first metacarpal with involvement of the first carpometacarpal joint. When the impact is severe, subluxation of the carpometacarpal joint may be present. This fracture is often the result of jamming the thumb and also occurs when a softball strikes the end of the thumb with a great deal of force (Fig. 6–77).

Colles' Fracture

Colles' fracture most often affects older adults and can be described as a forked fracture of the distal radius and a chip fracture of the ulnar styloid. This is sometimes referred to as the ***dinner fork deformity.*** When placed in the lateral position, this fracture presents a ***posterior*** or ***backward*** displacement of about 30 degrees (Fig. 6–78).

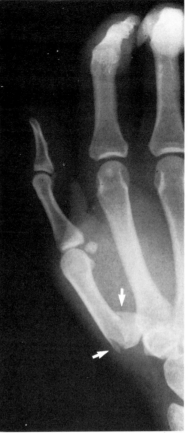

Figure 6–77. Oblique fracture of the base of the first metacarpal, with angulation of the fragments relative to each other, in a 28-year-old man. This is referred to as Bennett's fracture.

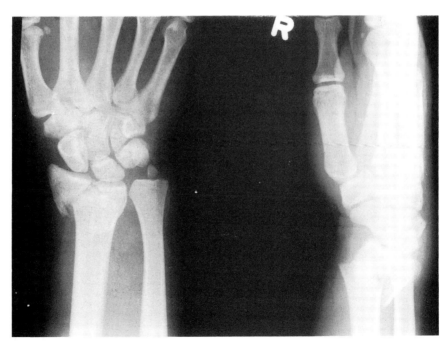

Figure 6–78. Colles' fracture, which is a forked fracture of the distal radius with backward displacement and a chip fracture of the ulnar styloid. This 62-year-old woman fell on her outstretched hand.

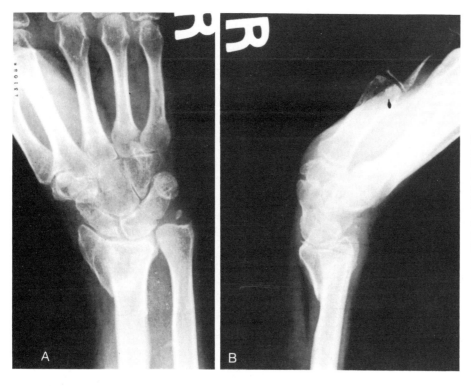

Figure 6–79. *(A)* Posteroanterior and *(B)* lateral views reveal a forked fracture of the distal radius, with forward displacement and a chip fracture of the ulnar styloid, in a 58-year-old woman. The forward anterior displacement of the fractured distal radius is what differentiates a Smith's fracture from a Colles' fracture.

Smith's Fracture

Smith's fracture is identical to Colles' fracture except that when the wrist is placed in the lateral position, the distal radius is displaced ***anterior*** or ***forward*** about 30 degrees (Fig. 6–79).

Supracondylar Fracture

Supracondylar fracture is a common pediatric fracture in which there is an alteration in the alignment of the condyles to the humeral head and the condyles may come to lie directly under the shaft of the

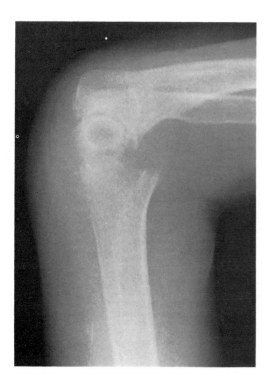

Figure 6–80. Supracondylar fracture of the left distal humerus in a 65-year-old woman.

humerus. Another indication of elbow fracture is visualization of the *fat pad sign.* The joint capsule of the elbow is inserted into the hollows of the distal humerus, and each of these hollows contains a fat pad that acts as a buffer between the humerus and the olecranon and coronoid processes. If an effusion occurs, these fat pads, which are normally not visible, appear. If the fat pads are visible on the lateral view following trauma to the elbow, a supracondylar fracture should be suspected. A fat pad sign in adults may indicate a radial head fracture. AP and oblique views demonstrate supracondylar fractures. An internal or medial oblique view will best demonstrate radial head fractures (Figs. 6–80 and 6–81).

Carpal Navicular Fracture

Carpal navicular fracture is usually caused by falling on one's hand. The pain and loss of motion are often indicative of wrist fracture, although the usual deformity such as is present with a Colles' or Smith's fracture is not apparent. Routine AP, lateral, and oblique views may not demonstrate the fracture because of the foreshortening of the navicular. Ulnar flexion views are recommended with the hand in the PA position. In the Stecher method, the wrist is elevated to a 20-degree incline while the central ray is directed perpendicular to the navicular bone or the hand is pronated and the central ray directed 20 degrees toward the elbow (Fig. 6–82).

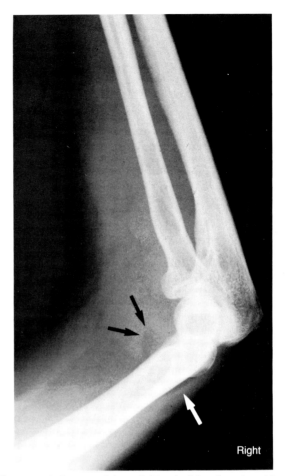

Figure 6–81. Fracture of the radial head of the elbow in a 49-year-old woman. The lateral view reveals an abnormal fat pad sign anteriorly.

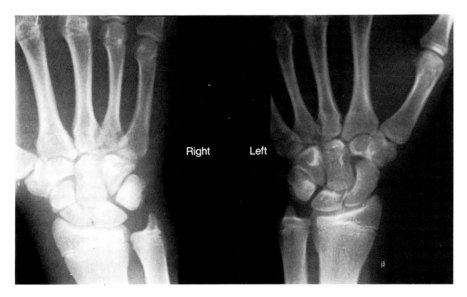

Figure 6–82. Complete transverse fracture of the navicular bone of the right wrist in a 13-year-old boy. As is the case with pediatric patients, the opposite wrist is used for comparison.

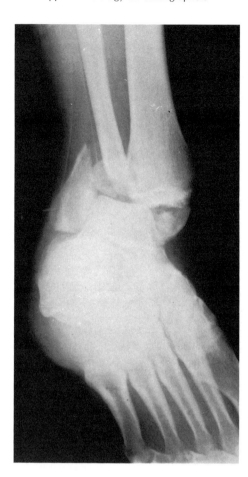

Figure 6–83. Trimalleolar Pott's fracture of the right ankle.

Figure 6–84. Moderately displaced subcapital fracture of the right hip, which is not recent, in a 90-year-old woman.

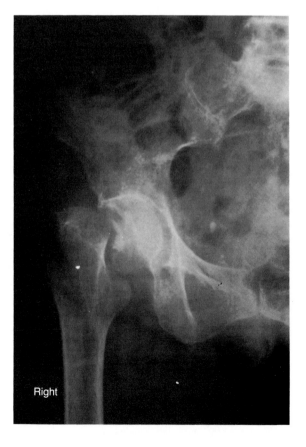

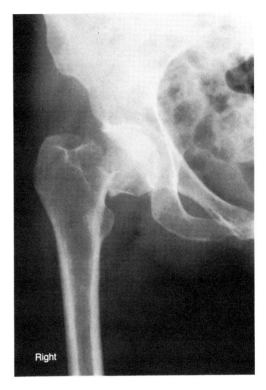

Figure 6–85. Transcervical neck fracture of the right hip in a 62-year-old woman.

Pott's Fracture

A Pott's fracture is a complete break of the medial malleolus, with possible derangement of the ankle mortice. This is a type of avulsion fracture. The malleolar fragment is usually displaced. A metallic screw or pin has to be surgically inserted in order for the fragment to remain in contact with the distal fibula (Fig. 6–83).

Figure 6–86. Intertrochanteric fracture of the right hip in an 87-year-old man.

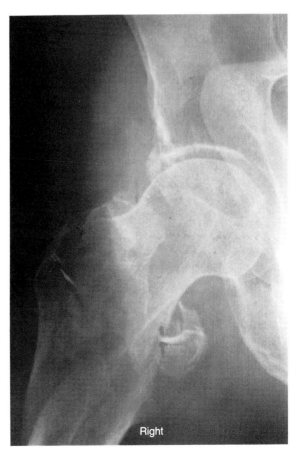

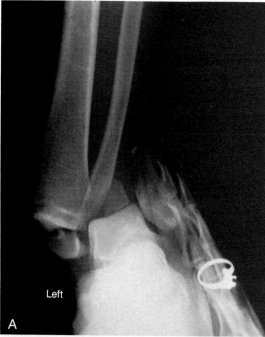

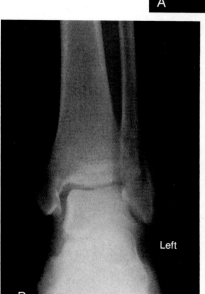

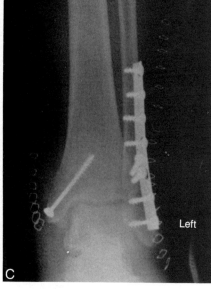

Figure 6–87. *A,* Trimalleolar fracture-dislocation, with marked lateral displacement, in a 58-year-old woman. *B,* Marked improvement in position of the fragments after reduction. The talus dislocation has been reduced. The medial and posterior malleolus are mildly displaced. There is still slight widening of the medial side of the ankle mortise. *C,* An open surgical reduction film reveals the presence of a single screw through the medial malleolus and a plate with several screws inserted into the lateral malleolus and distal fibula. The fractured fragments are in good position and alignment. The ankle mortise is within normal limits.

Hip Fractures

The exact location and severity of a hip fracture depend on the direction of the forces involved. The most common types of hip fracture include *subcapital,* *transcervical,* and *intertrochanteric.* In elderly women, osteoporosis is the predisposing cause (Figs. 6–84, 6–85, and 6–86).

Bimalleolar Fracture

A bimalleolar fracture is a fracture of the lateral and medial malleolus (Fig. 6–87).

Trimalleolar Fracture

A trimalleolar fracture has three components: the medial and lateral malleolus and the posterior distal tibia (Fig. 6–88).

Fracture of the Base of the Fifth Metatarsal

Fracture of the fifth metatarsal is a common transverse fracture that occurs when the foot is suddenly twisted when the ankle pronates (Fig. 6–89).

Stellate Fracture

Stellate fracture occurs when a person falls directly on the patella, shattering it. Radiographically, the

Figure 6–88. Trimalleolar fracture-dislocation of the left ankle in a 44-year-old woman. Transverse fracture of the medial malleolus with slight separation of the fractured fragments. Oblique comminuted fracture of the distal fibula, with posterior angulation of the distal fragments. Posterior dislocation of the talus, with a posterior lip fracture of the distal tibia.

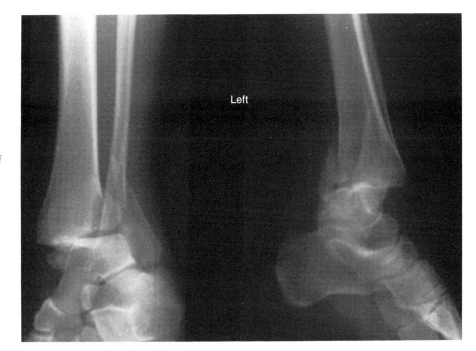

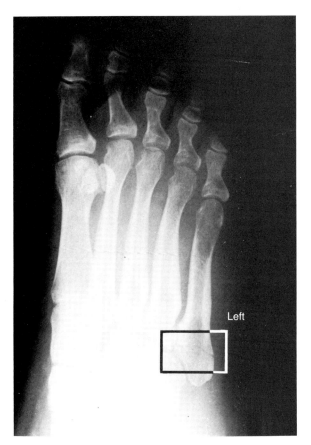

Figure 6–89. Nondisplaced transverse fracture of the base of the right fifth metatarsal in a 32-year-old woman.

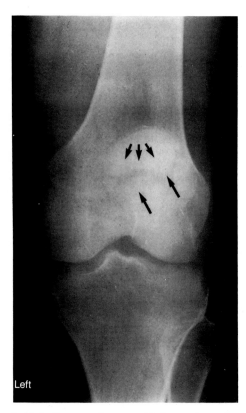

Figure 6–90. Stellate-type fracture with fracture lines distributed throughout the patella in a 47-year-old man. All fragments remain in good position.

patella is comminuted without separation. The fractures form a star-like image, sometimes also referred to as the shattered glass effect (Fig. 6–90).

Dislocation

Traumatic dislocation most frequently involves the shoulder joint when a person falls on a hand or elbow. The most common shoulder injury is a **subcoracoid** dislocation. When performing a shoulder series, it is best to position the patient erect, either sitting or standing. Although it is quite apparent when a shoulder is out of the joint capsule, an axial view helps differentiate an anterior from a posterior dislocation (Fig. 6–91).

Dislocation and subluxation of the acromioclavicular are not that difficult to demonstrate with the patient in the erect position. It is important to place the patient erect in the PA position, maintaining a close relationship between the part and the film. Two exposures are taken of both joints simultaneously, with and without weights. Sandbags or other suitable weights are grasped, and the arms are gently released with the humerus in anatomical position. External rotation of the shoulder is useful in demonstrating subluxation. The patient will be able to assume this

position with weights for only a moment, so another radiographer should be poised to make the exposure (Fig. 6–92).

Internal Fixation and Its Radiographic Evaluation

Once the orthopedic surgeon has determined that an open reduction with internal fixation is necessary, several factors must be considered: (1) the type of internal fixation device and its biomechanical characteristics; (2) the type and position of the fracture; the degree of dislocation; the appearance of bony defect and its significance in the stability of the internal device; (3) the quality of the bone; the degree of atrophy, osteoporosis, and any preexisting or post-traumatic pathological conditions; and (4) stability; whether the fracture site will bear weight or not.

Once the open reduction is complete and the internal fixation device is in place, the following must be considered and evaluated: (1) bone healing; an assessment of callus formation; and (2) bone reaction; observing any changes that may be signs of infection, atrophy, and so on. Stable internal fixation can be performed with the use of intramedullary nailing, interfragmentary compression by insertion of screws or plates, or a tension band plate. The advantages of these methods are that the fracture can be returned to reasonable alignment so that healing can occur. Complications after healing often include muscle atrophy, stiff joints, and circulatory disturbances due

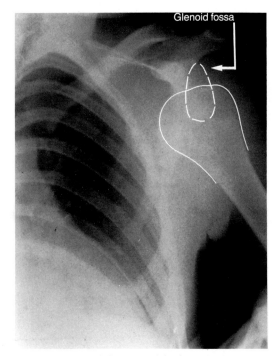

Figure 6–91. Anterior dislocation of the humerus in a 17-year-old.

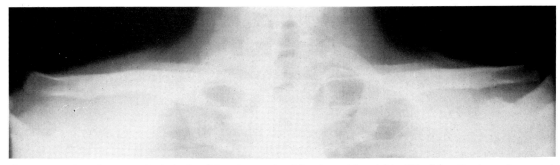

Figure 6–92. Complete acromioclavicular dislocation on the right taken with weights. This dislocation is most apparent when the right and left sides are compared.

to long-term immobilization by a plaster cast or bandages. There is a trend to immobilize the extremity externally and to initiate physiotherapy as soon as possible.

Intramedullary nailing was first performed in 1940. Since that time, many advances have improved this procedure. The use of the C-arm mobile fluoroscope in surgery now permits television viewing of procedures as they take place. Because of this, the length of the surgical procedure has been significantly reduced. When internal fixation devices immobilize the fractures so that bone margins are in contact with each other, a direct method of healing takes place. A second type of healing is referred to as indirect healing. This is the presence of callus formation that begins from the periosteal tissues and includes the periosteum, the marrow, and the haversian canals. New osteoblasts are formed, mature, and begin to remodel the area in and around the fracture site.

The materials used in the manufacture of internal fixation devices today include noble austenitic steel with chromium, nickel, molybdenum, manganese, and silicon. Some of these metals have been known to corrode, loosening at the fracture site. Chemical corrosion has caused nails and screws to slip out of the insertion site and even fracture. Thus, continual radiological follow-up is required when internal fixation devices are used.

The actual healing time varies with the age and physical condition of the patient. Bone healing is rapid in children, slower in middle-aged persons, and extremely slow to absent in the elderly.

Self-Assessment Quiz

For each of the following questions, select the one best response and circle the letter that precedes it.

1. Congenital clubfoot is also known as
   a. fibrous dysplasia
   b. achondroplasia
   c. talipes equinovarus deformity
   d. toeing in

2. Congenital hip dysplasia is a malformation of the
   a. acetabulum
   b. femoral head
   c. metaphysis
   d. diaphysis

3. Ortolani's and Trendelenburg's signs are indicative of
   a. congenital clubfoot
   b. achondroplasia
   c. congenital hip dysplasia
   d. dwarfism

4. Achondroplasia is the most frequent cause of
   a. congenital heart disease
   b. dwarfism
   c. congenital hip dysplasia
   d. osteomalacia

5. The brittle bone disease is also known as
   a. Köhler's disease
   b. achondroplasia
   c. Marfan's syndrome
   d. osteogenesis imperfecta

6. The upper half of the body is shorter than average whereas the lower half is longer than average in the disorder known as
   a. Osgood-Schlatter disease
   b. achondroplasia
   c. Marfan's syndrome
   d. rickets

7. *Marble, chalk,* and *ivory bones* are terms used to describe
   a. osteoporosis
   b. osteopenia
   c. osteopetrosis
   d. osteomalacia

8. A condition characterized by loss of bone is referred to as
   a. osteoporosis
   b. osteomalacia
   c. osteopetrosis
   d. osteotomy

9. Osteoporosis affects the young as well as the elderly.
   a. true
   b. false

10. Overproduction of the growth hormone may produce a condition known as
    a. mongolism
    b. achondroplasia
    c. osteogenesis imperfecta
    d. acromegaly

11. Rickets and osteomalacia are the results of a
    a. hormone imbalance
    b. metabolic problem
    c. vitamin deficiency
    d. calcium excess

12. Fractures are a complication of
    a. osteogenesis imperfecta
    b. rickets
    c. osteoporosis
    d. osteomalacia
    e. all of the above

13. Osteomyelitis is correctly characterized as
    a. the result of bacteria
    b. pyogenic
    c. a bone infection
    d. a postoperative complication
    e. all of the above

14. The initial radiographic sign of osteomyelitis is soft tissue swelling with loss of the fat planes.
    a. true
    b. false

15. Brodie's abscess may be found in the
    a. proximal long bones
    b. flat bones
    c. distal long bones
    d. sacrum

16. A septic and suppurative form of arthritis is described as
    a. juvenile
    b. senile
    c. gouty
    d. acute

17. Rheumatoid arthritis afflicts adults only.
    a. true
    b. false

18. Still's disease is also called
    a. gout
    b. senile arthritis
    c. juvenile rheumatoid arthritis
    d. osteomyelitis

19. Marie-Strümpel disease and bamboo spine are synonyms for the condition known as
    a. ankylosing spondylitis
    b. spondylolisthesis
    c. spina bifida
    d. scoliosis

20. Urate deposits in the joints are a major sign of
    a. rheumatoid arthritis
    b. gout
    c. senile arthritis
    d. spondylitis

21. The most common form of arthritis is
    a. senile or osteoarthritis
    b. gout
    c. rheumatoid
    d. acute

22. Bouchard's and Heberden's nodes are pea-shaped nodules in the proximal and distal interphalangeal joints of the hands as a complication of
    a. gout
    b. senile arthritis
    c. juvenile arthritis
    d. acute arthritis

23. Partial to total joint replacement with a prosthesis is called
    a. arthrodesis
    b. laminectomy
    c. osteoplasty
    d. arthroplasty

24. An osteotomy is performed to change bony alignment to relieve stress.
    a. true
    b. false

25. In the elderly, a skull deformity that involves thickening of the calvarium is known as
    a. osteomalacia
    b. hyperostosis
    c. Paget's disease
    d. acromegaly

26. Which of the following diseases are examples of aseptic necrosis?
    a. Legg-Calvé-Perthes
    b. Köhler's
    c. Kienböck's
    d. Osgood-Schlatter
    e. all of the above

27. Legg-Calvé-Perthes disease affects the
    a. tarsal scaphoid
    b. femoral head
    c. tibial tubercle
    d. carpal lunate

28. Osgood-Schlatter disease affects the
    a. tarsal scaphoid
    b. femoral head
    c. tibial tubercle
    d. carpal lunate

29. In fibrous dysplasia, radiographs usually reveal well-defined zones of rarefaction surrounded by narrow rims of sclerotic bone.
    a. true
    b. false

30. A condition in which there is a loss of bony continuity involving the neural arch of a vertebra is known as
    a. spondylitis
    b. spondylolysis
    c. spondylolisthesis
    d. spina bifida

31. The forward movement of one vertebra on another describes
    a. spondylitis
    b. spondylolysis
    c. spondylolisthesis
    d. spina bifida

32. Which of the following are complications of fracture?
    a. nonunion
    b. osteomyelitis
    c. infection
    d. emboli
    e. all of the above

33. Which of the following described a compound fracture?
    a. open
    b. closed
    c. comminuted
    d. complex

34. Which of the following types of fractures occur at right angles to the long axis of the bone?
    a. oblique
    b. transverse
    c. spiral
    d. impacted

35. A fracture in which a bone fragment is driven into another is known as
    a. twisted
    b. angled
    c. compound
    d. impacted

36. In which of the following types of fractures is a fractured bone separated into two or more and often numerous fragments?
    a. compound
    b. simple
    c. comminuted
    d. torus

37. Which type of fracture is most common in the mid-metatarsal region?
    a. complete
    b. comminuted
    c. incomplete
    d. stress

38. Osteolytic bone metastases may result in which type of fracture?
    a. incomplete
    b. oblique
    c. fatigue
    d. pathological

39. Colles' and Smith's fractures occur in the
    a. hip
    b. wrist
    c. patella
    d. ankle

40. Supracondylar fractures can be found in the
    a. humerus
    b. ulna
    c. femur
    d. radius
    e. humerus and femur

41. Lateral bending and ulnar flexion are movements that are useful in demonstrating fractures of the
    a. navicular
    b. lunate
    c. base of the fifth metatarsal
    d. ankle

42. Most fractures of the hip in elderly women are the result of
    a. osteopetrosis
    b. osteomalacia
    c. rickets
    d. osteoarthritis
    e. osteoporosis

Study Questions

1. What is thought to be the reason why congenital clubfoot and other foot and leg deformities occur?

2. What are some of the differences between an achondroplastic dwarf and a midget?

3. In what ways can pathogens invade bone and produce infection?

4. Describe the process of bone healing following fracture.

5. Describe the process that causes bone to demineralize or lose calcium.

6. What are some of the most common fixation devices used in fracture repair?

7. Which body organs are most affected secondarily by bone and joint disease?

8. Which bone and joint diseases most frequently can be imaged via nuclear medicine?

9. What bone diseases can be effectively demonstrated with computed scanning and magnetic resonance imaging?

Seven

Central Nervous System

Related Terminology

aneurysm
apoplexy
arteriovenous malformation
ataxia
bruit
chemonucleolysis
choroid plexus
circle of Willis
concussion
contusion
digital subtraction angiography
dysphagia
epidural
falx
hemiparesis
hydrocephalus
mannitol
meningioma
meningocele
metrizamide
myelocele
myelomeningocele
spina bifida
subarachnoid
subdural
transient ischemic attacks
ventriculovenous shunt

Objectives

Upon completion of Chapter 7, the reader will be able to

- Explain the ways in which the central nervous system can be imaged.

- Identify the radiological characteristics of hydrocephalus.

- Identify the factors that precipitate stroke, aneurysm, and hemorrhage.

- Describe the primary types of skull fractures that are observed on the finished radiograph.

- List the three most common malformations of the spinal cord.

- List and describe the primary methods of treatment of central nervous system disorders.

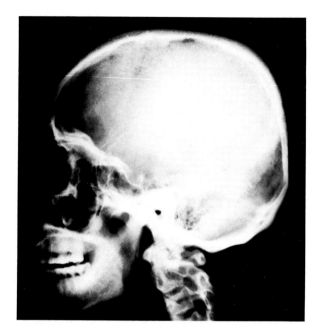

Figure 7–1. Normal lateral skull view, revealing the meningeal channels and diploic veins.

Imaging the Central Nervous System

There are several methods of imaging the central nervous system: plain films, computed tomography (CT), magnetic resonance (MR) imaging, sonography, angiography, radionuclide brain scanning, and myelography.

Plain films of the cranium usually involve several projections: posteroanterior (PA), semiaxial (Grashey/ Towne's method), submentovertical, verticosubmental (Schüller method/cranial base), and right and left lateral. It is most important for the radiographer to be familiar with the normal anatomy visualized in each projection to be able to differentiate and distinguish normal/abnormal conditions and normal variants of the cranial vault. Blood vessels can cause impressions on the bones of the cranial vault. These impressions are usually linear or star-shaped radio-

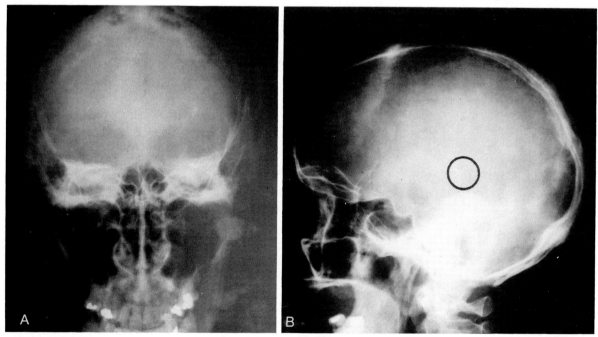

Figure 7–2. *A,* Frontal skull view revealing a calcified pineal gland situated in the midline. *B,* Right lateral skull view revealing a calcified pineal gland.

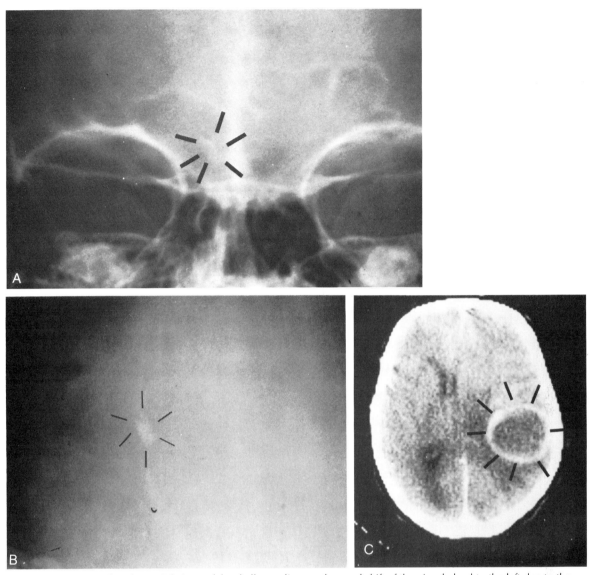

Figure 7–3. (A) Frontal and (B) axial views of the skull revealing an abnormal shift of the pineal gland to the left due to the presence of a space-occupying lesion in a 68-year-old woman. The CT scan (C) demonstrates a large tumor in the right cerebral hemisphere.

lucencies. These markings may be mistaken for fractures. It is most important to visualize vascular markings from two points of view, namely frontal and lateral. The vascular markings should be equally prominent in both projections. These prominent markings serve as grooves for the middle meningeal arteries, which course through the inner skull table. These grooves are located just anterior of the coronal suture up to the skull vertex. Meningeal veins usually accompany the middle meningeal arteries. Smaller veins lying within the diploic space (between the inner and outer tables) vary in number and size. The diploic veins are usually seen in the parietal region and are bilateral. Visualization of the meningeal arteries and diploic veins can be pathologically signifi-

cant, especially if there is enlargement only one side. This often suggests an underlying meningioma (Fig. 7–1).

A common skull finding that is normal is the appearance of a calcified pineal gland, situated in the midline on plain films. This finding occurs in about 60% of adults. It must be seen in two projections and especially on the lateral view. In the presence of a space-occupying lesion, the pineal gland may be displaced. The midline shift, if pathological, will usually exceed 3 mm. Shifts of less than 3 mm may represent a normal variant (Figs. 7–2 and 7–3).

It is not uncommon to observe calcification of the choroid plexus. The choroid plexus lies on the floor of the skull, within the body of the lateral ventricles.

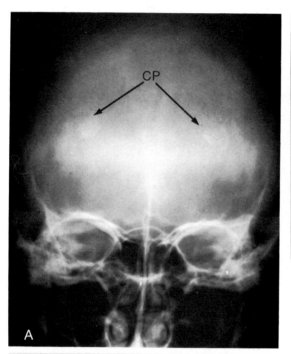

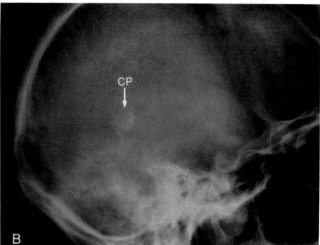

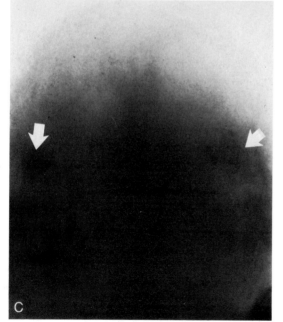

Figure 7–4. Bilateral calcified choroid plexuses (CP) seen on *(A)* frontal, *(B)* left lateral, and *(C)* axial views of a man's skull.

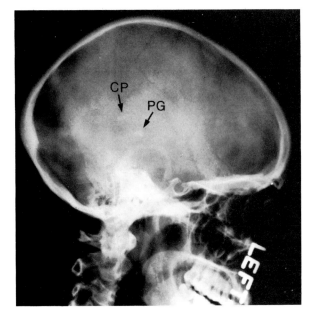

Figure 7–5. Left lateral view of a woman's skull revealing the presence of a calcified pineal gland (PG) lying anterior and inferior to a calcified choroid plexus (CP).

The lateral ventricles are responsible for the production of cerebrospinal fluid, which circulates throughout the ventricular pathways and into the subarachnoid space. For the most part, the calcifications occur bilaterally and can best be observed in a frontal view of the skull. It is not uncommon for the pineal gland and one or both choroid plexuses to appear simultaneously on a frontal or lateral skull view. On the lateral view, the pineal gland is located somewhat anterior and inferior to the choroid plexus (Figs. 7–4 and 7–5).

The falx cerebri and falx cerebelli are folds of dura mater that separate the cerebral and cerebellar hemispheres. These are also normal variants that may be present on skull radiographs of older adults, especially on the semiaxial view. These calcifications typically are not clinically significant (Fig. 7–6).

Lesions of the cranium often result in areas of focal

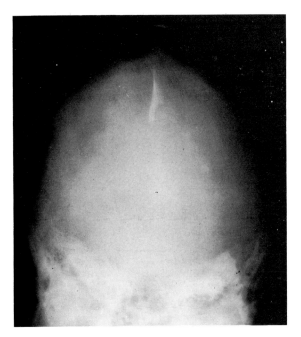

Figure 7–6. Calcified falx cerebri as seen on an axial view of the skull of a 64-year-old man.

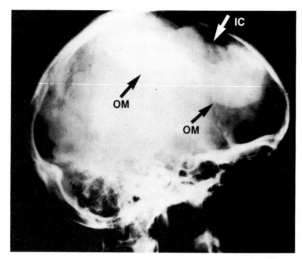

Figure 7–7. Invading carcinoma (IC) and osteoblastic metastases (OM) seen over much of the lateral skull in a 44-year-old man.

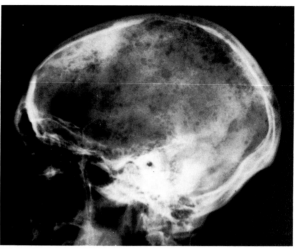

Figure 7–8. Osteolytic metastases of the skull, consistent with multiple myeloma, in a 78-year-old woman.

or diffuse osteoblastic sclerosis or focal or diffuse osteolytic lucency (Figs. 7–7 and 7–8).

One of the more important aspects of routine skull radiography is the visualization and evaluation of the sella turcica. The sella turcica or hypophysis houses the pituitary gland. Pituitary tumors are the most common cause of sellar enlargement. The sella turcica is typically somewhat ovoid and usually measures about 8 to 12 mm in width and 6 to 8 mm in height when seen on a lateral view. The sphenoidal sinuses lie immediately below the sella turcica and are identifiable by their aeration. The floor of the pituitary fossa forms the roof of the sphenoidal sinus. The early stages of a pituitary adenoma produce an *asymmetrical* enlargement of the pituitary fossa. On the lateral view of the skull, a double line forming the floor is often observed, indicating the enlargement. Visualization of the sella turcica may also reveal decreases in bone density or the presence of erosion, which may be indicative of intracranial pressure as a result of the developing space-occupying lesion (Fig. 7–9).

Plain films of the spine are most useful in demonstrating and evaluating congenital anomalies of the spine, abnormal curvatures, spondylosis, spondylitis, spondylolysis, osteomyelitis, and trauma. Although the spinal cord cannot be directly visualized, secondary causes of cord compression can readily be identified. These secondary causes include fracture, dislocation, and metastasis.

CT makes possible the visualization of the brain. With the infusion of an iodinated contrast medium,

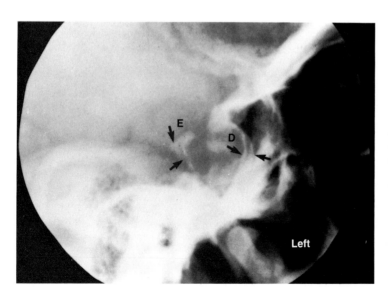

Figure 7–9. Moderate enlargement of the sella turcica, with a double-wall sign (D) in the floor and some erosion (E) of the posterior wall, in a 43-year-old woman. This is suggestive of a space-occupying lesion of the sella turcica. There is increased calvarial bone density.

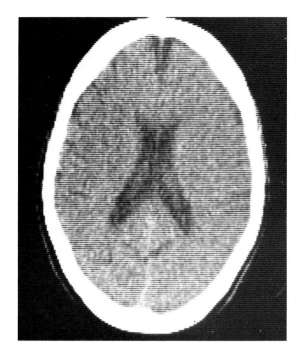

Figure 7–10. Normal preinfusion CT scan.

enhanced fresh blood can be seen as an opaque substance. Blood may lie within the brain itself in various locations or reside outside of the brain. The major disadvantage of CT is that the exact source of the hemorrhage usually cannot be visualized. CT of the spine is excellent for evaluating conditions of the vertebrae, spinal canal, and paravertebral soft tissues. Because its density is greater than the usual contents of the spinal canal, a herniated disk is often clearly revealed. Currently, CT is the method of choice for demonstrating spinal cord abscesses and neoplasms (Figs. 7–10 and 7–11).

MR imaging, formerly known as nuclear magnetic resonance, is the newest imaging modality. MR imaging of body structures employs theories of magnetism and does not use ionizing radiation. So far, the use of MR for imaging the head and neck has produced encouraging results, but imaging of thoracic and abdominal structures has proved less promising. Proponents of CT scanning and MR imaging are competing for recognition within the medical community. However, it appears that there are applications for both modalities. CT has produced excellent images of the brain, but MR is said to be more

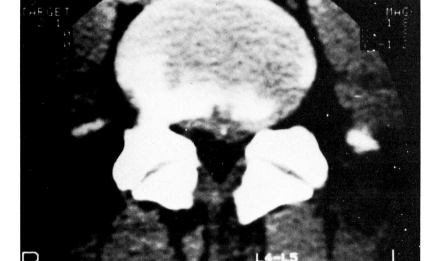

Figure 7–11. Herniated or bulging disk at the level of L4-5 and extending to the left side in a 33-year-old man.

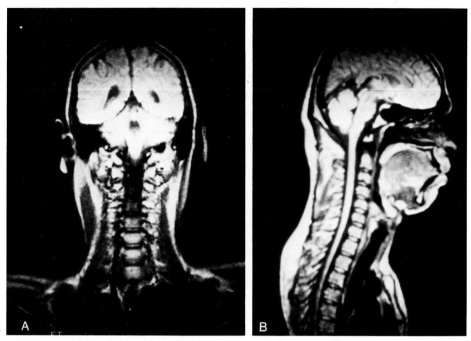

Figure 7–12. *(A)* Negative posterior and *(B)* lateral views of the brain and spinal cord as seen in magnetic resonance imaging.

sensitive in the detection of brain lesions. Because of its increased sensitivity, MR is better able to discriminate soft tissues whereas CT may tend to miss a lesion within the soft tissues. This increased sensitiv-

ity may lead to earlier detection of a brain lesion. On the other hand, it has been found that MR may be less successful in distinguishing a tumor from surrounding edema and in detecting calcification. With

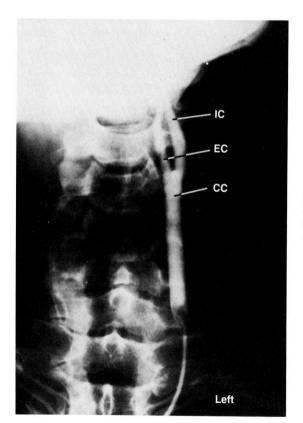

Figure 7–13. An essentially negative anteroposterior carotid arteriogram of a 47-year-old man. Identified are the common carotid (CC), internal carotid (IC), and external carotid (EC) arteries.

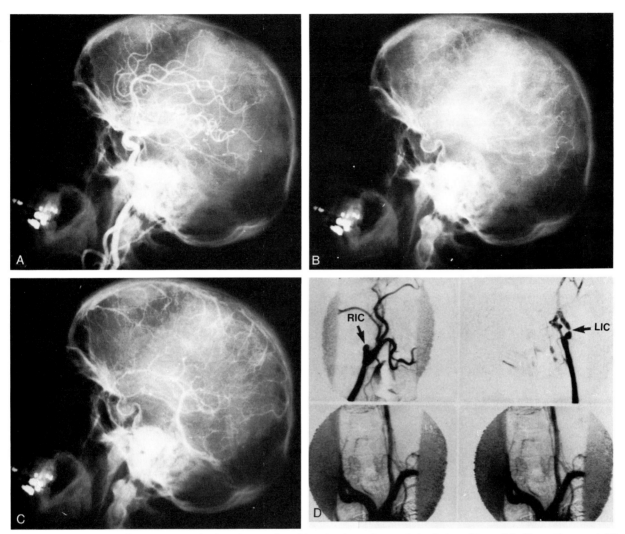

Figure 7–14. An essentially negative cerebral angiogram describing the three phases of circulation: *(A)* arterial, *(B)* capillary, and *(C)* venous phases. *D,* Complete obstruction of the right internal carotid artery (RIC) and 95% stenosis of the left internal carotid artery (LIC).

MR imaging, tumor margins are better visualized than with contrast-enhanced CT scans (Fig. 7–12).

Sonography is of limited application for delineating brain lesions. However, it is most useful when examining children because of the openings provided by the fontanelles, which permit excellent images while avoiding the high levels of radiation associated with CT.

Angiography is used to demonstrate many types of brain lesions. It is especially useful for locating aneurysms, as well as for identifying specific abnormal cranial vessels and for evaluating the quality and direction of intracerebral circulation. Angiography is used in diagnosing extracranial carotid disease, arteriovenous malformations, intracranial mass lesions, and various forms of hemorrhages and aneurysms. Currently, digital subtraction angiography or digital vascular imaging is being employed as an alternative to arterial angiography. In digital subtraction angiography, an iodinated contrast agent is injected into an arm vein rather than through the femoral artery. This procedure allows the subject to be treated as an outpatient. The risks and costs of digital angiography have been greatly reduced, but the medical community has been less than satisfied with the amount of venous opacification that it provides. The concept of digital subtraction is being combined with venous angiography. With this imaging method, an accurate diagnosis is made with the least amount of risk (Figs. 7–13 and 7–14).

Radionuclide brain scanning is effective in imaging intracerebral processes that affect the blood-brain barrier. Primary brain tumors, abscesses, and metastatic disease are demonstrated as focal areas of increased isotope activity or uptake. A disadvantage of nuclear brain scanning is that the specific cause of

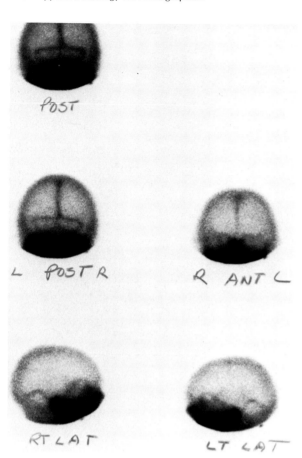

Figure 7–15. Normal isotope scan of the brain of a 40-year-old woman.

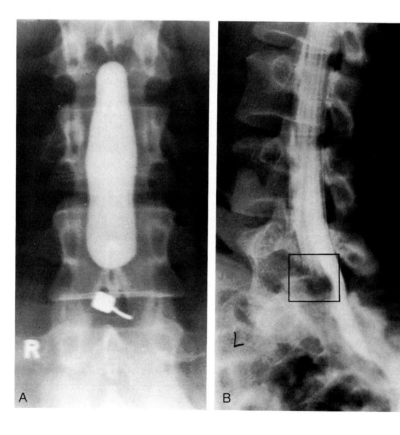

Figure 7–16. *A,* An essentially normal lumbar myelogram using an oil-based contrast agent. *B,* A large ventral-extradural defect on the left of L5-S1, compatible with a herniated disk in an adolescent. A water-soluble contrast agent was used.

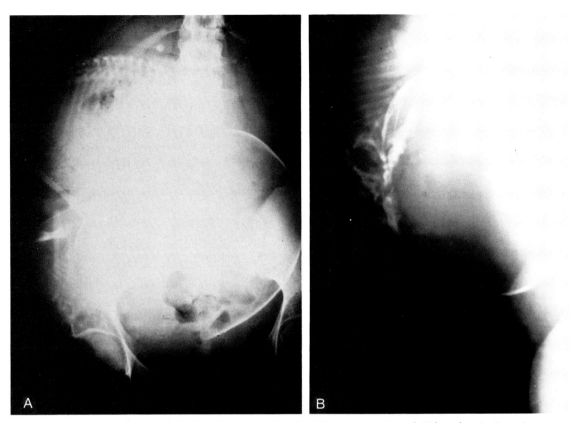

Figure 7–17. A full-term hydrocephalic fetus demonstrated in the *(A)* anteroposterior and *(B)* lateral projections, in a 31-year-old woman.

the increased activity cannot be identified. Radioisotope brain scans have largely been replaced by CT (Fig. 7–15).

Myelography makes possible visualization of the spinal cord and nerve roots by injection of radiopaque agents, such as oil-based Pantopaque or water-soluble metrizamides. Oily Pantopaque must be removed from the subarachnoid space after completion of the procedure. Metrizamide is absorbed by the body and generally has fewer side effects. It is less opaque but allows better visualization of nerve roots (Fig. 7–16).

The Brain

Congenital Disorders

Hydrocephalus

General Information. The nervous system has an unusually long maturation period, which is thought to predispose to malformations of the brain and spinal cord. Approximately 10 to 20% of developmental defects are due to this long period of maturation. The factors that have been identified as those that produce malformation include maternal infections, fetal infections, fetal hypoxia, irradiation, nutritional deficiencies and excesses, chemical agents, and mechanical forces.

Hydrocephalus is an excessive accumulation of cerebrospinal fluid within the ventricles, in the subarachnoid space about the brain, or in both. The degree of hydrocephalus is measured by the increased size of these structures rather than by measurement of fluid. Hydrocephalus affects about 1 of every 1000 newborns.

Prior to sonography, this condition was only detected when an anteroposterior (AP) radiograph of the abdomen was taken for fetal age or position. In the later stages of pregnancy, the fetus advances into the birth canal. In the past, a woman might have had a protracted labor because of her inability to give birth vaginally to a hydrocephalic fetus. A radiographic procedure known as a pelvimetry was ordered to determine the measurements of the pelvic inlet and outlet. This procedure caused the patient significant discomfort, since she was in active labor and had to be positioned for at least three exposures. It also resulted in a great deal of radiation to the fetus. If the measurements indicated that the birth canal was too narrow to accommodate the fetal head, a cesarean section was performed (Fig. 7–17). With sonography, we can now detect most congenital anomalies much earlier. Hydrocephalus can occur as a complication secondary to cerebral trauma or can be associated with many diseases affecting the brain.

Internal hydrocephalus is characterized by an ac-

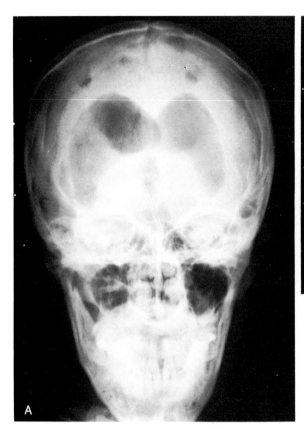

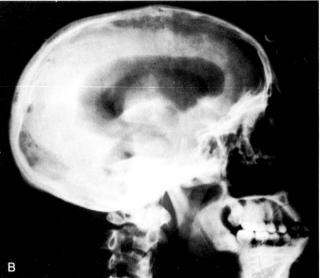

Figure 7–18. *(A)* Posteroanterior and *(B)* lateral views of a man's skull demonstrating communicating hydrocephalus as the result of adhesive arachnoiditis.

cumulation of cerebrospinal fluid that is limited to the ventricles. *External* hydrocephalus is the presence of excess fluid in the enlarged subarachnoid space over an atrophied brain. Hydrocephalus is also classified in terms of communication. In the communicating form, the flow of cerebrospinal fluid is free between the ventricles and the subarachnoid space about the cauda equina. In this form, the infant's head is of normal size but there is bulging of the frontal fontanelles. This is typically caused by faulty absorption of spinal fluid (Fig. 7–18).

When there is an obstruction between the ventricles and the cauda equina, the hydrocephalus is considered to be **noncommunicating.** The cerebro-

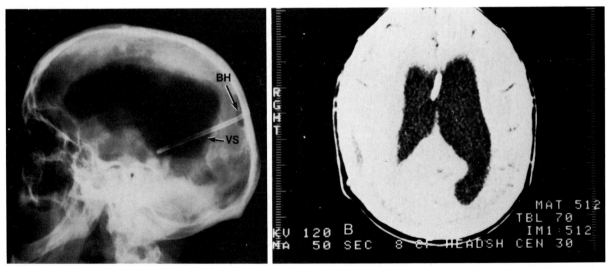

Figure 7–19. *A,* Obstructive hydrocephalus in a 41-year-old man, caused by the presence of a tumor. BH = bur hole; VS = ventriculovenous shunt. *B,* Marked obstructive hydrocephalus with a neoplasm in the posterior portion of the third ventricle in a 42-year-old man.

spinal fluid is produced by structures in the ventricles called choroid plexuses. The cerebrospinal fluid flows from one ventricle to another through interventricular passageways and into the subarachnoid space. The majority of the cerebrospinal fluid is returned to the venous system through the arachnoid villi, which lie in the several venous sinuses (Fig. 7–19).

Hydrocephalus is thought to develop from some abnormality along the route described. Of all forms of hydrocephalus, the form characterized by overproduction of spinal fluid is least common. Obstruction of the flow of spinal fluid is a common cause of hydrocephalus. The obstructing lesion can be developmental, neoplastic, inflammatory, or mechanical and can occur almost anywhere in the tract. However, the most common form of obstructive hydrocephalus results from an abnormality between the third and fourth ventricles. Specifically, the defect involves a malformation of the cerebral aqueduct or iter of Sylvius. This is a form of internal noncommunicating hydrocephalus. The pattern of ventricular enlargement can usually help determine the site of the obstructing lesion. Dilated ventricles are indicative of acute obstructive hydrocephalus. Once growth is complete, the fontanelles are closed. Thus all the spaces of the brain are of a fixed size. When conditions exist in which there is a loss of brain tissue, there is a compensatory increase in fluid within the spaces of the brain and spinal cord. Referred to as *compensatory* hydrocephalus, this is the most common form of hydrocephalus.

Diagnosis. The cranial size is clearly enlarged disproportionate to age. The scalp veins are distended, indicating increased venous pressure. The skin of the scalp is extremely thin, fragile, and shiny. The neck muscles are underdeveloped. In severe cases, the orbital roofs are depressed, the eyes are displaced downward, and the sclera is prominent. In the adult forms, the common signs include altered levels of consciousness, ataxia, incontinence, and decreased intellectual capabilities. PA projections of the skull reveal separation of the sutures and widening of the fontanelles. The ventricles are substantially distended (Fig. 7–20).

Treatment. The most effective treatment is a ventriculovenous *shunt.* This method allows for the passage of excess cerebrospinal fluid back into venous circulation via a catheter with one end placed in the lateral ventricle and the other end entering the common facial vein and passing into the internal jugular vein. Other shunts are also used. In a ventriculoatrial shunt, communication is made between the lateral ventricle and the cardiac atrium. In the ventriculoperitoneal shunt, a catheter is passed from the lateral ventricle to the peritoneum.

Cerebrovascular Disease

Cerebrovascular Accident (Stroke)

General Information. A cerebrovascular accident or stroke is a sudden impairment of cerebral circulation in one or more blood vessels supplying the brain. This interruption of blood flow, referred to as ischemia, results in a diminished supply of life-giving oxygen and leads to necrosis or death of the vital brain tissue. This area of ischemic necrosis is referred to as an infarct. A cerebral infarct or stroke is a serious condition that causes total disability in 50% of those who survive an initial episode. Recurrent strokes may affect the survivors in a matter of weeks,

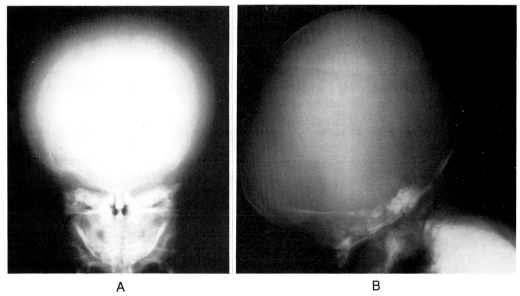

| A | B |

Figure 7–20. *(A)* Anteroposterior and *(B)* lateral views of the skull of a 1-day-old girl, revealing marked progressive hydrocephalus.

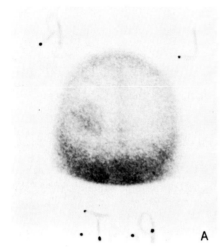

Figure 7–21. *(A)* Brain scan and *(B)* flow demonstrating large areas of increased nuclide activity in the right posterior hemisphere, consistent with cerebrovascular accident and cerebral hemorrhage, in a 38-year-old woman.

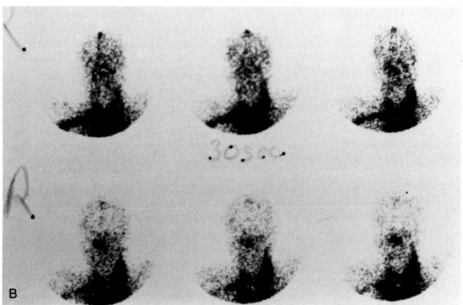

months, or years. Cerebrovascular accident is the third leading cause of death, the second leading cause of early death, and the most common cause of neurological disability. Approximately 500,000 people annually suffer from an initial stroke, and 50% of first-time strokes are fatal.

There are three major causes of stroke: thrombosis, embolism, and hemorrhage. Of the three, *thrombosis* is the leading cause, and it primarily affects the extracerebral arteries of middle-aged and older adults. The ischemic injury results from obstruction of a vessel. What circulation remains is usually collateral. Ischemia usually results in congestion and cerebral edema. There is a tendency for the stroke to occur during sleep, shortly after awakening, during surgery, or following myocardial infarction. The risk of cerebral thrombosis increases with obesity, smoking, and the use of oral contraceptives. In most cases, there is a history of transient ischemic attacks (TIAs), which followed a variable and gradual course. The symptoms occur intermittently. Most thromboses causing strokes are associated with a history of atherosclerosis, hypertension, or diabetes. Death is usually caused by massive cerebral damage.

Cerebral *embolism* is the second leading cause of stroke and is the result of vascular occlusion precipitated by several types of emboli, such as a clot, fat, a tumor, bacteria, a foreign body, or even air. The majority of cerebral embolic strokes are the result of a clot that breaks off the wall of the atrium during fibrillation. Fibrillation is an uncoordinated, ineffective type of heart rhythm originating in the right ventricle. This type of stroke can occur in any person of any age. However, individuals with a history of rheumatic heart disease, endocarditis, posttraumatic vascular disease, myocardial fibrillation and other cardiac arrhythmias, or postcardiac surgery are at increased risk. The middle cerebral artery is the artery most often obstructed by an embolism. Together, thrombosis and embolism account for 60% of all cerebral infarcts. If the embolus is septic, an abscess may form and encephalitis may develop later. It is also possible for the infarct to develop within the wall of a vessel, commonly producing an aneurysm and subsequent cerebral apoplexy or hemorrhage.

The third leading cause of stroke is *hemorrhage.* Cerebral hemorrhage may occur suddenly without warning, affecting any age-group. The precipitating causes are chronic hypertension or aneurysm that causes a gradual weakening of the vessel wall and subsequent hemorrhage of a major cerebral artery or one of its branches. Of those persons suffering a cerebral hemorrhage and stroke, 75% will succumb within 30 days of the initial incident.

Cerebrovascular accidents are classified according to their course of progress. TIAs are actually considered to be small strokes. They usually affect individuals older than 50 years, and the highest incidence is in black males. TIAs temporarily interrupt the arteries of the carotid and vertebrobasilar systems. The symptoms are sometimes minimal and are overlooked. On other occasions, the symptoms may last for 12 to 24 hours. In either event, the attacks are intermittent and are a warning of an impending thrombotic cerebrovascular accident. It has been reported that TIAs have occurred in approximately 50 to 80% of individuals who later suffered a stroke. In a TIA, minute microemboli are released from a mural thrombus and temporarily limit blood flow in the smaller distal branches of the cerebral arterial tree. The predisposing factors for TIA are similar to those of a stroke. In most cases, the incidents are episodic and the patient's symptoms disappear in a short time. The symptoms usually correspond to a specific arterial location. A progressive stroke or stroke in evolution is a condition that often occurs like the beginning of a TIA, in which there are some minimal deficits; however, in a couple of days the condition worsens. As the condition continues to worsen, it is evident that the neurological deficits are not transient, and their effects are considered to be maximal.

Diagnosis. The symptoms of strokes of all types depend on the arterial involvement. The internal carotid, anterior cerebral, middle cerebral, and vertebrobasilar arteries and their branches are most commonly affected. Severe headaches are often the earliest symptom. Other deficits include aphasia, dysphagia, hemiparesis, paralysis, numbness, vision disturbances, poor coordination, confusion, incontinence, personality change, dyslexia, and coma. Individuals with a history of TIAs, atherosclerosis, hypertension, diabetes, heart disease, or gout have a higher incidence of stroke. Persons who are obese, smoke cigarettes, do not exercise, have high serum triglyceride and cholesterol levels, use oral contraceptives, or have a family history of stroke are at increased risk (Fig. 7–21).

Treatment. Besides surgery, methods are usually preventive and palliative. Medications such as stool softeners, anticonvulsants, steroids, and certain analgesics are sometimes used. Aspirin is contraindicated since it increases the tendency for hemorrhage, but it is useful in the treatment of TIAs.

Hemorrhage

General Information. Hemorrhage is the escape of blood from a ruptured artery or vein. Massive brain hemorrhages are a common cause of death in patients with severe hypertension. The hemorrhages in fatal cases almost always have ruptured into the adjacent ventricle, with evidence of the presence of blood in the cerebrospinal fluid. Brain displacement with herniations and resultant brain stem hemorrhage are common. The part of the brain surrounding the hemorrhage is greatly swollen and edematous.

Four primary types of hemorrhage are identified. *Epidural* hemorrhage is an accumulation of blood in the temporal region as a result of traumatic rupture of the middle meningeal artery or its branches. Epidural hemorrhage commonly results from blunt skull trauma and is associated with recent skull fractures. The fracture line courses across a meningeal groove, causing separation of the dura from the inner table of the calvarium and tearing the artery. A clot forms within this space, causing compression of the underlying brain tissue. Because arterial hemorrhage is rapid, the patient is neurologically symptomatic almost immediately. Unless surgery is undertaken almost immediately, death can result from brain compression, with displacement, edema, and herniation (Fig. 7–22).

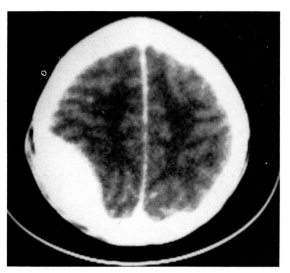

Figure 7–22. A curvilinear area of increased density in the right posterior lateral aspect of the right occiput, consistent with epidural hematoma, in a 21-year-old man involved in a motorcycle accident.

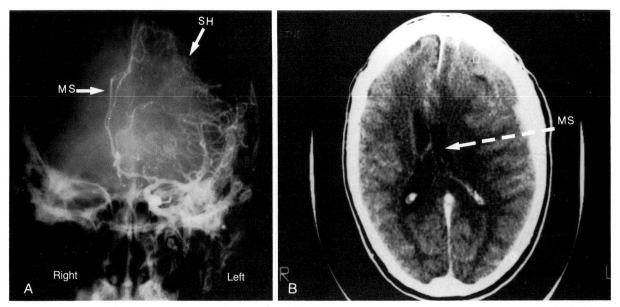

Figure 7–23. *A,* Cerebral angiogram, large subdural hematoma on the left with evidence of transfalx and hippocampal herniations in a 59-year-old man. MS = midline shift; SH = subdural hematoma. *B,* CT scan reveals considerable midline shift (MS) to the right.

Subdural hemorrhage refers to a slow, leaking type of venous hemorrhage occurring between the dura mater and the arachnoid membranes. This hemorrhage results from blunt trauma to the skull, with no evidence of fracture. On some occasions, this condition can occur in the absence of trauma. This is especially true of elderly patients with brain atrophy, in whom sudden anterior or posterior head movements may tear a small vein. The clot accumulates after a bridging vein is torn at the point where the vessel leaves the subdural space to enter the dura. This leaking of blood can be acute as well as chronic.

Most are found in the temporoparietal region and occur bilaterally. Subdural hematomas are associated with brain displacement, herniation, fatal brain stem hemorrhages, and neurogenic pulmonary edema (Figs. 7–23 and 7–24).

Subarachnoid hemorrhage results from blunt skull trauma, with or without fracture. Although hemorrhage can be the sole result of the trauma, postmortem examinations have revealed that the hemorrhages can be directly related to contusions and lacerations. Berry aneurysms often are the cause of subarachnoid hemorrhage. Berry aneurysms are fatal

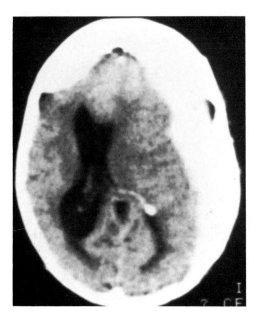

Figure 7–24. A very large left subdural hematoma, 3.3 cm in greatest dimension, extending all the way to the vertex in an 86-year-old woman.

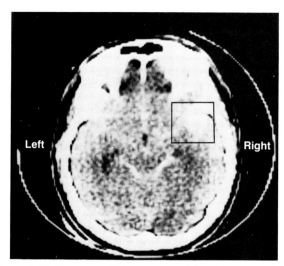

Figure 7–25. Subarachnoid hemorrhage of the right temporal region (square) in a 22-year-old man. A cerebral angiogram revealed the middle cerebral artery to be the source of the hemorrhage.

30% of the time and often occur at points of bifurcation along the circle of Willis. Postmortem examinations reveal that approximately 3% of subarachnoid hemorrhages involve a defect of the media of one of the cerebral arteries. Of all subarachnoid hemorrhages, 85% are found in the circle of Willis. The most commonly affected arteries include the anterior cerebral, the anterior communicating, and the posterior communicating arteries (Fig. 7–25).

Intracerebral hemorrhage often is caused by hemangiomas, a rupture of vessels weakened by long-term hypertension, or nonpenetrating skull trauma. This form of hematoma is common in the frontal lobe but can be found in the cerebellum, midbrain, and pons. The larger hemorrhages are usually fatal (Fig. 7–26).

Diagnosis. The diagnosis is usually confirmed by the clinical history, symptoms, signs, and laboratory and radiology test results. Signs and symptoms of hemorrhage and increased intracranial pressure are corroborated by spinal fluid analysis. CT and cerebral angiography are imaging modalities that demonstrate the lesion.

Treatment. In the presence of intracranial pressure, a surgical craniotomy is indicated. In the event of trauma, cerebral angiography is performed to determine the extent of intracerebral circulation. Except for surgery, treatment is mostly conservative. Mannitol may be given to reduce cerebral edema. The patient is maintained on strict bed rest, and the vital signs are checked regularly. If a compound depressed skull fracture is present, infection is a possible complication. Meningitis is an especially serious complication. Early coma is common with epidural hemorrhage, and delayed coma is common with subdural hemorrhage.

Aneurysm

General Information. An aneurysm is a localized, abnormal, persistent expansion, dilatation, or outpouching of a vessel, usually an artery. It is caused by a weakness in the vessel wall and is often described as a pulsating tumor or a bruit heard over the swelling. An aneurysm generally involves all three layers of a vessel wall and may be congenital or acquired. Most aneurysms tend to enlarge with time. They can be classed according to the composition of the wall of the dilatation (a true aneurysm versus a false aneurysm), by shape, or by the pathogenic mechanism.

A *true* aneurysm includes all three layers of the arterial wall and is closely associated with atherosclerosis. A *false* aneurysm contains a fibrous wall and is the result of a vessel rupture, with the formation of a cavity contained by the outer adventitial and perivascular tissues. False aneurysms are associated with trauma.

Saccular and fusiform aneurysms are the two most common forms. Fusiform aneurysms are found in various locations of the aorta and peripheral arteries. The focus of this discussion will be confined to the saccular aneurysm, which is most common in the cerebrovascular system.

A *saccular* aneurysm is a spherical protrusion with a reasonably defined neck or origin that affects a part of the vessel circumference. Cerebral aneurysms for

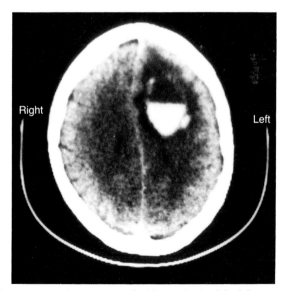

Figure 7–26. A huge intracerebral hemorrhage of the left frontoparietal area in a 67-year-old man. Fluid level is identified within the hematoma. A low density about the hematoma suggests edema. There is a midline shift to the right.

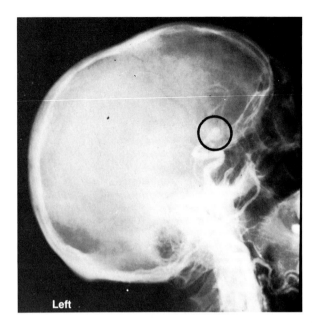

Figure 7–27. Berry aneurysm of the left internal carotid artery.

the most part involve the arteries of the circle of Willis. These aneurysms may be classified as berry or congenital, atherosclerotic, inflammatory, mycotic, or traumatic. The berry or congenital aneurysm is a developmental defect and is of the greatest clinical significance. These aneurysms are found in 5 to 6% of all adults at postmortem examinations. This finding is twice as common in women as in men, although there is no apparent reason why this is so. Of the aneurysms found during postmortem examinations, 40% show evidence of hemorrhage or rupture, 30% are multiple, and about two-thirds are bilateral. A history of hypertension is present in 60% of those

with aneurysms both with and without hemorrhage. The average age at the time of rupture is 50 to 55 years. There is a 25 to 50% mortality rate on the first rupture. In those with fatal ruptures, 50% succumb within 24 hours, the vast majority within the first hour, and approximately 95% within 2 weeks. The cerebral vessels of the anterior portion of the circle of Willis are involved about six times more frequently than those vessels of the posterior part of the circle of Willis. The bottom, or fundus, of the berry-shaped aneurysm is the weakest portion of the aneurysm and the most likely location of rupture. In most cases of rupture, the hemorrhage takes place into the sub-

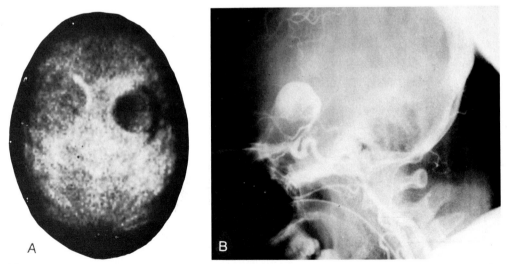

Figure 7–28. *A*, A 7-cm giant aneurysm of the right middle cerebral artery as demonstrated on CT scan of a 42-year-old woman. *B*, Right lateral view of a cerebral angiogram showing the same lesion.

arachnoid space. There may be adjacent extension of hemorrhage into the ventricles. Cerebral displacement, herniation, and brain stem hemorrhage are common secondary complications (Fig. 7–27).

Elderly patients frequently have aneurysms involving the first or second major bifurcations of either middle cerebral artery. Age-related vessel weakening, hypertension, and advanced arteriosclerosis are frequent causes of aneurysm formation. This aneurysm may also be associated with meningitis, a brain abscess, or a cerebral infarct. Leakage or rupture of the aneurysm into the subarachnoid space is common (Fig. 7–28).

Diagnosis. Several tests and procedures are used in the diagnosis of cerebral aneurysms. A lumbar puncture may detect the presence of blood in the cerebrospinal fluid, as well as increased intracranial pressure. If there is calcification of the walls of an aneurysm, it may be seen on plain radiographs of the skull. CT scanning, cerebral angiography, and MR imaging offer three methods of imaging. After a history is taken and a physical neurological examination is performed, the baseline CT scan is obtained as soon as possible, even if the diagnosis is obvious from a clinical standpoint. The CT scan usually provides confirmation by demonstrating subarachnoid hemorrhage and also provides information on the location of the ruptured aneurysm. An angiogram can indicate the specific vessel involved, but the decision to use this technique is primarily made by the neurosurgeon. Angiography is necessary when one of four situations exists: (1) when there is a question about the diagnosis, (2) when early clipping of the aneurysm is being considered, (3) prior to the removal of a hematoma, or (4) in cases of hematoma of the temporal lobe from aneurysm of the middle cerebral artery. When the CT scan reveals a definite subarachnoid hemorrhage, a lumbar puncture is not necessary. If CT shows marked ventricular enlargement or a hematoma, a lumbar puncture would be a most dangerous procedure. The CT scan may also reveal swelling of the brain caused by edema (Fig. 7–29). If the initial diagnosis of subarachnoid hemorrhage from an aneurysm is in doubt, then a cerebral angiogram is indicated at the outset, to visualize the aneurysm. When evacuation of an intracerebral hematoma is planned, angiography must be performed to show the location of the aneurysm. Cerebral angiography is preferred in cases of aneurysms of the middle cerebral artery because clots are common within the aneurysm. In the presence of clots, the patient's condition may deteriorate, and draining the clot becomes necessary.

Treatment. Angiography with biplane filming is indicated just prior to surgery to demonstrate the vessel responsible for feeding the aneurysm. Angiographic filming usually includes both carotids and vertebrals. This is necessary because of the high frequency of multiple aneurysms, which are present

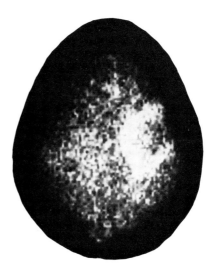

Figure 7–29. Contrast-enhanced CT scan revealing a lesion of the right parietal lobe in a 39-year-old man. There is a 4-cm area of decreased density (D), which is compatible with edema, and there is a 1.5-cm area of enhancement (E).

about 25% of the time. Once the feeder vessel is identified, additional projections are obtained to demonstrate the relationship of the vessels in the vicinity of the aneurysm. Surgical repair, when possible, involves clipping, ligation, or wrapping the aneurysm with muscle.

Head Injuries

The large majority of head injuries are due to traffic accidents. Head injuries are present in 65% of all injured persons and account for 71% of all traffic-related fatalities, including passengers and pedestrians. The remaining 39% occur at home and in violent criminal acts. Head injuries are associated with a mortality rate of 6.5%.

In 25% of persons who die of head injuries, there are no signs of skull fracture. It is important to note that despite the fact that skull x-rays are taken for the majority of head injuries, radiological demonstration of skull fractures is of secondary importance. Trauma to the brain and brain stem is of primary importance. There is often no direct correlation between the severity of brain damage on one side and the degree of an existing skull fracture on the opposite side. The skull series (x-rays) is used to determine if this correlation exists. The greatest danger is from *shock* and not from fracture. X-ray studies may be postponed and primary measures initiated to treat or prevent shock, cerebral edema, hemorrhage, central nervous system respiratory depression, and aspiration.

Since the advent of CT scanning, skull x-rays have taken a further secondary role in diagnosis. A CT scanning department operates 24 hours a day, and a technologist frequently is on site or only minutes away. Since a CT scan can detect early hemorrhage, it is invaluable for early diagnosis. Although CT is now preferred, skull x-ray films are still performed if the patient's condition permits.

The skull series usually includes an AP semi-axial projection (Grashey/Towne), direct PA, PA with 15-degree caudal angle, parietoacanthial (Waters'), submentovertical or verticosubmental cranial base, and both lateral projections. Stereoscopic views are occasionally ordered on the Waters' and Towne's methods and on the lateral projections. Accuracy of positioning in the lateral projections can be assured by observing the superimposition of the mandibular rami and supraorbital plates. The lateral views reveal fractures of major bones of the skull and face and structures such as the orbits, sinuses, and sella turcica. The AP semi-axial projection is useful in observing the occipital bone, foramen magnum, and petrous ridges. The direct PA projection of the skull delineates the frontal bone to best advantage, as well as the petrous ridges, nasal cavities, and posterior part of the skull. The angled PA projection gives a clear evaluation of the medial, lateral, and superior borders of the orbits, ethmoidal sinuses, and nasal cavities. The cranial base projections (Schüller's method) best reveal the cranial floor (Fig. 7–30). Stereo views are advantageous for observing penetrating foreign bodies.

In performing skull radiographs, it is important to review the form, shape, and symmetry of the skull and the internal and external contours, including the density of the tables, the distinction of sutures, the vascular channels, and potential fractures. The vascular channels may be differentiated by size. The venous channels are wider than the arterial channels. It is important to check the form and delineation of anatomical landmarks such as the sella turcica, petrous bones, orbits, mastoids, and the possibility of a shift of the pineal gland, which could indicate an epidural or subdural hematoma. The sinuses should be delineated. Sinus cavity transparency versus opacity and air-fluid levels are clinically significant. An opaque appearance may imply a tear in the dura, a fracture, an exudate, or a hemorrhage. Air may also be observed in the subarachnoid space. One must pay attention to the facial contour, including the temporomandibular joints. In the lateral view, a visibly opaque sphenoidal sinus could indicate a fracture of the sellar floor (roof of the sphenoidal sinus). The presence of soft tissue swelling may indicate the extensiveness of the trauma. A fracture line crossing the groove of the middle meningeal artery may be indicative of an epidural hemorrhage or hematoma.

Radionuclide scanning is another diagnostic method that has in large part been replaced by CT scanning. This method of brain scanning requires intravenous injection of a radioactive isotope (technetium). The isotope accumulates in the lesion and is seen as an area of increased uptake.

Cerebral angiography, although not performed routinely, is used when there is a need to discern the level of cerebral circulation. Angiography can demonstrate complete stasis of brain vessels, which, along with a flat electroencephalograph, is the current criterion for determining brain death. Angiography may also establish the presence of a hematoma and may indicate whether or not it can be surgically approached. Generally, if the patient shows signs of severe functional central nervous system loss, this procedure is not necessary.

When there is evidence of severe trauma of the skull and brain, there is often an audible **bruit** of the eye. The eye may pulsate and protrude (exophthalmos), with marked dilatation and arterialization of veins in the eye (conversion of venous blood to arterial blood with high oxygen content). These findings may be diagnostic of an arteriovenous fistula between the internal carotid artery and the cavernous sinuses (which are irregular-shaped venous channels between layers of the dura mater of the brain, one on either side of the body of the sphenoid bone that communicates across the midline). These findings are usually evident in the most severe head injuries resulting from vehicular accidents. Angiography reveals simultaneous opacification of the internal carotid artery and an abnormally enlarged cavernous sinus, together with the petrous sinus and internal jugular vein. This condition is not without complications. Vascular occlusion, fat embolism, saccular aneurysms, a draining abscess (from penetrating wounds), and meningitis all are possible complications. In this type of severe traumatic head injury, cerebrospinal fluid may leak from the nose and ear. When this fluid is found on the bed linen as a yellowish stain, it is referred to as the **halo sign** and may indicate a skull fracture that extends through the anterior base of the skull or posterior wall of the frontal sinus. This drainage occurs when there is a tear of the dura, which is common in cranial base fracture. Angiography reveals the presence of an epidural or subdural hematoma by displacement of

Figure 7–30. Routine projections of the skull. *A,* Posteroanterior. *B,* Semiaxial (Grashey/Towne's). *C,* Right lateral. *D,* Left lateral. *E,* Parietoacanthial (Waters'). *F,* Submentovertical.

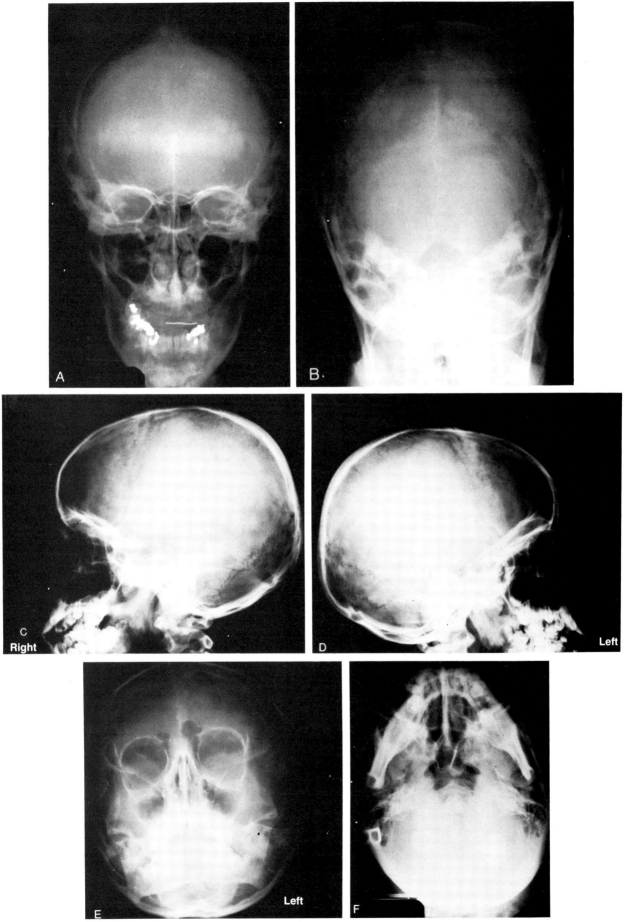

Figure 7–30 *See legend on opposite page*

vessels away from the skull, with a free space of vasculature between the contrasting vessels of the brain surface and the inner table of the skull. When the anterior cerebral artery displaces toward the opposite side despite a proven hematoma, another hematoma may be pressing on the opposite side.

Of all brain hematomas and hemorrhages, about 65% are subdural, about 25% are epidural, and about 10% are intracerebral. If the location of the hemorrhage is anterior, the artery is displaced toward the opposite side (epidural and subdural) and forms an arch toward the opposing side. If the hemorrhage is posterior, the anterior cerebral artery is displaced in parallel fashion. Unilateral brain edema is also usually evident. Recent statistics have shown that patient with skull fractures have a subdural hematoma on the opposite side of the fracture 65 to 75% of the time. With fractures intersecting the middle meningeal artery, epidural hematoma is found on the side having a fracture.

Concussion

General Information. A *concussion* is a violent blow to the head that causes the brain to shift within the vault and strike the adjacent cranial wall, resulting in loss of consciousness. This is the most common head injury, and it is less severe than a cerebral contusion. Most patients recover within 24 to 48 hours. Headaches may be severe but will abate with time. Analgesics are usually not given with any type of head injury, since they may mask the symptoms. This type of injury is common in child abuse, falls occurring in the home, vehicular accidents, and fights in which the individual is punched in the head. The signs and symptoms include short-term loss of consciousness, headache, vertigo, and vomiting. The patient usually cannot recall the incident itself or the events leading up to it. Behavioral changes such as lethargy and irritability are sometimes noted.

Diagnosis. The diagnosis is typically made by taking the history of the incident and by performing a complete neurological examination. This examination determines the patient's level of consciousness, mental state, cranial nerve and motor function, deep tendon and abdominal reflexes, and orientation as to name, time, place, and so on. CT scans and skull x-ray films are usually indicated to rule out hemorrhage or fracture.

Treatment. The treatment for concussion is very conservative. The major emphasis is placed on maintaining bed rest, checking vital signs, and checking for any signs of hemorrhage or hematoma. The patient is often admitted to the hospital for 24 to 36 hours.

Contusion

General Information. In *contusion,* the brain is bruised but the skin is not broken. This injury is far more serious than a concussion and may involve broken blood vessels, possibly resulting in an epidural or subdural hematoma. This may disrupt normal nerve function in the affected area and may result in loss of consciousness, hemorrhage, edema, and possibly death. A contusion usually results from direct impact, often by a blunt object, and occurs in vehicular accidents and acts of violence. The injury is characterized by acceleration of the brain, when it moves forward suddenly, and deceleration, when it rebounds backward. The brain is injured where it strikes a bony prominence inside the skull, especially the sphenoidal ridge, resulting in hemorrhage or hematoma followed by tentorial herniation (the brain stem forcefully presses against or herniates into the foramen magnum). Cerebral edema is also usually present.

Diagnosis. Brain contusion may be associated with scalp and facial lacerations and on some occasions with labored respiratory function. The patient is usually unconscious from minutes to as long as 1 hour. On regaining consciousness, the patient is usually drowsy, confused, disoriented, agitated, or violent. Transitory hemiparesis or unilateral numbness is common, and the pupils may be unequal. Unequal pupils are indicative of intracranial pressure, usually the result of tentorial herniation. The origin of the intracranial pressure is often an epidural or subdural hematoma. Because epidural hemorrhage is arterial, the neurological signs rapidly become evident. In subdural hemorrhage, which is venous, the bleeding is slow and neurological signs may not be evident for 24 to 36 hours. CT scans indicate findings such as cerebral edema, ischemia, hemorrhage or necrosis, and skull fracture. Skull x-ray films primarily reveal the presence of fracture. Angiography determines the patency of cerebral vessels and the presence of a hematoma. Obviously, a full neurological examination should be conducted. Signs of impending hematoma and increased intracranial pressure may be noted.

Treatment. The treatment is usually quite conservative. Bed rest is imperative, and intravenous feedings can help prevent shock. Medications such as mannitol may be given to control cerebral edema. If the patient is unconscious, insertion of a nasogastric tube can help prevent aspiration. At regular intervals, the nose and ears should be inspected for central nervous system leaks (cerebrospinal fluid). If a hematoma is present, a craniotomy is performed to control bleeding and to aspirate blood.

Fractures

General Information. Skull fractures are considered a neurosurgical condition because of the potential for damage to the brain. Skull fractures are classified according to their location: Calvarial fractures occur in the bones of the cranial vault. Basilar fractures may be found in the bones of the cranial base or floor. Facial fractures are those afflicting any of the facial structures.

Fractures of the skull and face are revealed as irregular *radiolucent* lines on x-ray films, except for depressed fractures, which may appear as a curvilinear density as a result of overlapping fragments. Fractures usually appear more radiolucent than vascular markings since they traverse the full thickness of the bone. Fractures usually have jagged edges, and it is usually possible to see how the jagged edges fit together. Fractures branch or may abruptly change direction. Venous channels are *wider* and have more undulating grooves. They appear to course back and forth in a sinuous (bending) fashion. Arterial grooves have *parallel* sides that are nonundulating and are often mistaken for a fracture. Fractures of the skull can be open or closed. They may vary from those producing no displacement to those producing severe displacement.

The usual cause of skull fractures is direct violence or trauma to the head, often from a blunt object. The three most common causes of skull fractures, in their order of frequency, are motor vehicle accidents, severe falls, and premeditated violence. Skull fractures are often accompanied by other types of head wounds such as abrasions, contusions, lacerations, and avulsions. The head is very vascular, and even the most minor wound can result in hemorrhage. In many cases, the hemorrhage is quite profuse. It is common to find injuries of both the face and skull simultaneously, with lacerations and fractures being very common.

Diagnosis. Skull fractures present a variety of signs and symptoms. In addition to the usual scalp and soft tissue injury, varied amounts of hemorrhage are possible. In severe cases, evidence of hypovolemic shock (shock produced by loss of blood volume) and signs of brain injury must be dealt with immediately. Some of the signs of brain injury include agitation and irritability followed by unconsciousness and changes in respiration (labored). These altered states of consciousness may last hours, days, weeks, or indefinitely. Cerebral edema may impair the flow of impulses to the brain, resulting in respiratory distress. Metal fragments may rupture blood vessels, resulting in subdural, epidural, or intracerebral hemorrhage or hematoma.

In cases of severe skull injury, fractures of the cranial base are most common. About 75% of cranial base fractures involve the middle cranial fossa. For the most part, midfossa fractures are not demonstrated on survey films of the skull. They often result in hemorrhage from the ears, mouth, and nose. If the dura mater is torn, cerebrospinal fluid drainage from the nose and ears commonly is noted. Permanent neurological deficits result from 50% of midfossa fractures.

About 25% of all fractures of the cranial base involve the anterior cranial fossa, specifically the cribriform plate and frontal sinuses. Fluid levels are present 33% of the time when cranial base fractures are present. To view fluid levels (assuming the patient is recumbent) requires a horizontal x-ray beam. Leakage of cerebrospinal fluid indicates a cranial base fracture, even if the fracture is not identified on the skull radiographs. Cerebrospinal fluid leaking from the ear usually implies that there is a fracture of the petrous portion of the temporal bone.

Besides the described signs and symptoms, other complications may be in evidence. Convulsive (jacksonian) epilepsy may be noted. The radiographer should be aware that any posttraumatic skull injury can result in convulsive seizures at any time; thus it is recommended that a second person be present to give assistance. A method of summoning emergency personnel should be established. A patient wtih a head injury should never be left unattended. Other complications include hydrocephalus and infections such as meningitis or brain abscess.

As a rule of thumb, brain injury should be suspected in all skull fractures until clinical evaluation indicates otherwise. The most immediate and important diagnostic procedures include CT scans, skull x-ray films, neurological examination, and electroencephalogram. An angiogram is necessary only when neurosurgery is contemplated. Analyzing spinal fluid for gross blood and observing for the *halo sign* on the bed sheets are two other methods of diagnosis. The halo sign is a blood-tinged spot surrounded by a lighter ring of spinal fluid.

Treatment. The treatment of skull fractures is usually supportive and is directed at the signs and symptoms that are present. Ongoing treatment for shock is mandatory. With cranial vault fractures, hemorrhage is of major concern. Thus, a craniotomy may be performed to aspirate blood and remove bony fragments and necrotic tissue, to relieve pressure, and to prevent infection. When a significant amount of bone has been destroyed by the injury or removed during surgery, a cranioplasty is performed and a tantalum mesh or acrylic plate is sewn in place. Antibiotic therapy is used, especially in fractures of the cranial base. Intravenous feedings are given to reduce cerebral edema and decrease inflammation.

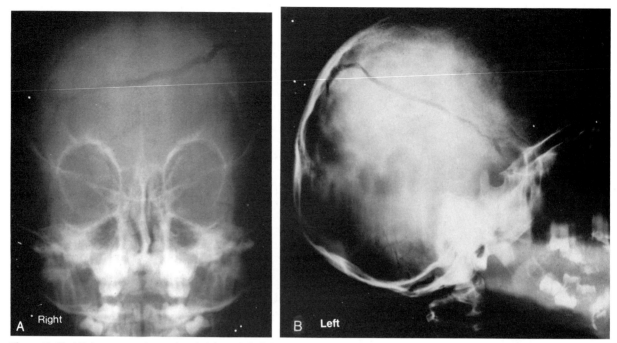

Figure 7–31. (A) Anteroposterior and (B) left lateral skull films demonstrating a long linear fracture extending across the temporoparietal region as the result of direct blunt trauma in a 7-year-old boy.

Linear

A linear fracture is a common hair-like break, usually without any displacement. It is best visualized with the affected side closest to the film. It is always best to attempt to align the affected part as parallel to the film as possible. Linear fractures must be delineated from sutures and vascular markings (Fig. 7–31).

Comminuted

A comminuted fracture is one in which the bone is splintered or crushed into many fragments. This type of fracture is usually the result of direct massive trauma. Comminution of bone fragments is often associated with depressed and penetrating fractures due to missiles. On occasion, a particular bone may have two or more individual fractures. For example, the parietal bone often has more than one fracture line (usually linear), but the fragments are large rather than splintered. In all skull fractures and especially in those of the comminuted variety, it is important to determine if the fractures penetrated into cavities such as the sinuses or crossed over vascular grooves. Fractures often tear vascular structures when crossing their grooves. This is especially true of the middle meningeal groove and correspond-

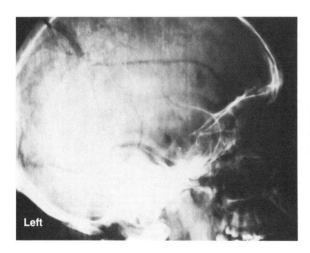

Figure 7–32. Multiple comminuted linear fracture of the frontal, parietal, temporal, and occipital bones in a 24-year-old man. The injuries were sustained when his motorcycle struck a utility pole. The patient was not wearing a protective helmet.

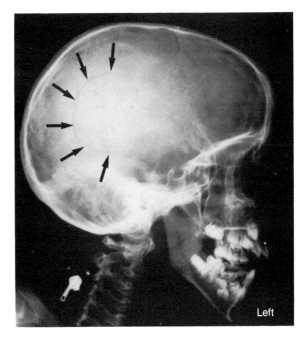

Figure 7–33. Left lateral skull view demonstrating a depressed curvilinear fracture of the left midparietal region without displacement in an 8-year-old girl who was struck with a baseball bat. This is sometimes referred to as an eggshell fracture.

ing artery, which if torn can produce epidural hemorrhage or a hematoma (Fig. 7–32).

Depressed

Depressed fractures usually present a *curvilinear* appearance due to blunt trauma. Causes of this type of fracture include weapons such as baseball bats, lead pipes, and hammers. Falls from ladders and roofs commonly cause this type of injury. Depressed fractures usually present overlapping fragments. Correct and rapid recognition is of greatest importance,

because injury may require immediate surgical intervention. In a less severe form, the area of fracture may resemble a broken eggshell. In an eggshell fracture, the bone may be comminuted but no displacement or severe depression is evident. Radiographically, tangential, lateral, and anterior views demonstrate this type of fracture to best advantage (Fig. 7–33 and 7–34).

Projectile/Penetrating

Projectile/penetrating fracture is most common as a result of gunshot incidents and industrial accidents

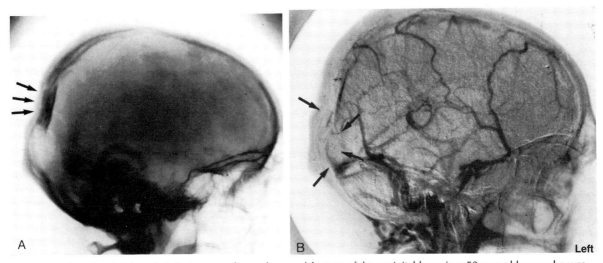

Figure 7–34. *A*, Subtraction left lateral skull view revealing a depressed fracture of the occipital bone in a 52-year-old man who was struck from behind with a gun butt. For 2 weeks after initial emergency treatment, the patient complained of headaches. *B*, A cerebral angiogram revealed that the fractured fragments compressed the sagittal sinus, resulting in partial occlusion, as demonstrated on the venous phase.

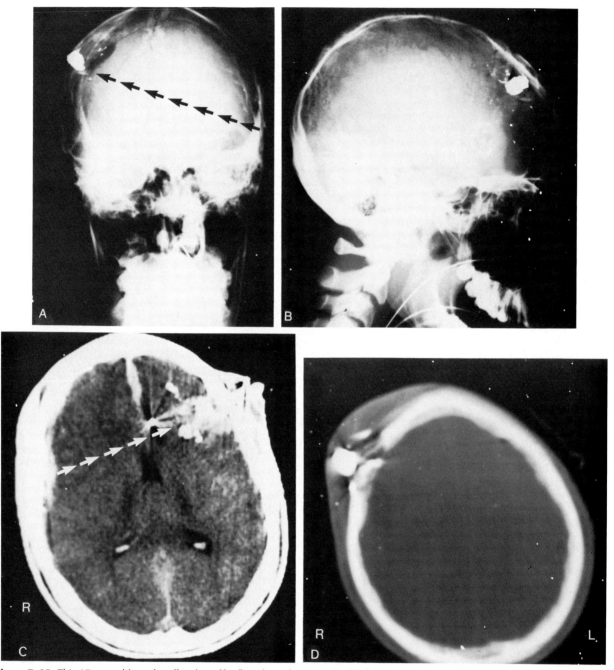

Figure 7–35. This 17-year-old youth suffered a self-inflicted gunshot wound while playing Russian roulette. *(A)* Posteroanterior and *(B)* lateral skull films reveal multiple metallic fragments in the bony calvarium anteriorly, with a large bullet fragment in the right temporal region and an obvious bullet tract extending from the left side and traversing upward and exiting on the right side of the skull. The bullet entered on the left side of the skull. *C,* CT scan revealing the bullet fragment tracking from the left temporofrontal area obliquely upward to the right frontal region. There is associated subarachnoid bleeding, and there appears to be generalized edema. *D,* A small extracerebral hematoma is also present on the right, with posttraumatic pneumocephalus.

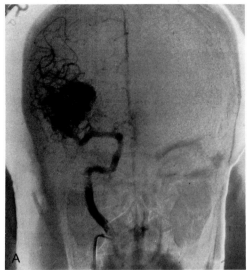

Figure 7–36. This 55-year-old man with developing headaches and seizures had suffered a gunshot wound in 1951 while in Korea. *(A)* Frontal and *(B)* lateral cerebral angiogram views reveal an arteriovenous malformation of a frontoparietal branch of the middle cerebral artery.

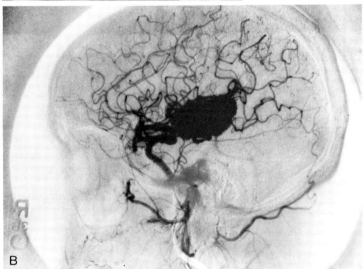

in which metal bolts and fragments enter the skull as missiles. This type of injury often combines linear, depressed, and comminuted fractures in a single wound. The locations of the entrance and exit wounds are most important. Fragmental shattering of metal produces multiple foreign bodies scattered throughout the brain substance (Fig. 7–35).

Arteriovenous Fistula/Malformation

General Information. Arteriovenous fistula is a direct communication between an artery and a vein. It is usually the result of trauma and is often associated with a direct blow to the frontal region. It can also be associated with fracture of one of the bones of the paranasal sinuses. This fistula is the result of a disruption of the internal carotid artery where it passes through the lamina of the cavernous sinuses. Once the arteriovenous fistula has been formed, the veins in this area become engorged with arterial blood.

Diagnosis. Arteriovenous fistulas/malformations frequently originate from a branch of the middle cerebral artery, which consists of a tangle of dilated vessels (Fig. 7–36).

Treatment. Surgery is the treatment of choice for most arteriovenous fistulous communications/malformations.

The Spinal Cord

Congenital Malformations

Spina Bifida

General Information. Spina bifida is one of the most common malformations of the spine, involving the neural arch. This condition occurs in about 5%

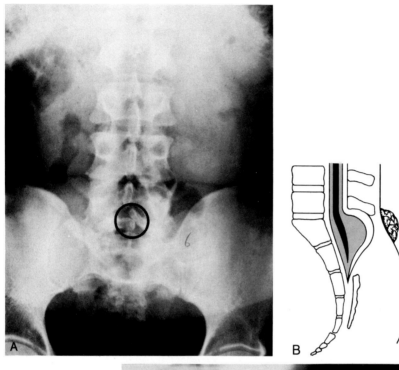

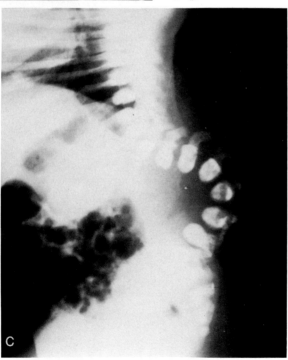

Figure 7–37. *A*, Spina bifida occulta of L6, a transitional (extra) vertebra. Anteroposterior view of the lumbar spine of a 53-year-old man. *B*, Spina bifida occulta, lateral view. *C*, Stillborn girl with acute spina bifida.

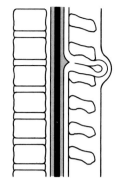

Figure 7–38. Meningocele.

of live births. Annually more than 12,000 people are born afflicted with some form of spina bifida. The incidence is highest in those of Welsh or Irish ancestry. If a defect occurs during the development of the embryonal mesodermal tissues, a gap may occur in the neural arch or the lamina, through which the spinal contents may or may not protrude. In spina bifida occulta, there is incomplete closure of the neural arch, resulting in a gap of the lamina but no protrusion of the spinal contents. Spina bifida occulta most frequently is found in the lumbosacral region, the levels of L-4 to L-5 and L-5 to S-1 being the most common locations. It is the most common but least serious spinal cord defect (Fig. 7–37). In spina bifida cystica, a cystic swelling of the meninges or spinal cord protrudes through the defect. Spina bifida with meningeal protrusion is referred to as ***meningocele,*** which is actually a local defect in the bone and dura (Fig. 7–38). Spina bifida with protrusion of the spinal cord is referred to as ***myelocele*** (Fig. 7–39). The most serious variety of spina bifida is ***myelomeningocele,*** in which both the meninges and spinal cord protrude (Fig. 7–40).

Diagnosis. Spina bifida occulta is often accompanied by a depression or dimple, tuft of hair, soft fatty deposits, or port-wine mole or a combination of these on the skin over the spinal defect. It is possible that all visible signs may be absent. Ordinarily, spina

bifida occulta does not cause neurological dysfunction, but foot weakness or bowel and bladder disturbances are occasionally present during the phases of rapid growth when the spinal cord's ascent within the vertebral column may be impaired by its abnormal adherence to other tissues. Although they are often overlooked, AP radiographs of the lumbosacral spine reveal the bony defect. CT scans and myelograms may be obtained to rule out other spinal cord diseases and tumors. In patients with large open lesions, bilateral leg paralysis is not uncommon. The prognosis varies with degree of neurological deficit.

Treatment. In the most serious cases, surgical closure of the protruding sac is attempted. However, the neurological deficit is permanent and cannot be reversed. Most of the measures taken are supportive rather than corrective and include vigorous physical therapy, other physical supports, braces, and splints.

Spinal Disk Disease

General Information. The intervertebral disks consist of a dense ring of fibrous tissue called the anulus fibrosus, which surrounds a soft pulp-like center referred to as the nucleus pulposus. When subjected to heavy pressure, the nucleus may force itself through a weakened or torn anulus. When the disk prolapses backward, it protrudes into the spinal canal and may impinge on the cauda equina or a nerve root as it passes downward toward its intervertebral foramen. It may then cause pain that can be felt in the distribution of the nerve root and weakness in the muscles supplied by it. Disk disease may be related to aging and advanced arthritic disease, as well as to trauma and strain.

Diagnosis. The neurosurgeon or orthopedic surgeon obtains a detailed patient history. Among the diagnostic tests for disk herniation is the straight-leg raising test. In this test, the patient lies supine and the physician applies support to the pelvis while placing the other hand under the ankle and slowly raising the leg. If the patient complains of pain down

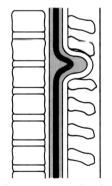

Figure 7–39. Myelocele.

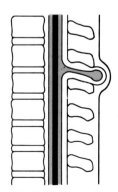

Figure 7–40. Myelomeningocele.

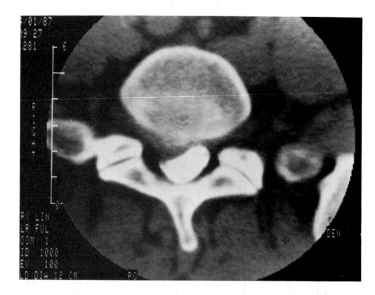

Figure 7–41. CT scan showing a large herniated disk, which is notably deforming the thecal sac. The disk material is extruded somewhat inferior to the level of the disk space. The patient is a 27-year-old man.

the posterior buttock and thigh, disk disease is a diagnostic consideration. Radiographs are useful for demonstrating joint narrowing and for ruling out other obvious causes. CT scans and myelography currently provide the most definitive diagnosis of disk disease (Figs. 7–41, 7–42, and 7–43).

Treatment. At first, the treatment is conservative: bed rest, traction, physical therapy, analgesics, and steroid therapy. If the patient's pain is not relieved, surgery is indicated. Laminectomy with spinal fusion is the usual surgical procedure. This is followed up with about 2 weeks of postoperative bed rest, and

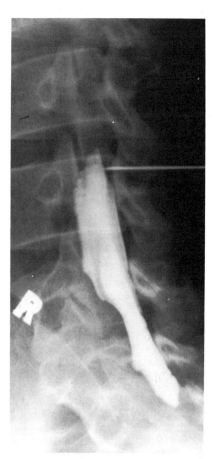

Figure 7–42. Lumbar myelogram revealing a herniated disk at the L5-S1 level in a 42-year-old man. An oil-based contrast medium was employed.

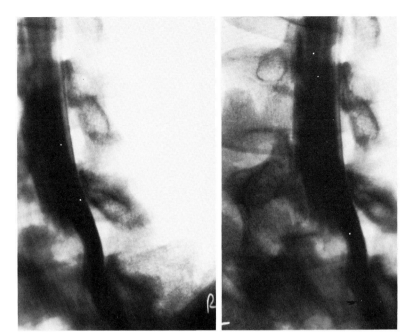

Figure 7–43. A large extradural defect on the left side of L5-S1, compatible with a herniated disk, in a 17-year-old female. A water-soluble contrast medium was employed.

then careful mobilization with a back support. When strict criteria for surgery are established, the success rate is high. Since a large majority of patients are younger than 50 years, there is a good chance of an acceptable recovery.

A relatively new procedure, chemonucleolysis, is actually a diskogram that includes the injection of an enzyme known as chymopapain directly into the bulging disk. When the technique is successful, the enzyme shrinks the swollen disk and thereby reduces the prolapse. Although this procedure is not indicated for all types of disk disease, it has offered eligible candidates an alternative to a surgical laminectomy and spinal fusion (Fig. 7–44).

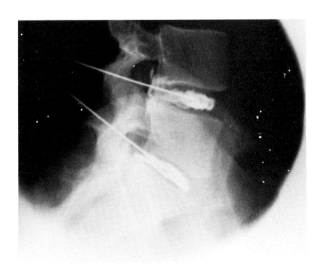

Figure 7–44. Diskogram and injection of chymopapain into the L4-5 and L5-S1 disk levels in a 26-year-old man.

Self-Assessment Quiz

For each of the following questions, select the one best response and circle the letter that precedes it.

1. The pineal gland is found
   a. to the right of the midline
   b. in the midline
   c. to the left of the midline

2. In relation to the choroid plexus, the pineal gland is located somewhat
   a. anterior and inferior
   b. anterior and superior
   c. posterior and inferior
   d. posterior and superior

3. Computed tomography is currently the method of choice for demonstrating spinal cord abscesses and neoplasms.
   a. true
   b. false

4. The most sensitive technique for detecting brain lesions is
   a. computed tomography
   b. pneumoencephalogram
   c. magnetic resonance imaging
   d. skull x-ray

5. Excessive accumulation of cerebrospinal fluid within the cerebral ventricles is termed
   a. meningocele
   b. myelocele
   c. hydrocephalus
   d. Down's syndrome

6. Most cases of hydrocephalus result when there is a congenital defect of the
   a. third ventricle
   b. fourth ventricle
   c. cerebral aqueduct
   d. brain stem

7. Which of the following are major causes of stroke?
   a. thrombosis
   b. embolism and hemorrhage
   c. thrombosis and embolism
   d. thrombosis, embolism, and hemorrhage

8. Which of the following is the leading cause of stroke?
   a. thrombosis
   b. embolism
   c. hemorrhage

9. Which type of hemorrhage most often occurs in skull fracture?
   a. subarachnoid
   b. epidural
   c. intracerebral
   d. subdural

10. A slow leaking of venous blood following blunt head injury is
    a. subarachnoid
    b. epidural
    c. intracerebral
    d. subdural

11. Saccular and fusiform are types of
    a. brain tumors
    b. blood clots
    c. aneurysms
    d. hemorrhages

12. Which of the following are examples of aneurysms?
    a. berry
    b. mycotic
    c. congenital
    d. traumatic
    e. all of the above

13. Which artery is commonly associated with aneurysms in elderly patients?
    a. anterior cerebral
    b. internal carotid
    c. middle cerebral
    d. posterior cerebral

14. Angiography is necessary
    a. when there is a question about the diagnosis
    b. when early clipping of an aneurysm is being considered
    c. when a hematoma is to be removed
    d. when a hematoma is present in the temporal lobe involving the middle cerebral artery
    e. in all of the above instances

15. The majority of head injuries result from
    a. vehicular accidents
    b. home accidents
    c. acts of violence
    d. work accidents

16. Which of the following types of hemorrhages is most common?
    a. subarachnoid
    b. epidural
    c. subdural
    d. intracerebral

17. Which of the following has occurred when the brain is bruised but the skin is not broken?
    a. contusion
    b. concussion
    c. infarct
    d. fracture

18. A violent blow to the head that causes the brain to shift within the vault and strike the adjacent cranial wall resulting in unconsciousness is known as
    a. a contusion
    b. a concussion
    c. an infarct
    d. edema

19. Most depressed skull fractures have overlapping fragments.
    a. true
    b. false

20. In a wound by a penetrating missile, the exit wound is usually larger than the entrance wound.
    a. true
    b. false

21. In cases of severe injury, fractures of which part of the skull are most common?
    a. cranial base
    b. frontal bone
    c. occipital bone
    d. parietal region

22. What body fluid is found in the halo sign?
    a. vomitus
    b. blood
    c. cerebrospinal fluid
    d. urine

23. Incomplete closure of the neural arch is called
    a. myelocele
    b. meningocele
    c. myelomeningocele
    d. spina bifida

24. Spina bifida with meningeal protrusion is referred to as
    a. meningocele
    b. myelocele
    c. myelomeningocele
    d. sacroiliitis

Study Questions

1. *List all the methods of imaging the head, skull, and brain.*

2. *Describe the advantages and disadvantages of each method of imaging the head, skull, and brain.*

3. *What are the complications of head injury?*

4. *What is the purpose of a ventriculovenous shunt?*

5. *What conditions must exist for a patient to have a craniotomy?*

6. *What are some of the differences between oil and metrizamide myelography?*

7. *What criteria exist in determining whether a patient is eligible for chemonucleolysis?*

Eight

Neoplasia

Related Terminology

adenocarcinoma
astrocytoma
cachexia
chondroma
chondrosarcoma
craniopharyngioma
ependymoma
Ewing's sarcoma
fibroadenoma
fibrocystic disease
fibrosarcoma
glioblastoma
Hodgkin's disease
hypernephroma
leiomyoma
lymphosarcoma
medulloblastoma
multicameral
multiple myeloma
neurilemoma
oligodendroglia
osteosarcoma
pedunculated
schwannoma
sessile
transitional cell carcinoma
Wilms' tumor

Objectives

Upon completion of Chapter 8, the reader will be able to

- Explain the significance of cancer in the general population.

- Describe the standards of measure relating to cancer statistics.

- List and describe the four major types of cancer.

- List several manifestations of cancer.

- Explain the TNM system of cancer staging.

- Identify on radiographs abnormalities that suggest neoplasia affecting the lungs, bone, liver, esophagus, stomach, colon, brain, breast, and lymphatic system.

- Describe the three primary methods of cancer treatment.

- Describe the three major routes of metastasis.

- Describe the short- and long-term effects of cancer.

Cancer comprises a large group of diseases in which the growth and spread of the disease process are uncontrolled. A great deal of pain and suffering and eventual death are the outcome of cancer when it is not detected early. In the United States, cancer is the second leading cause of death, killing more than 400,000 Americans annually. The mortality rate of cancer is second only to heart disease. For women between the ages of 30 and 54 and for children between 3 and 14 years, cancer is the leading cause of death. Cancer has the ability to strike at any age. It kills more children between the ages 3 and 14 than any other disease. There were an estimated 3.5 million cancer deaths in the 1970s. During the 1970s, more than 6.5 million new cancer cases were documented, and more than 10 million people were receiving medical care for cancer. Current estimates by the American Cancer Society suggest that about 74 million Americans now living will eventually have cancer, or 30% of the U.S. population. This means that over the next several years cancer will strike three out of four families.

More than 5 million Americans with cancer are alive today, and 3 million of these have survived for 5 years. The survival rate is established between 5 and 10 years, but depending on the type of cancer, the patient can be considered cured after a symptom-free interval of 1 year. This is especially encouraging, because there was little chance for survival in the early 1900s, and fewer than one in five cancer patients were alive 5 years after treatment. In the 1940s, only one in four survived, and in the 1960s, one in three. Despite the fact that about 965,000 people will have been diagnosed as having cancer in 1987, it is estimated that 385,000 of that group, or 4 of 10, will be alive 5 years after diagnosis. In comparison with the 1960s, when only 1 of 3 survived, about 4 of 10 survived in 1987. This represents an increase of about 65,000 persons in 1987. To gain a more realistic assessment and evaluation of the progress against cancer, we now use the relative or age-adjusted survival rate. The age-adjusted survival rate takes into account life expectancy and age-related factors that influence the mortality rate. Elderly patients with cancer may also have other organ or organ-system diseases involving the heart, liver, kidneys, and so on. Patients also suffer from the effects of arteriosclerosis and other diseases and conditions of aging. Because of age-related diseases, it is sometimes impossible to pinpoint the exact cause of death. Thus, the age-adjusted rate seems to be a more realistic measurement of the extent of success in the battle against cancer.

It is estimated that 170,000 people will die of cancer in 1987. Breaking these estimates down further, daily deaths number 1323, one every 65 seconds. Considering all the possible causes of death, one in five will be from cancer. The American Cancer Society has reported the following estimated statistics on cancer deaths: 472,000 in 1986; 462,000 in 1985; and 453,492 in 1984.

The national death rates for cancer continue to climb, and the primary reason for this is the continual rise in lung cancer. In 1930, the number of cancer deaths per 100,000 population was 143. In 1984, this rate was 170. Overall, 50% of all patients having cancer will die of that cancer. Fifty percent of all cancer deaths occur in persons older than 65. From age 20 to 40 years, cancer is more common in women, but between the ages of 60 and 80, cancer is more prevalent in men. Overall, more men than women die of cancer. In women, the principal fatal cancers are found in the breast, colon, rectum, lung, ovary, and uterus. These account for 60% of all cancer deaths in women. In men, the principal cancers involve the lung, colon, rectum, and prostate. For both men and women combined, lung cancer causes more deaths than any other cancer. Because of increased public awareness and advances in medical science and diagnostic procedures, one in three patients is cured of cancer. The key to cancer cure is *early detection*. The significance of mortality is underscored by the 50% cancer mortality rate, which is greatly influenced by when the cancer is detected.

Causes of Cancer

The work environment often exposes workers to caustic industrial chemicals, many of which have been designated as possible *carcinogens* and are used in the manufacture of food, cosmetics, plastics, and many other home-related products, including building materials. Exposure to air and water pollution have been cited as potential causes of cancer. Radiation, primarily from exposure to sunlight, rates as a significant cause of basal cell and squamous cell carcinoma of the skin. *Skin cancer* is the most common cancer throughout the world.

Changes in the immune system lead to a decreased resistance to all forms of infections. The body can also produce antibodies that react negatively and attack the body. These *autoimmune* diseases are thought to be potential direct or indirect causes of cancer.

Viruses have long been suspected as being precursors of cancer. Because it is difficult to isolate a virus, its exact relationship in the development of cancer is uncertain.

An individual has a much greater chance of acquiring cancer if there is a positive family history. Some pregnant women were at one time treated with synthetic estrogen (diethylstilbestrol, or DES), and several had female offspring who later developed cancer. Agent Orange, a chemical defoliant, is thought to have contributed to birth defects in the offspring of Vietnam veterans who were exposed to this chemical.

Many types of drugs, including narcotics, analgesics, and steroids, are often toxic to cells and have produced abnormal structural changes in cells. It is thought that this may be the result of decreased antibody production and the destruction of circulating lymphocytes.

Tobacco smoking, especially of cigarettes, has been linked to lung cancer—85% of lung cancer cases among men, 75% among women, and 83% overall. Smoking is related to 320,000 deaths annually and about 30% of all cancer deaths.

In the past 10 to 15 years, stress has been thought to be an agent that is contributory to cancer. Research indicates that anxiety brought about by everyday stresses greatly alters hormone production and the function of the endocrine organs. Biofeedback techniques, in addition to medical approaches, have received considerable attention. It is thought that if people could control their emotions, heart rate, and so on that they might be able to reduce tension and anxiety. Stress is also a factor in heart disease, in that it can cause hypertension and the precipitation of blood lipids, which adhere to the intima of the artery and eventually reduce blood flow.

Characteristics of Cancer

Neoplasia is a process of unexpected proliferation of cells in the parent tissue. Sometimes this lesion may be simply referred to as hyperplasia. Typically, both neoplasia and hyperplasia arise as a result of exposure to some form of stimulus. A hyperplastic condition usually recedes when the stimulus is removed, such as occurs in a localized infection. However, for the most part, the stimulus causing neoplasia has yet to be identified. That is why most cancers are classed as *idiopathic*.

The growth that takes place in abnormal lesions is certainly not part of the normal process. Most tumors start long after normal growth has ceased and when tissues are undergoing atrophic changes due to age. Excessive growth is the most obvious feature of a neoplasm. Neoplasms can typically be distinguished by their growth potential. A benign tumor or neoplasm usually presses on adjacent structures but remains discrete to a particular tissue boundary. A malignant neoplasm has no particular respect for tissue boundaries. It invades and destroys surrounding tissue and obstructs body passageways. It has been proved that no tumor is ever beneficial to the host. The tumor growth is uncontrolled and is uncoordinated with the local environment. Malignant tumors are usually larger than benign tumors, but some benign tumors grow increasingly large. Neoplasms acquire the blood supply from host tissue and compete with the host's cells for nutrients, usually resulting in anemia. The neoplasm is related to the tissue type from which it arose.

The tumor situation, or where it is located, determines the potential for surgical removal. The time involving regional and distant spread is expressed as duration. Histology is the process of cell differentiation and anaplasia. The radiosensitivity of a tumor is the predicting level of success of radiation treatments in cure or determining prognosis.

Basic Structure of Neoplasms

Neoplasms typically comprise two components. The *parenchyma* consists of tumor cells from the host cell. The tumor grows in the *stroma*, which consists of connective tissue, and depends on the blood supply.

Types of Cancer

Four types of cancer have been identified. *Carcinomas* arise from epithelial cells and tend to be solid tumors. The large majority of malignant neoplasms are carcinomas. *Sarcomas* arise from connective tissue and are the second most common malignant neoplasm. *Lymphomas* originate in lymphoid tissues, and the many subtypes are classified according to the specific tissue involved. *Leukemia* is cancer of the hematopoietic system and blood-forming organs.

Cell Differentiation

Cell differentiation is a process in which a cell matures into a functionally and structurally specialized cell. Differentiated cells are often nondividing and may be thought of as end cells. The degree of differentiation of the tumor cells from the normal cell and the estimated rate of growth of the tumor are considered when attempting to grade the cancer.

Grading of Cancer

Grading is an attempt to estimate the degree of malignancy of a neoplasm based on histological criteria, including the degree of differentiation and the projected growth rate of the tumor. The degree of differentiation is estimated from the resemblance of the tumor to the normal tissue of origin. For example, a squamous cell carcinoma that forms considerable keratin and intracellular bridges is considered well differentiated. The estimated growth rate is based on the number of mitoses per unit of tissue. A rapidly growing tumor has more mitotic figures than a slowly growing tumor. Cancers are usually classified into three or four grades, designated by Roman numerals. The higher the grade, the greater the degree of anaplasia. The greater the degree of anaplasia, or the loss of resemblance to normal cells (undifferentiation of the cell), the greater the degree of malignancy. The criteria for each grade varies for different types of cancer. Although it is useful for determining the type of treatment, grading is more valid when applied to groups of cases than for predicting the behavior of individual cases. Generally, the higher the grade, the poorer the prognosis but the greater the radiosensitivity of the tumor. The grades are as follows:

- *Grade I:* Marked tendency (¾) to differentiation
- *Grade II:* ¾ to ½ differentiated
- *Grade III:* ½ to ¼ differentiated
- *Grade IV:* ¼ to undifferentiated (anaplasia—most severe; tumor undergoes rapid growth toward malignancy)

Staging of Cancer

Staging is an evaluation of the extent of a cancer based on clinical findings. Treatment protocol is based on this finding. Staging uses the *TNM System* devised by the International Union Against Cancer.

T = Size of the primary tumor
N = Regional lymph node involvement
M = The presence or absence of distant metastasis
CIS = Cancer in situ (confined to its original site)

Numerical staging is usually designated from one through four. One refers to the smallest size (T1), four to the largest size (T4). The least amount of regional metastasis is M1, and the largest amount of distant metastasis is M4.

Spread of Malignant Tumors

Spread of cancer through the bloodstream is termed *hematogenous* and is characteristic of most sarcomas. Tumor cells form a thrombus, fragment, and are transplanted as emboli along the route of travel. This is also a late feature of carcinoma (distant metastases).

Lymph nodes are located in great numbers throughout the body. Most carcinomas spread from a primary site to the regional lymph nodes, to distant lymph nodes, and into the bloodstream via the pulmonary artery. *Lymphatic* metastasis involves passage of cancer cells through lymphatic vessels and nodes and eventually to many major organs.

Transcoelemic spread involves a seeding of cells through body cavities and passageways. Cancer of the stomach and colon penetrates the walls of these structures and seeds into the peritoneum. Cancer of the bladder often seeds into the ureteral pathway and eventually produces obstruction.

Sites of Metastasis

Perhaps the most common metastatic site is the liver. Liver metastases are received from almost any site, either as an early or late occurrence. Liver cancer is usually fatal and in many cases is the terminal site of distant metastases. The lungs are common sites for most early metastases. Most sarcomas metastasize to the lungs, and carcinomas from the breast, thyroid, and kidney also metastasize to the lungs. Carcinomas frequently metastasize to bone (distant metastases) and are thought to be the most common malignancy of the skeleton. Primary bone sarcoma can metastasize to the lungs. The brain is another recipient of metastases. Malignant neoplasms from the lung and breast spread to the brain even before the primary lesions are apparent. Brain metastases are most often fatal. Carcinoma of the breast can metastasize almost anywhere. Initial spread is to the axillary lymph nodes, followed by spread to the lungs, brain, bone, and liver.

Significance of Metastasis

Metastasis is a disastrous complication of a primary malignant neoplasm, and it is often unmanageable. The sites and extent of metastases determine the patient's fate. The patient's chances for survival are greatly diminished once the cancer extends beyond the lymph nodes. For example, carcinoma of the colon usually has about a 5-year, 70% survival rate if confined to the primary site. On the other hand, the survival rate decreases to about 37% when it has spread away from the primary site. Again, the importance of public awareness, diagnostic screening, physical examinations, and self-examinations cannot be overemphasized.

Effects of a Malignant Neoplasm

Several changes take place in body tissues, organs, and systems as a result of malignancy. A loss of function may be incurred through the obstruction of body passageways. This is most common with carcinoma of the colon, esophagus, and urinary bladder. Ulceration is most evident when the tumor is near the mucosal surface. Destruction of tissue is evident when the tumor deeply infiltrates the subserosa and muscularis. Infection predominates when the blood supply is diminished. Bacterial infection arises from the accumulation of toxic wastes during stasis. *Pain* is a symptom that occurs in the late stage of cancer and occurs when the nerve endings are infiltrated by the growing neoplasm. The pain is agonizing and is difficult to control, even with the most powerful drugs. *Hemorrhage* is caused by erosion of a blood vessel and is considered an early sign of cancer of the colon, kidney, and urinary bladder. Because hemorrhage occurs early in the life of some cancers, it can serve as a sign for early detection. The highest rate of cure takes place when cancer is detected during this stage. Other cancers such as those found in the mouth present with bleeding, such as a late stage of oral cancer. *Cachexia* is defined as an emaciated and debilitated state present in persons with advanced cancer. Weight loss and muscle atrophy are due to the patient's inability to maintain proper diet and the loss of nutrients vital to the body. Part of this condition is due to the cancer itself, but significant contributory factors are the effects of radiation and chemotherapy. The almost constant nausea caused by these treatment modalities makes it nearly impossible for the patient to eat. What little is eaten is usually lost by vomiting. Various types of hormonal changes are evident in cancer patients. These changes vary according to the type of cancer and the sex and age of the patient.

Signs and Symptoms of Cancer

Pain is not usually an early sign of cancer, but abnormal bleeding from a body passageway usually is an early sign. Hemorrhage can assume many forms. *Melena* is the passage of dark, tarry stools due to bleeding somewhere in the gastrointestinal system. The blood is black because it has been altered by the digestive enzymes. *Hematochezia* is bright red blood in the stool, and it is almost always the result of hemorrhage from the colon, most likely the rectosigmoid region. Colonoscopy provides clues about the site of bleeding. Blood in the sputum, referred to as *hemoptysis*, is the result of an active process from the bronchi. Blood present in vomitus is referred to as *hematemesis*. This hemorrhage is usually from the stomach. When the blood vomitus resembles coffee grounds, it has been altered by the stomach acids. Any form of an abnormal growth is usually referred to as a lesion. A lesion may be characterized by changes in skin color, pruritus, weeping, or a change in size or swelling of an area. Other signs and symptoms include persistent coughing or hoarseness, altered bowel habits (diarrhea and constipation), difficult or painful urination (dysuria), loss of appetite (anorexia) and subsequent weight loss, increased hormone production, and general malaise.

Diagnosis

Health counseling and cancer checkups for men and women over 20 years of age should be conducted every 3 years. Adults older than 40 should arrange for an annual physical examination. In addition to routine blood chemistries and hematological tests, the examination should include screening for common types of cancer, such as those of the thyroid gland, testicles, breast, ovaries, lymph nodes, oral region, and skin.

The American Cancer Society recommends a sigmoidoscopic examination for adults over 50 every 3 to 5 years after two negative examinations 1 year apart. An annual occult fecal blood test is recommended for adults over 50. A digital rectal examination is recommended for adults over the age of 40. A Pap smear is recommended for women between the ages of 20 and 65 (and before age 20 if sexually active) at least every 3 years after two negative results 1 year apart. A pelvic examination every 3 years is recommended for women 20 to 40 years of age and annually for women over 40. An endometrial tissue sample is recommended at menopause for women of high risk. Direct family history of cancer, history of infertility, obesity, failure of ovulation, abnormal uterine bleeding, and estrogen therapy are factors that increase risk. Mammography is a diagnostic tool in which radiation is used to visualize early lesions of the breast. This is especially important, because lesions are radiographically visible long before they can be felt by physical examination. The recommended frequency of mammography is still being debated in medical circles. Because of technological advancements, the radiation dose received by the patient is significantly less than in the past. The American Cancer Society recommends a baseline mammogram between the ages of 35 and 40. Between the ages 40 and 50, the woman should consult her personal physician. Annual mammograms are recommended for women with history of breast cancer in the immediate family. Annual breast examinations should be conducted by a physician for women over 40, in addition to monthly self-examinations. Chest x-ray films and sputum samples are no longer recommended for asymptomatic patients.

Diagnostic Imaging

Advances in medical imaging have enhanced the accuracy of diagnosis and also provided essential information for establishing a reasonable treatment plan. Computed tomography (CT) makes possible cross-sectional viewing of a tumor, revealing its shape and location with a high degree of accuracy. Pinpointing the margins of a tumor results in a more accurate radiation dosage while sparing normal tissue. Magnetic resonance (MR) imaging uses a huge electromagnet to detect tumors by sensing the vibrations of the different atoms in the body. It is predicted that MR imaging will revolutionize the diagnosis of cancer and other diseases. A significant amount of funding is being directed toward the advancement of specialized radiopharmaceuticals for cancer diagnosis. Monoclonal antibodies are tailored to seek out chosen targets on cancer cells.

Cancer Treatment

There are currently three primary methods of treating cancer. These methods can be employed individually or in combination, depending on the type of cancer and the extent of metastasis present.

Surgery seeks to eradicate the tumor by removing all cancerous and precancerous tissue, excising the entire lesion and any surrounding regional lymph nodes. Some tumors are removed when they are detected, even if they are not cancerous. Lesions such as polyps of the colon or larynx have a tendency to become malignant, thus the surgery is preventive. Some cancers can be cured by surgery alone, especially those in an early stage of development. Other cancers require surgery followed immediately by radiation treatments.

Radiation alters the membranes of cancer cells and destroys them while damaging normal cells as little as possible. X, gamma, and beta radiation are the most common types. Beta radiation produces the least skin damage. In addition to eradicating radiosensitive cancers, radiation therapy is often used palliatively to shrink the tumor, giving the patient a psychological lift, and the tumor can be reduced in size prior to resection. The general side effects include weakness, fatigue, nausea, vomiting, anorexia, anemia, and diarrhea.

Chemotherapy is indicated in combination with radiation therapy if the lesion has spread to stage 2 and beyond. In certain instances, chemotherapy can be used by itself, especially if the patient cannot tolerate radiation treatments. Chemotherapy can be used for both curative as well as palliative therapy. Some success has been noted with prostatic and breast carcinomas, as well as certain leukemias. Common lung, breast, and colon cancers do not usually respond to chemotherapy as well as to radiation therapy. Chemotherapy produces severe injury to cancer cells. A combination of several drugs has been most successful in treating Hodgkin's disease and Wilms' tumor of the kidney when combined with radiation.

Immunotherapy is a mode of treatment currently being investigated. The goal of immunotherapy is to use the body's own disease-fighting systems to control cancer. Interferon, interleukin-2 and monoclonal antibodies are currently being studied. Other new concepts being researched include tranfusion of blood components, bone marrow transplants, and hyperthermia.

Lung Tumors

General Information. Benign lung tumors are uncommon and include the hamartoma, which is a lobular mass consisting of hyaline cartilage and other cellular components; the lipoma, a tumor consisting of adipose tissue; and the leiomyoma, a smooth muscle tumor. However, among lung tumors, the most significant is *lung cancer*, which thus is the focus of this discussion.

Lung cancer represents 7 to 8% of all cancer deaths and is the leading cause of death in men, accounting for 35% of all cancer-related deaths. Lung cancer accounts for 9% of all cases of cancer in women and is responsible for 20% of cancer-related deaths in women. The age-standardized lung cancer death rate for women is higher than that of any other cancer. It has surpassed breast cancer as the leading killer of women.

Only 13% of lung cancer patients live for 5 or more years after diagnosis. Eighty percent of lung cancer deaths occur in people who smoke tobacco. It is estimated that in 1987 there will be 150,000 new cases and 136,000 deaths as the result of lung cancer. Although the incidence of lung cancer is appreciably lower in women, the most striking fact of the 1987 statistics is the marked increase in incidence in women. The percentage of change in the incidence of lung cancer during the period from 1947 through 1967 was 133% for men and 108% for women. The average age of onset is 60 years, with only 1% occurring before the age of 30 years. Worldwide statistics imply that lung cancer is most frequent in industralized countries. The United States currently has the world's ninth highest mortality rate due to lung cancer (19 per 100,000). In comparison, Scotland's mortality rate of 113 per 100,000 is the highest in the world. Lung cancer is 10 times more common in tobacco smokers. Other leading causes include exposure to asbestos, mining of radioactive metals, atmospheric pollution, and mining of nickel and silver.

Lung cancer is grouped into four histological types: squamous cell or epidermoid carcinoma, adenocarcinoma/bronchogenic carcinoma, anaplastic/undifferentiated/large cell carcinoma, and anaplastic/oat cell/small cell carcinoma. Of the four, *squamous cell* is the most common malignant tumor of the lung. It involves the lining of the smaller bronchi within the pulmonary parenchyma. Fifty percent to 60% involve the hilum and tend to grow into the lumen of the bronchi, producing a narrowing of the bronchi and eventual endobronchial obstruction with associated pneumonia. Squamous cell carcinoma is less likely to metastasize early. Regional spread involves the lymph nodes and distant metastasis via the bloodstream.

Adenocarcinoma/bronchogenic carcinoma arises in the more peripheral areas of the lung and is known to metastasize frequently and widely to the opposite lung, as well as to the liver, kidney, bone, and brain. Bronchogenic carcinoma occurs equally often in both sexes and is associated with chronic diseases and

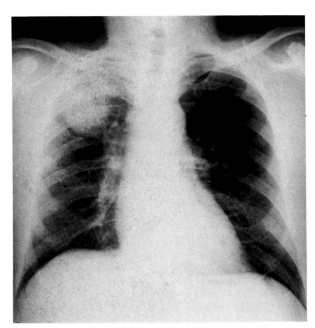

Figure 8–1. Primary bronchogenic carcinoma of the right upper lung in a 51-year-old man.

infections. This generally is a slower growing tumor and tends to have a more favorable prognosis.

Anaplastic/oat cell/small cell carcinoma usually has already spread when it is discovered. It is a very aggressive and rapidly growing tumor. It readily metastasizes to the regional and distant lymph nodes, liver, adrenal glands, bone, brain, and bone marrow.

Anaplastic/large cell carcinoma is similar in behavior to bronchogenic carcinoma. It metastasizes to the mediastinal lymph nodes, pleura, adrenals, brain, and bone.

Diagnosis. The high mortality rate of lung cancer is largely the result of the lack of symptoms in the early stages of the disease. A thorough physical examination including a complete patient history is the first step in establishing a diagnosis. The clinical manifestations are vague and varied and often mimic other pulmonary conditions. Changes in pulmonary habits are the most significant clinical signs. A productive cough with rust-streaked purulent sputum, chest pain, hemoptysis, and dyspnea are the most common signs and symptoms. Routine chest radiographs can detect a lesion as early as 2 years before symptoms occur and is the most valuable means of diagnosis when bronchogenic carcinoma is suspected. The radiologist must decide if the tumor is confined to the lung or if the pleura or mediastinum has been invaded. The radiographs may reveal the tumor as well as its effects, such as obstruction and atelectasis, but cannot predict with any certainty the cell type. Tumors are most often located in the larger and central bronchi (hilar) or peripherally (Fig. 8–1). Tomography is valuable in revealing the outline of the mass projecting into the lung, the extent of

primary tumor in the major bronchi, and especially the hilar and mediastinal nodes. Tomography is useful in identifying the narrowing of a bronchus and demonstrating cavitation. A narrowing is usually diagnostic of carcinoma (Fig. 8–2). Sputum specimens taken from the tracheobronchial tree are positive in about 75% of cases of bronchogenic carcinoma. Bronchial washings/brushings at the time of bronchoscopy are another way to obtain a specimen, but the results are not as satisfactory as collecting sputum following bronchoscopy. Percutaneous needle biopsy under fluoroscopic and ultrasonic guidance and CT scanning control is most useful and highly accurate. Some risks of percutaneous needle biopsy include hemorrhage and pneumothorax. These risks have been minimized by the increased visibility provided by the imaging equipment, the increased flexibility of the needles, and increased competency of physicians. CT scanning is helpful in determining if the tumor is limited to the lung or has invaded the chest wall or mediastinum. In addition, CT can detect metastatic lesions in distant locations such as the brain, liver, and adrenal glands. Radioisotope procedures such as gallium scans are most accurate as a preoperative screening tool in the diagnosis of mediastinal nodes. Xenon gas is used to yield information regarding lung ventilation and perfusion, but it does not provide information regarding malignancy. Bone scans using technetium 99 are used to diagnose occult metastases. Bone metastases are revealed as areas of increased isotope uptake or as hot spots (Fig. 8–3). Plain radiographs of the skeleton often indicate metastases by revealing osteolytic lesions. Bone marrow aspira-

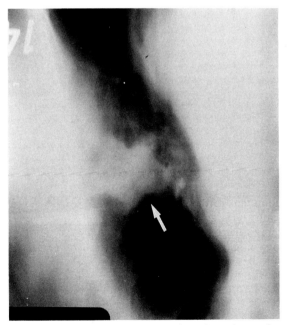

Figure 8–2. Tomogram demonstrating a bronchogenic neoplasm of the left upper bronchus, with distal pneumonia, in an 88-year-old woman.

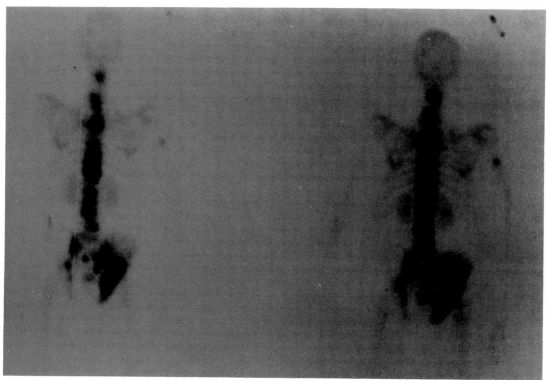

Figure 8–3. Multiple areas of increased isotope activity of the spine and pelvis, consistent with spreading metastatic bone disease, in a 60-year-old man.

tion and biopsy are essential for the diagnosis of small cell/anaplastic carcinoma. Thoracentesis permits chemical and cytological examination of pleural fluid. Cancer cells from numerous sites can enter the pulmonary circulation and be distributed throughout the lungs. Each lesion is revealed as a separate tumor on the posteroanterior (PA) chest film (Fig. 8–4).

Treatment. The extent of malignant disease determines the surgical procedure to be performed. Lobectomy, pneumonectomy, and segmental resection are the surgical options. The goal is to remove all the tumor while preserving as much of the normal tissue as possible. The 5-year survival rate for stage 1 is 50%. The survival rate for a stage 3 lesion is 15%. Most stage 3 lesions are inoperable. In the presence of distant metastases, surgery is contraindicated. Radiation therapy is used (1) to treat a localized carcinoma (inoperable), (2) in conjunction with surgery, and (3) palliatively (to relieve distressing symptoms). The optimum dose is 5000 to 6000 rads over a 5- to 6-week period. There is often a compromise between the required tumor dose and the normal tissue tolerance. CT scans more precisely define the volume of tissue to be treated and properly locate the positions of thoracic organs and structures. The success or failure of radiation therapy depends on the extent of distant metastases. Chemotherapy is widely used because of the fact that metastasis is present 50% of the time on initial diagnosis, and metastasis develops in about 90% of all lung carcinomas. Despite the wide range of use of chemotherapy, only small gains

have been achieved with large cell and bronchogenic carcinoma. However, chemotherapy has proved to be effective, with partial to total remissions being reported, in small cell anaplastic carcinoma. In primary lung cancer, the number of agents available and the diversity of possible theraputic schedules have generated a great number of chemical combinations that may include from two to seven drugs. Chemical toxicity usually increases when the number of drugs used is increased. Most long-term survivors have received a combination of chemotherapy and radiation. As with bone cancer, experimental immunotherapy is being used with some level of success in the treatment of lung cancer. Some initial success has been achieved but has not been duplicated in further testing, thus this treatment remains quite controversial.

The lungs are frequent recipients of metastatic disease, especially from primary cancers of the **breast** and **prostate**. The usual causes of death are attributed to the combination of pneumonia, obstruction, bronchiectasis, hemorrhage, and metastasis.

Alimentary Tract Tumors

Esophagus

General Information. Cancer of the esophagus accounts for about 2% of all cancer deaths in the United States and is responsible for 7% of all cancer deaths in men. It is most common in black men over

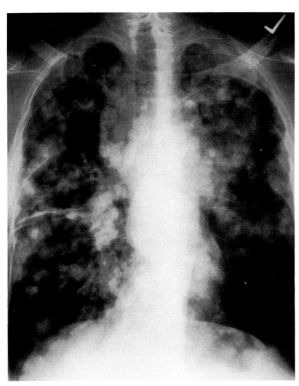

Figure 8–4. Diffuse pulmonary and mediastinal metastases in a 61-year-old man.

the age of 60 years. Cancer may occur in younger persons in association with achalasia or hiatal hernia. Incidence is highest in the Orient, where there is a mortality rate of 46.3 per 100,000 in men older than 35. In contrast, Sweden and Finland report that 45 to 50% of esophageal cancers afflict women. There is no obvious reason for this difference. In comparison, the United States reported a mortality rate of 10 per 100,000. In the United States, the southern coastal states have the highest mortality rate, most likely involving elderly black males. It is estimated that 9700 new cases were diagnosed in 1987 and that 8800 individuals died from the disease in that year. Men are affected three times more often than women.

Long-standing use of **tobacco** and **alcohol** predisposes the patient to esophageal carcinoma. This cancer is common in middle-aged women with Plummer-Vinson syndrome, in which there is a vitamin B complex deficiency with stenosis of the esophageal mucosa. It is to be noted that this type of carcinoma is almost nonexistent in Seventh-Day Adventists. In this religious group, smoking and alcohol use are forbidden.

Diagnosis. When describing esophageal cancer, three regions are considered: the proximal/upper third, the middle third, and the distal/lower third. Twenty percent of cases of esophageal carcinoma are located in the upper/proximal third (level of the cricoid membrane), which is the most lethal location. Thirty-seven percent of cases are found in the middle

third, at the level of the tracheal bifurcation, and 43% involve the lower third of the esophagus, which is at the level of the diaphragm and is the most treatable location of esophageal cancer. Ninety percent of patients with esophageal cancer complain of **dysphagia.** They often have left vocal cord paralysis, a persistent cough from a fistulous tract leading from the esophagus to the trachea, and hemoptysis, which may indicate a communication with the aorta. The prognosis is favorable when there are early signs of obstruction, indicating that surgery can correct the problem before metastasis occurs. When the condition occurs over a longer interval and severe weight loss and muscle wasting are evident, the prognosis is poor. This form of cancer is invasive and has spread before being detected. Squamous cell carcinoma is the most common form of esophageal cancer and accounts for 98% of cases, which are equally divided between the proximal and distal halves of the esophagus. Adenocarcinoma is usually found in the lower third of the esophagus and accounts for only 2% of cases of esophageal carcinoma. Involvement of the lower third is usually suspected to be an extension of a lesion from the fundus of the stomach. Dynamic fluoroscopy and radiography of the barium-filled esophagus (barium swallow or esophagogram) often delineate an irregular **polypoid filling defect** or ulcerative **stricture** involving the esophageal lumen (Fig. 8–5). This is accomplished with the use of thick barium, which typically consists of four parts barium to one part water, but currently is available in a tube or suitable container. Radiographs of the esophagus

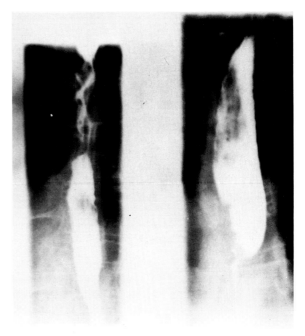

Figure 8–5. Barium swallow revealing a 2- to 3-cm polyp-like filling defect at the left about the level of T-7 in a 63-year-old man.

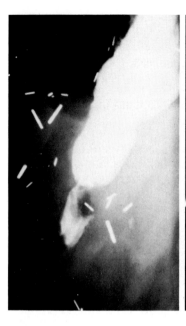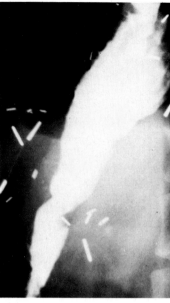

Figure 8–6. Barium swallow with Gastrografin evaluating the patency of the anastomosis of the upper esophagus and stomach in a 50-year-old man. The lower esophagus has been resected. The contrast material flowed freely through the upper esophagus and through the anastomotic site, with no signs of extravasation. The major portion of the stomach lies above the hemidiaphragm, with the area of the esophageal hiatus located in the region of the antrum of the stomach.

are taken in the following positions: PA, both anterior obliques, and lateral. For each view, the patient is given at least two mouthfuls of barium to swallow. This allows the barium to coat the entire esophagus. It is not necessary to have the patient suspend respiration, since inspiration is achieved during swallowing. When the esophagus is full of barium, it should reveal a smooth outline and show the indentation of the aortic arch. When the esophagus is empty, the barium usually lies between the folds of mucosa, which appear as three or four long, straight parallel lines. Laryngoscopy and bronchoscopy are employed to determine the extent of spread beyond the esophagus. An overpenetrated (exposed) PA chest radiograph is useful in describing mediastinal nodes. CT can reveal the extensions of the tumor into adjacent tissue. For advanced lesions, radioisotope scans are usually indicated.

Treatment. The site of origin of the neoplasm is the single most important factor in selecting the course of treatment. Cancer in the proximal/upper third of the esophagus has the poorest prognosis, despite the fact that it readily responds to theraputic radiation. Lesions in the lower third have a better prognosis and are best treated surgically. The procedure of choice is a esophagogastrectomy with jejunal or colonic bypass grafts. This reconstructive surgery is completed by anastomosing the esophagus within the chest for lesions of the lower third (Fig. 8–6). The success of treatment relies greatly on the depth of invasion. Lack of serosa in the esophagus facilitates the spread of the lesion to adjacent structures and limits the chance of surgical resection. Embolization in the submucosa and muscular lymphatics is quite common and results in inadequate surgical removal, with recurrence at the line of resection. Also of significance is the relationship between nodal spread to the size of the lesion. Half

of the patients with a lesion that is less than 5 cm have metastasis. Nodal disease will be present in 90% of patients with lesions greater than 5 cm. Lymphatic invasion is more common than vascular invasion. The patient usually succumbs before distant metastases occur. Squamous cell carcinoma in the lower/distal third is better corrected surgically and is not as responsive to radiation. Generally, chemotherapy is not helpful in the treatment of esophageal carcinoma. Metastatic spread primarily takes place in the liver, lungs, and lymph nodes. The prognosis is extremely poor, with approximately a 5 to 7% average survival rate for all sites.

Stomach

General Information. Adenocarcinoma is the most significant malignant tumor of the stomach and accounts for 97% of all malignant lesions in the stomach. Lymphosarcoma and leiomyoma account for the remaining 3%. The most common symptom of gastric carcinoma is **hemorrhage**, which may be present in the emesis (hematemesis) or feces (melena). The incidence is highest in Japan (105.1 per 100,000) and Chile (95.3 per 100,000). In comparison, the United States experienced a mortality rate of 13.6 per 100,000. The mortality rate appears to be higher in low socioeconomic groups and in persons whose diet is high in starch plus low in fresh fruits and vegetables. Two reasons have been suggested for the decrease in the United States: (1) increased consumption of foods containing ascorbic acid (vitamin C), which acts as a chemical antagonist for gastric carcinogens such as nitrites and nitrates, and (2) decreased use of pickled, highly salted, and smoked foods because of better refrigeration.

It is estimated that in 1987 nearly 14,200 people died as a result of gastric carcinoma. Of that total, more than 50% of cases involved the pylorus; more than 25% the lesser curvature; less than 10% the cardia; 10% the body and fundus; and 2 to 3% the greater curvature. When the greater curvature is afflicted, this area is first a site of ulceration. In the United States, the peak incidence is during the fifth decade of life, and males predominate over females by a 2:1 ratio. Gastric carcinoma accounts for 10% of all cancer deaths. Several factors have been suggested as possible precursors of gastric carcinoma: (1) genetics—individuals with *type A blood* have a higher incidence, (2) gastric atrophy, (3) achlorhydria or hypochlorhydria, (4) gastric polyps, (5) pernicious anemia, and (6) a history of gastric ulcer. Gastric carcinoma is classified into four distinct types: (1) the fungating or polypoid type, which has the best prognosis; (2) the ulcerating type, which arises as a growth away from the lumen and may be confused with a benign ulcer; it appears in the early life of the cancer and is the most common type of cancer, accounting for 30% of all stomach cancers; (3) the superficial spreading type; and (4) a diffuse spreading type, referred to as linitis plastica/scirrhous carcinoma, which accounts for 10% of all gastric carcinomas. It is common for the diffuse type to infiltrate the walls before the layers bulge into the lumen. The involved part becomes contracted, thick walled, and firm. It begins and encircles the pylorus and causes obstruction. The prognosis is extremely poor, and cure is rare because of the early disease advancement prior to detection. Gastric carcinoma metastasizes very early to the liver and other organs and structures, including the lungs and bone. Metastases grow in the liver, and emboli are discharged and spread via the portal venous system to the lungs and eventually to the bone.

Diagnosis. Symptoms quite often are vague, and the patient may wait months before seeking medical advice. This explains why many carcinomas are inoperable. Typically, the patient complains of tiredness and perhaps some weight loss. Initial blood tests may indicate anemia. A stool examination is essential for diagnosing occult blood. A gastric analysis may indicate that achlorhydria is present, which means that carcinoma is a distinct possibility. The upper gastrointestinal series is the most complete and accurate means of diagnosing any abnormality of the stomach. A combination of fluoroscopic spot views is usually taken by a radiologist, with the patient in erect and recumbent positions, and PA, right anterior oblique (RAO), and lateral views are taken in the recumbent position by a radiographer. These views are routine regardless of the type of pathology present. Both sets of radiographs reveal the barium coating the mucosal lining of the stomach, and they usually detect most forms of pathology. Carcinoma of the stomach usually is revealed as an irregular, usually rounded *filling defect*, with alteration of the

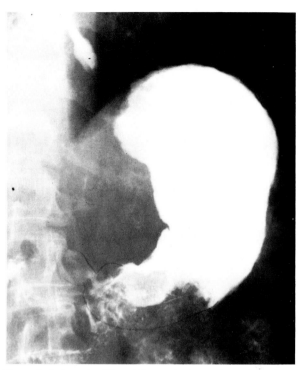

Figure 8–7. Irregular filling defect and a large, deep ulceration, with the ulcer cavity diminishing the major portion of the pyloric antrum. The findings are compatible with ulcerating gastric carcinoma.

normally smooth mucosal pattern (Fig. 8–7). The radiologist is usually able to distinguish between benign and malignant disease on the finished radiographs. Radionuclide scans indicate the degree of distant metastases.

Treatment. A radical subtotal gastrectomy is usually the initial treatment of choice. This procedure involves the surgical removal of a large part of the stomach. It is indicated for gastric ulcers, which have a significant predisposition for eventually developing into cancer. At the same time, the surgeon may remove the spleen and resect the associated lymph nodes. Reconstruction is accomplished by a gastrojejunostomy or gastroduodenostomy. The remaining part of the stomach is anastomosed onto that of the jejunum. One of the more common procedures is the Billroth II gastrojejunostomy. As a rule, radiation therapy is not effective in the treatment of gastric carcinoma. The therapeutic radiation dose is quite high, the tolerance level would be reached very fast, and the side effects would be significant. Carcinoma of the stomach recurs in 50 to 80% of persons who have had a previous gastrectomy. Radiation therapy (4500 rads) is usually administered after the second resection. Thus far, chemotherapy has been somewhat successful when administered postoperatively or in cases that are inoperable. More success has been noted in the stomach, as compared with the limited success in the colon. However, it is much too

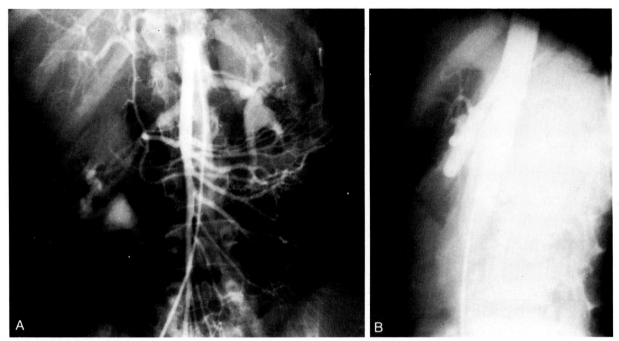

Figure 8–8. Biplane filming, selective superior mesenteric artery arteriogram, which was essentially within normal limits and negative for hemorrhage. *A,* Anteroposterior; *B,* lateral.

early to determine if the addition of chemotherapy postoperatively results in an improved disease-free interval or in overall survival.

Small Intestine

General Information. Cancers of the small intestine are unusually rare, accounting for an estimated 800 cancer deaths in 1987. The incidence is about equal in both sexes. The most frequent lesion is the adenomatous polyp, most often found in the duodenum.

Diagnosis. The most obvious symptom of small bowel cancer is *obstruction*. Most symptomatic patients are diagnosed via radiographic barium studies; however, it is most difficult to evaluate this condition by any diagnostic means. Bleeding usually occurs in about 50% of patients who are symptomatic. Endoscopic procedures may locate the exact site of hemorrhage and distinguish this condition from other inflammatory disorders. A superior mesenteric angiogram is also useful in locating the site of hemorrhage (Fig. 8–8). Radiographically, an infarct of the mesenteric artery can be observed by distension of the small intestine, as seen in Figure 8–9.

Treatment. Surgical resection of the obstructing lesion is the primary treatment. Radiation therapy is typically ineffective with carcinomas, thus is not often employed unless the lesion is unresectable and extensive. Chemotherapy is most often used palliatively. Carcinoma of the small intestine initially infiltrates the regional lymph nodes and liver.

Colon and Rectum

General Information. In 1987, an estimated 145,000 new cases of cancer of the colon (102,000) and rectum (43,000) were expected. Colorectal cancer is second in frequency only to lung cancer. It is estimated that 60,000 people succumbed to colorectal cancer in 1987. In the United States, men and women are affected equally often. The rectum is the site of 42% of all colorectal cancers, and the sigmoid colon is the site of 20%. Thus, the majority, or 62%, of all colorectal cancers are found in these two locations. In the remainder of the colon, 16% is found in the cecum and ascending colon, 8% in the transverse colon and splenic flexure, and 14% in the descending colon. Two out of every three patients are over 50 years of age. Colon cancer occurs in younger patients with a family history of the illness or in the presence of chronic ulcerative colitis. It has been found that younger patients typically have a more aggressive lesion and greater malignant potential. Although it has not been proved, the high incidence of cancer in the distal colon is thought to be due to inadequate movement of fecal matter in the distal sigmoid colon and rectum.

In addition to hereditary factors and a history of ulcerative colitis, the environment and, more specifically, the diet are thought to play a role. Carcinogens have been found in both food and water supplies. Many natural and synthetic food ingredients are suspected carcinogens. Foods that are high in animal fat and proteins are thought to increase the risk of colon cancer.

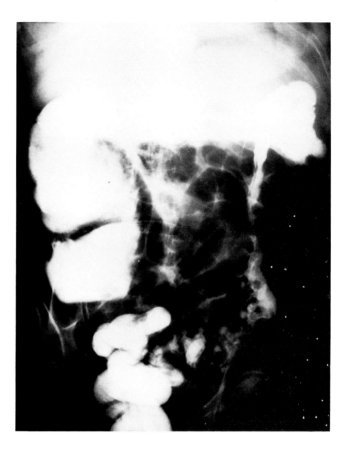

Figure 8–9. Marked small bowel distension with no colonic obstruction in a 71-year-old woman. Confirmed mesenteric artery ischemia.

The *polyp*, which is typically a benign *adenoma*, has malignant potential. Polyps arise mostly in the rectosigmoid area. The adenoma characteristically arises from the mucosal surface on a stalk. A stalk-like polyp is referred to as *pedunculated* (Fig. 8–10). A *sessile* or broad-surfaced adenoma may have many villous or thread-like projections covering its surface. The probability of malignancy is much greater with a villous adenoma than with the simple polyp.

Diagnosis. The symptoms of colorectal cancer depend on the site of the cancer. Altered bowel habits involving diarrhea and constipation with rectal bleed-

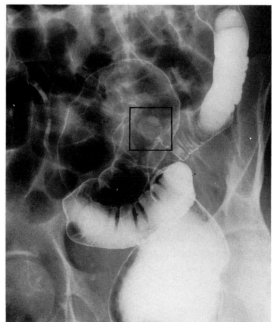

Figure 8–10. Air contrast of the colon revealing a 2-cm pedunculated polypoid lesion in the sigmoid colon of a 50-year-old man.

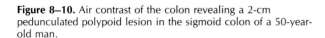

ing are among the earliest symptoms. It is important to note that the colonic mucosa is extremely vascular and bleeds when irritated. Early detection of this bleeding is essential to a good prognosis. The 5-year survival rate for colon cancer is 86%, and 77% for rectal cancer prior to lymph node invasion. When the lesion invades into adjacent tissue, the survival rate decreases. When there is lymph node involvement, the survival rates decrease to 39% and 21%, respectively. The survival rate when involvement entends beyond the regional lymph nodes depends on the extensiveness of the lymphatic/hematogenous metastasis. Distant metastasis most commonly involves the *liver* and then the *lungs*. Blood from the left side of the colon is typically bright red, whereas blood from the right side of the colon is dark red and contains mucus. Anemia is usually present in right-sided lesions and is absent in left-sided lesions. However, in either event, the presence of rectal bleeding and/or blood-laden stool may be an early sign of cancer. Annual digital rectal examinations are recommended for persons older than 40. A stool guaiac slide test is used to demonstrate *occult* blood in the feces. The guaiac slide test should be performed annually on all persons age 50 and older. At age 50, proctosigmoidoscopy should be performed every 3 to 5 years following two initial negative sigmoidoscopic examinations 1 year apart after age 50. Approximately 70% of cases of colon cancer are diagnosed via a sigmoidoscopic examination and biopsy. Twenty percent of colon cancers are diagnosed via a barium enema and biopsy. However, because of the inconsistency of patient preparation and the patient's inability to cooperate during the procedure, diagnosis is often compromised. The barium enema is indicated in evaluation of any unexplained abdominal mass or evidence of rectal bleeding, whether occult or overt. The barium enema, like other radiopaque procedures, often demonstrates abnormalities such as narrowing or stricture of the lumen, ulceration, dilatation, and filling defects. Narrowing of the lumen may be due to spasm, stricture formation, or compression by an extrinsic mass. Dilatation of the colon can be caused by many conditions, including obstruction, paralytic ileus, volvulus, ulcerative colitis, or Hirschsprung's disease. Various degrees of filling defect are possible in the presence of carcinoma. Radiographically, the sigmoid region often reveals an *apple-core/napkin-ring* deformity (Fig. 8–11). A double-contrast barium enema is helpful in distinguishing tumors from fecal matter.

Treatment. Following cytological confirmation, the primary treatment involves surgical resection of the lesion with intestinal anastomosis or abdominoperineal resection and permanent colostomy, depending on the extent of the cancer. Radiation is administered both pre- and postoperatively. The success of therapy depends on the amount of metastasis. Radiation can be helpful when a tumor is inoperable. It can reduce the size of the tumor, decrease the pain, and relieve obstruction and hemorrhage. Chemotherapy is administered when there is metastasis, however it has not significantly affected the survival rate. A great deal of experimentation is being done with terminal cancers of the colon in which there is distant metastatic spread.

Hepatobiliary System Tumors

Liver

General Information. Primary carcinoma is rarely found in the liver. In the United States, primary liver cancer accounts for only 2% of all cancers. Liver cancer is 6 to 10 times more common in males, and the average age of onset is between 60 and 70 years. Patients with cirrhosis are more apt to develop cancer of the liver. It is estimated that about 70% of patients with liver cirrhosis will develop liver cancer. Primary cancer of the liver is usually more frequent than

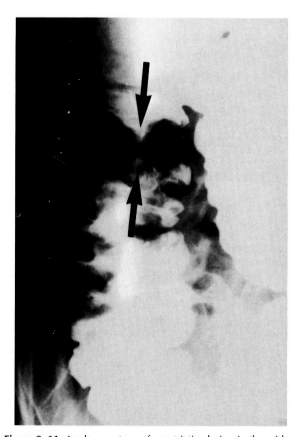

Figure 8–11. Apple-core type of constrictive lesion in the mid ascending colon in a 66-year-old woman. The lumen is markedly narrowed and irregular. There are overriding edges. These findings are consistent with carcinoma of the colon.

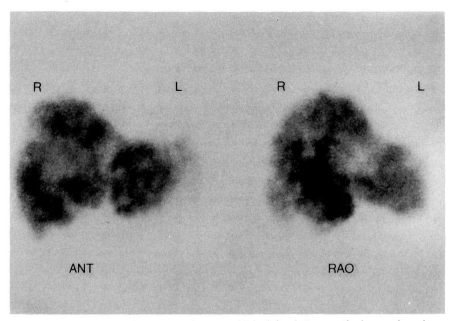

Figure 8–12. Radioisotope liver scan indicates multiple defined circumscribed parenchymal defects of both lobes of the liver, compatible with multiple metastatic lesions, in a 50-year-old man.

cancer of the bile ducts. There is also a significant association between hepatitis B virus and primary liver cancer. Metastasis takes place initially through the portal vein into the lymphatics. Distant metastasis takes place in the lungs and brain. The liver is also the leading recipent of metastasis from many other organs.

Diagnosis. Patients with primary liver cancer often present with vague symptoms such as anorexia, weakness, and abdominal fullness. There is progressive liver enlargement, or hepatomegaly. It is common for the abdominal distension and fullness to mask the signs of weight loss. The tumors grow rapidly. Primary cancer must first be differentiated from metastatic liver cancer. Radioisotope scans of the liver, which are 80 to 90% accurate, are most valuable in distinguishing between primary and metastatic disease. The lesions visualize as *filling defects* (Fig. 8–12). CT usually reveals the extent of the tumor and whether multiple lesions are present (Fig. 8–13). Afflicted persons are jaundiced, thus the serum bilirubin and alkaline phosphatase levels are elevated.

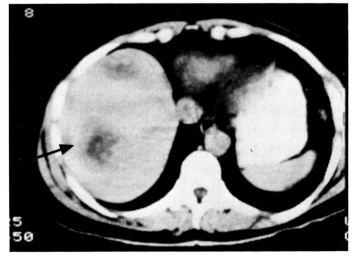

Figure 8–13. CT scan showing multiple defects in the liver parenchyma, consistent with metastases. This 54-year-old woman was diagnosed as having carcinoma of the colon.

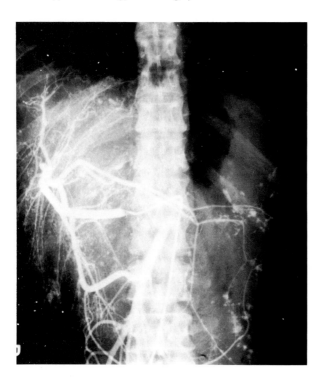

Figure 8–14. Selective hepatic angiogram revealing groups small of dilated spaces filling diffusely with contrast medium over both lobes of the liver. The liver in this 66-year-old man is considerably enlarged. The blood flow is extremely slow. There is evidence of considerable stretch of the branches of the left hepatic artery. The findings are consistent with cavernous hemangioma of the liver.

Hepatic arteriography will demonstrate increased arterial vascularity, which is a primary characteristic of liver tumors (Fig. 8–14).

Hepatic metastases frequently contain enough calcium to be visible on plain films of the abdomen (Fig. 8–15).

Treatment. Surgical resection is the treatment of choice and is only possible when the lesion is singu-

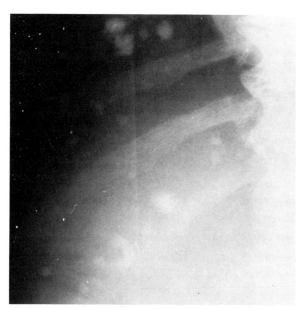

Figure 8–15. Flat plate of the abdomen revealing calcifications in the liver, consistent with hepatic metastases. This 79-year-old woman has a clinical history of primary carcinoma of the breast.

lar. There must be no evidence of lymphatic metastasis. Radiotherapy is not appropriate, because the lesions are not radiosensitive. Chemotherapy is somewhat successful at temporarily reducing the size of the tumor. Less than 1% of patients will survive 5 years when both lobes of the liver are involved. It has been reported that 33% have survived 5 years following resection of a solitary lesion.

Extrahepatic Bile Ducts

General Information. Carcinoma of the extrahepatic biliary ducts is quite uncommon, if not rare. It typically affects men in their 60s and is more common in patients having a history of cholelithiasis.

Diagnosis. The earliest sign of cancer is jaundice, although jaundice may be the result of other problems such as cholelithiasis, infection, and cirrhosis. It is known that jaundice occurs at some point in the life of the cancer and that calculi are found in 20% of patients with biliary tract cancer. Radiographically, the lesion is demonstrated as a *filling defect*, with the ampulla of Vater as the most common site. Several vague symptoms are apparent early, including weakness, anorexia, weight loss, and abdominal bloating. Sometimes the weight loss is not apparent because of the abdominal distension. Transhepatic cholangiography is able to demonstrate the site of obstruction and the irregular and ragged appearance of the tract (Fig. 8–16). Endoscopic retrograde cholangiopancreatography (ERCP) is useful in demonstrating the site of obstruction (Fig. 8–17). As in liver

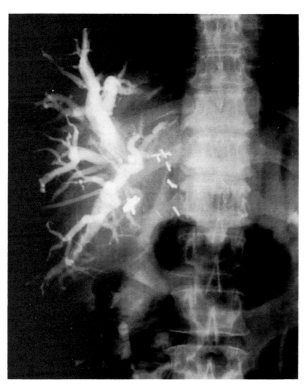

Figure 8–16. Percutaneous transhepatic cholangiogram showing a 4- to 5-cm narrowed segment of the common bile duct in the region of the porta hepatis. This most likely represents cholangiocarcinoma in this 60-year-old woman.

cancer, the serum bilirubin and alkaline phosphatase levels are abnormally elevated.

Treatment. Surgery offers the only possibility for a total cure, especially when the common bile duct or ampulla of Vater is involved. A lesion in the hepatic duct is inoperable because of the probable invasion of the liver. Radiation therapy is employed postoperatively in lesions that are not advanced. Information regarding the recent use of chemotherapy is incomplete and is being studied further.

Pancreas

General Information. Carcinoma of the pancreas is known as a *silent* disease because symptoms are not apparent until the cancer has significantly advanced. The late occurrence of symptoms also explains the high rate of mortality. It is estimated that 24,300 deaths resulted from pancreatic cancer in 1987. In the past 30 years, the death rate for pancreatic cancer has risen 21%, to 10.4 deaths per 100,000 men. During this same period, the death rates for women rose 25%, to 7.0 deaths per 100,000 women. It is estimated that there were 26,000 new cases of pancreatic cancer in 1987. Pancreatic cancer is the *fifth* leading cause of cancer deaths. The

incidence among blacks is about 1.5 times higher than among whites. To summarize these data, this cancer is 30% more common in men than in women and occurs about 50% more frequently in blacks than in whites.

The risk factors increase after age 30, and the rate of peak incidence occurs between ages 70 and 79. People who smoke have twice as great a chance of contracting cancer of the pancreas as nonsmokers. It has been suggested that high-fat diets may be a risk factor, and countries where people consume more fat have higher rates of pancreatic cancer. Although no formal evidence is available, coffee is being investigated as one of the possible causes of pancreatic cancer.

Diagnosis. Carcinoma of the pancreas is a rapidly progressive disease that usually has metastasized by the time it is diagnosed. As is with other cancers of the digestive and hepatobiliary tract, the early symptoms are vague. Loss of weight is the most common symptom, and 70 to 80% of patients complain of a dull epigastric pain. Three regions of the pancreas— the head, body, and tail—are susceptible to neoplastic growth. The large majority (70%) of the neoplasms arise in the head. When the body is involved, the tumor grows around a nerve plexus, resulting in back pain. The abdominal pain is usually persistent. When the tail is involved, the symptoms are the result of the already spreading metastasis. Cancer of the head of the pancreas has the most favorable prognosis. The prognosis worsens as the body and tail become in-

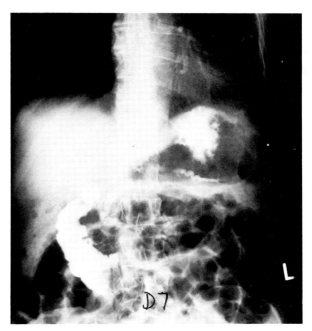

Figure 8–17. A ragged and dilated appearance of the pancreatic duct as revealed on endoscopic retrograde cholangiopancreatography, suggesting the possibility of duct obstruction or chronic pancreatitis in this 61-year-old man.

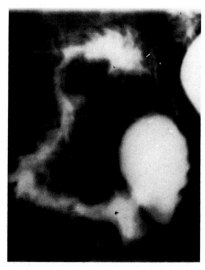

Figure 8–18. Small bowel series revealing an abnormal appearance of the duodenum in which its midportion is pulled to the left. The normal C-chaped configuration is altered to resemble a reversed number 3. This finding is consistent with annular carcinoma of the head of the pancreas. The patient is an 85-year-old man.

volved. Because approximately 90% of pancreatic cancers have metastasized when initially diagnosed, the prognosis is extremely poor. An upper gastrointestinal series may reveal distortion of the C loop of the duodenum in such a way that it resembles a reverse 3. Thus this is referred to as the **reverse 3** sign or syndrome. This finding only involves the head of the pancreas, which is compressing the duodenum (Fig. 8–18). Ultrasonography is an imaging modality with a reasonable degree of accuracy, however it is handicapped by gas surrounding the bowel. CT can identify the presence of metastatic lesions as well as the extent of the primary lesion. ERCP may be performed when CT scanning is inconclusive. Percutaneous needle biopsy is currently the only method of making a definitive diagnosis (Fig. 8–19). Other diagnostic tests include selective angiography, liver function tests, and laparotomy to assess the lymph node involvement.

Treatment. Because most pancreatic carcinomas have metastasized prior to diagnosis, surgery is not usually indicated. Resection is somewhat successful when only the head is involved. In the absence of metastasis, a total pancreatectomy has recently been recommended. Radiotherapy usually meets with unfavorable results because of the limited normal dose tolerance of adjacent structures such as the spinal cord, stomach, intestines, and kidneys. Neutron beam therapy has been somewhat successful in controlling the growth of the tumor and prolonging survival. In the event of widespread metastasis, chemotherapy is used palliatively. There has been some recent success with combining radiotherapy and chemotherapy, but a great deal of further research is

needed to increase the ratio of success. In 59% of cases, diagnosis is so late that none of these treatment methods are useful. The American Cancer Society reports that only 4% of patients live more than 3 years after diagnosis. The 2% of patients whose cancers occur in insulin-producing cells and not in the duct cells of the pancreas tend to survive longer. About 30% of these patients live more than 3 years after diagnosis.

Urinary Tract Tumors

Benign disease is relatively uncommon in the urinary tract. Renal cell carcinoma/**hypernephroma**/adenocarcinoma is an important malignant kidney tumor affecting adults. **Wilms'** tumor is the most important malignant kidney lesion in children. The kidney is also the recipient of metastatic lesions from many primary tumor sites in the body. Bladder carcinoma is the most frequently occurring malignancy of the urinary tract and accounts for 2.5% of all cancer deaths in the United States.

Many diagnostic procedures adequately demonstrate the urinary tract or identify abnormal conditions. The **urinalysis** is considered the most important laboratory test when evaluating the urinary tract. The excretory urogram or intravenous pyelogram (IVP) is valuable for demonstrating a space-occupying lesion or a filling defect anywhere in the urinary tract. Nephrotomography and ultrasonography are able to differentiate solid and cystic masses. Needle aspiration provides a means of obtaining information on the cellular contents of a renal cyst. CT provides information regarding renal size, density, and extent of a lesion. Selective renal angiography is excellent for demonstrating the hypervascularity and extent of hypernephroma and for identifying the preoperative blood supply. Venacavography reveals the extent of the lesion and information regarding the feasibility of resection or the type of surgery required. The rate

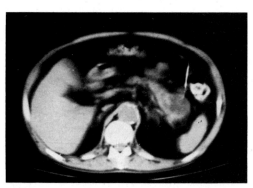

Figure 8–19. Under CT guidance, a percutaneous needle biopsy was performed on an irregular 3- to 4-cm cystic mass in the region of the tail of the pancreas in this 66-year-old man. No fluid was aspirated from the lesion. The findings were consistent with metastatic disease.

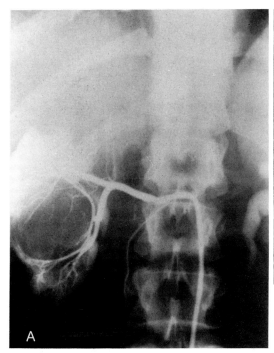

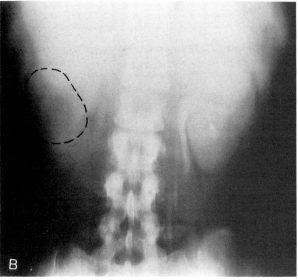

Figure 8–20. Right renal cyst demonstrated on *(A)* selective renal arteriogram and *(B)* nephrotomogram in a 34-year-old woman.

of survival of patients with urinary tract cancers depends on the extent of metastases.

Renal Cell Carcinoma

General Information. Renal cell carcinoma is the leading malignant lesion of the kidney. It accounts for 80% of all kidney cancers and has a 2:1 male predominance. The cause of this lesion is unknown, but chronic inflammation such as from nephro-lithiasis, tobacco smoking, chemical hydrocarbons, amines, amides, and certain compounds found in a variety of foodstuffs are thought to predispose individuals to its development. It is estimated that 21,900 new cases were reported and 9400 deaths resulted from renal cell carcinoma in 1987.

Diagnosis. The selective renal angiogram best demonstrates a mass of increased *vascularity*, irregular branching, and terminal blunting of renal vessels (Figs. 8–20 and 8–21). Because hypernephromas are very vascular, CT with contrast enhancement is use-

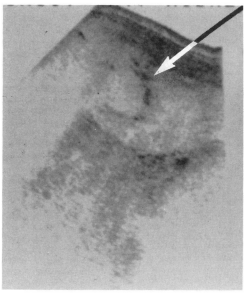

Figure 8–21. Sonographic visualization of a right renal cyst in a 51-year-old man.

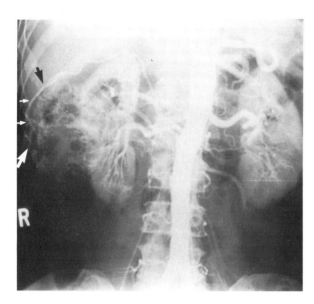

Figure 8–22. CT scan showing a large vascular tumor being primarily supplied from the upper pole, left renal artery, compatible with hypernephroma. The patient is a 58-year-old man.

ful in demonstrating this lesion and metastases (Figs. 8–22 and 8–23). Hypernephromas mainly metastasize through the bloodstream, but also through the lymphatic channels. The lungs, brain, bone, liver, and adrenal glands are most often affected. Approximately 95% of patients have evidence of metastasis at the time of death.

Treatment. Radical nephrectomy accompanied by lymph node resection is the preferred treatment for operative cases. Some evidence of total cure has been noted following total nephrectomy and removal of solitary metastatic lesions of the brain, liver, and bone, but these cases are few. Radiation therapy is limited to nonresectable tumors or is used immediately following resection. Chemotherapy has also had limited success. These tumors typically have a poor prognosis, with a 20% survival rate over a 10-year period because of the aggressive nature of the tumor and the fact that the patient is usually asymptomatic until the lesion reaches a large size and widespread metastasis has already occurred.

Wilms' Tumor

General Information. Wilms' tumor, or **nephroblastoma**, is the most common malignancy of renal origin affecting children. This tumor occurs equally often in both sexes and for the most part is diagnosed before the age of 5 years. Sixty-five percent occur before age 3 and 75% before age 5. The lesion is primarily unilateral, with only about 7% occurring bilaterally.

Diagnosis. The most obvious signs include a palpable abdominal mass, which is present in about 90% of patients, and hypertension, which is detected in about 75%. This lesion may also be part of one of several congenital malformations such as mental retardation, microcephaly, and spina bifida.

Wilms' tumor may be seen with conventional radiography of the kidney and sometimes is aided by nephrotomography. Sonography is helpful in ruling out other lesions such as cysts and hydronephrosis. Aortography and selective angiography, although dif-

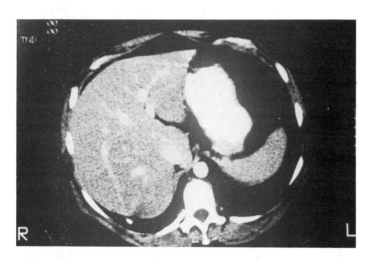

Figure 8–23. Large hypervascular tumor, left upper pole of the kidney, with a typical appearance of hypernephroma, in a 47-year-old woman.

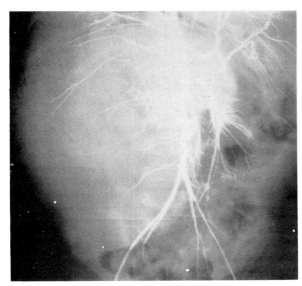

Figure 8–24. Wilms' tumor of the left kidney in a 1-year-old boy. This lesion typically presents a large abdominal mass with tumor vessels that are long and tortuous, resembling a creeping vine.

ficult to perform on pediatric patients, demonstrate a poorly *vascularized* lesion (Fig. 8–24). The paraaortic lymph nodes often are early sites of metastases. Commonly involved are the lungs, liver, adrenal glands, diaphragm, and bone.

Treatment. The treatment consists of surgical resection of the tumor, followed by radiation and chemotherapy. Wilms' tumor is very radiosensitive, and it is useful to radiate the paraaortic lymph nodes and lungs after surgery. Chemotherapy is used in combination with radiation to treat metastases. Generally, the younger the patient, the better the prognosis and survival rate. Children younger than 2 years have a good survival rate. Patients with distant metastases have the poorest prognosis.

Transitional Carcinoma of the Bladder

General Information. The American Cancer Society estimates that 45,400 new cases of bladder cancer were reported in 1987. Of those, 33,000 were males and 12,400 females. Bladder cancer accounts for 7% of new cancer cases in males and 3% in females. It is the 5th most common form of cancer in males and the 10th most common form of cancer in females. An estimated 10,600 deaths from bladder cancer will occur in 1987, and this lesion is the 8th leading cause of death among males and the 14th leading cause of death among females.

Smoking is the most significant risk factor, with bladder cancer twice as common in smokers as in nonsmokers. Smoking is thought to be responsible for an estimated 49% of the bladder cancers among men and 10% among women. Overall, the rate of bladder cancer is four times greater among men than

among women, and higher in whites than in blacks. Bladder cancer is more common in people living in urban areas and working in the leather and rubber industries. Aniline dyes, which are used in the manufacture of rubber and cable, have been linked to bladder cancer. Research into the possible effects of coffee and artificial sweeteners is inconclusive and is currently being debated.

Diagnosis. The most accurate means of identifying bladder cancer is with cystoscopy. Hematuria is present in about 75% of cases. The IVP is used to evaluate the upper urinary tract and bladder filling. Radiographically the bladder presents many variations in shape; however, a *filling defect* in the bladder shadow is almost always seen with this lesion (Fig. 8–25). Overlying bowel gas found in the sigmoid colon or rectum is difficult to distinguish from carcinoma. Oblique views of the bladder are taken in this event. Radioisotope scans of the liver and bone are useful in determining metastases, because these are the first metastatic sites. CT is especially useful when attempting to stage the invading lesion.

Treatment. The usual treatment of bladder cancer is either local resection or a total cystectomy, followed by radiation therapy. A total cystectomy is indicated when the tumor is invasive or anaplastic but has no metastasis outside of the pelvic region. The lesion may be treated in several ways, including intracavitary radium insertion or megavoltage irradiation of

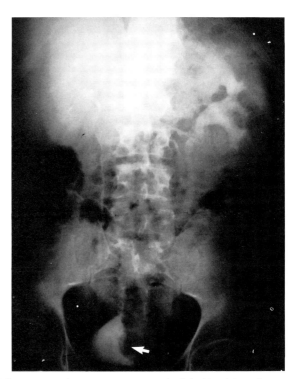

Figure 8–25. A 4 × 6-cm mass on the left side of the urinary bladder, causing obstructive uropathy of the left kidney in a 44-year-old man. This filling defect is consistent with transitional cell carcinoma of the bladder.

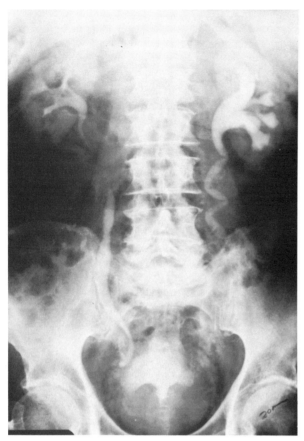

Figure 8–26. Filling defect at the bladder base, consistent with a markedly enlarged prostate gland causing a noticeable degree of bladder outlet obstruction in this 84-year-old man.

6000 rads in a 5- to 6-week period. Currently, there is no established method of chemotherapy used in treating transitional cell carcinoma of the bladder. Surgery alone or in combination with other treatments is used in 92% of the cases. When bladder cancer is detected early, 87% of patients will survive 5 years. In the advanced stages, the survival rate drops to 38%.

Reproductive System Tumors

The most significant tumor of the male reproductive system is *adenocarcinoma* of the *prostate* gland. More than 96,000 new cases and nearly 27,000 deaths were estimated for 1987. Men over the age of 66 are most susceptible to this type of cancer. Carcinoma of the *endometrium* is the leading gynecological cancer. More than 35,000 new cases and 3000 deaths were estimated for 1987. This condition is primarily diagnosed by pelvic and cytological examinations. Although many radiographic procedures are routinely performed, they are almost exclusively used to demonstrate distant metastases. Cancer of the cervix was expected to result in 6800 deaths in 1987. It is estimated that 16,000 new cases of invading cervical cancer are reported annually. This is the second most common malignancy in women between the ages of 15 and 34 years, but it can afflict women of any age. Leiomyoma is the most common uterine tumor associated with pregnancy and is often referred to as a *fibroid* tumor. These solid tumors are stimulated by pregnancy and can become quite large. Ovarian cyst is the most common cystic pelvis mass and is visually enhanced by sonography.

Adenocarcinoma of the Prostate

General Information. An estimated 96,000 new cases of adenocarcinoma of the prostate were expected in 1987. About 1 of every 11 men will develop prostate cancer during their lifetime. Prostatic cancer is the third leading cancer in men, following skin and

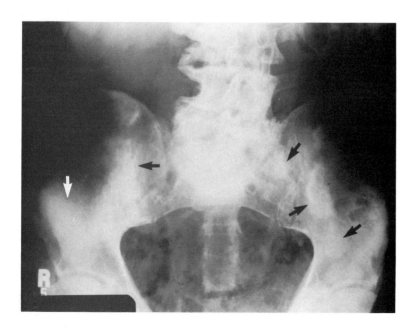

Figure 8–27. Marked osteoblastic metastases of the pelvis and lumbar spine. The patient, an 85-year-old man, was diagnosed as having primary carcinoma of the prostate gland.

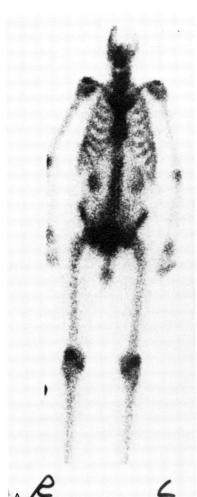

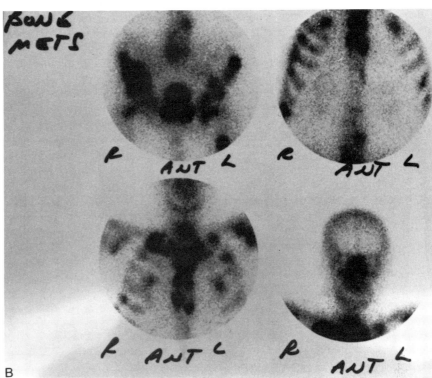

Figure 8–28. Radioisotope bone scan revealing metastases involving bones of the skull, spine, sternum, ribs, and pelvis. *A*, Anterior; *B*, posterior. This 54-year-old man was diagnosed as having primary carcinoma of the prostate gland.

lung cancer. It is estimated that 27,000 deaths occurred in 1987 as the result of prostate cancer. The incidence increases dramatically with age. About 80% of all prostate cancers involve men over the age of 65. For unknown reasons, black Americans have the highest rate of incidence in the world. Although there is some familial association, it is unclear whether this is due to genetic or environmental causes. Persons who work with cadmium are found to be at a slightly higher risk.

Diagnosis. The physician routinely performs a digital rectal examination. With prostatic hypertrophy, the enlargement is more anterior. A palpable prostatic nodule, associated with carcinoma, is usually located more posterior. Excretory urograms are usually ordered to rule out other forms of pathology. Radiographs of the contrast-filled bladder often reveal *diffuse* irregularity of the bladder as a result of an outlet obstruction due to prostate enlargement (Fig. 8–26). It is not uncommon to observe osteoblastic metastases of the pelvis when an excretory urogram is performed (Fig. 8–27). Sometimes, the metastases are apparent before the discovery of the primary lesion. A radionuclide bone scan using technetium

99m polyphosphate sometimes reveals an unsuspected area of activity when the bone films are negative (Fig. 8–28). The bone scan has practically replaced the radiographic bone surveys of the 1960s and early 1970s as a means of revealing the extent of bone metastases. CT of the pelvis assists in staging the disease.

Treatment. Prostate cancer can be treated with surgery alone or in combination with radiation, hormones, or chemotherapy. Surgery and radiation are indicated when the cancer is in an early stage of development and there is a good chance of cure. Hormone therapy and chemotherapy may be used to control the cancer for long periods of time by shrinking the size of the tumor and greatly relieving pain. Because of the overt symptoms, 63% of all prostate cancers are detected while still localized in the prostate. Eighty-three percent of patients with localized prostate cancer will survive 5 years following treatment. Because of the increased public awareness of the importance of a physical examination and the improved methods of detection and treatment, the survival rates for all stages combined have increased from 48 to 70% in the past 20 years.

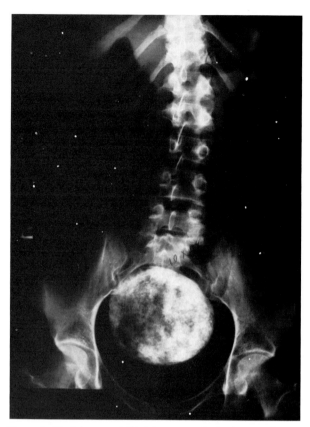

Figure 8–29. A large, calcified 9-cm mass in the lower pelvis, consistent with a benign leiomyoma or fibroid tumor of the uterus, in an 18-year-old female.

Leiomyoma of the Uterus

General Information. Leiomyoma, which is also referred to as a *fibroid* tumor, is a smooth muscle tumor of the uterus. It is the most common benign tumor in women and is associated with pregnancy, when it often increases in size because of hormonal stimulation. Leiomyomas are present in approximately 20% of all women older than 35. Fibroid tumors are typically benign, well circumscribed, rounded, firm, hard masses of gray-white tissue. They are often multiple and usually occur during the years of active reproductive life. This condition affects blacks three times more frequently than whites.

Diagnosis. Although bleeding is a usual early symptom and may be confirmed by a pelvic examination, many fibroids appear as incidental findings on abdominal radiographs. In this case, they can be calcified and most apparent (Fig. 8–29). When they are confirmed by a pelvic examination, a colon examination may be ordered to rule out carcinoma of the colon.

Treatment. The course of treatment depends on the severity of the tumor and symptoms. Frequent pelvic examinations are scheduled at periodic intervals. If a future pregnancy is anticipated, the tumor may be removed surgically. The tumor must not grow so large that it causes an intestinal obstruction. At a later time, a hysterectomy may be indicated.

Breast Tumors

There are three primary types of breast neoplasms. The *fibroadenoma* is the most common benign tumor of the breast. It may develop anytime after puberty, most often before the age of 30. A condition referred to as **mammary dysplasia** or *fibrocystic disease* is not neoplastic but is believed to be the result of estrogenic hormonal imbalance. It is the reason for more than half of all operations on the female breast. *Carcinoma* of the breast is the most common and most dreaded malignancy in women, and it commonly strikes in the prime of life. The course of breast carcinoma is unpredictable, and the risk of metastasis may last for 20 years or more. In 1987, an estimated 130,000 new cases and more than 41,300 related deaths were anticipated. The mortality rate is currently 92 deaths per 100,000 population. In 1981, breast cancer accounted for more than 27% of all cancers in females. The highest mortality is in the age-group between 55 and 74 years, and the survival rate is roughly 75%. Caucasian survival is presently 75%, as compared with that of blacks, whose rate is 63%. Worldwide statistics indicate that England and Wales have the highest mortality rate, 33.8 per 100,000. The United States currently has the 14th highest mortality rate of breast cancer, 27.1 per 100,000.

According to the Breast Cancer Detection Demonstration Project Data Management Advisory Group (BCDDP), the cancer is more frequent in the **left** breast and the most common location is the **upper outer** quadrant. One percent of breast cancer occurs in men. Breast cancer is five times more common in patients with a family history and in women with no children or whose first child was born after age 30. Cancer of both breasts occurs in 10% of cases, with 93% of these occurring sequentially and 7% simultaneously.

Although there is no known cause, there appear to be contributing genetic and hormonal factors such as viruses, diet, immunological factors, radiation of patients with tuberculosis, radiation treatments for mastitis, and estrogen levels.

Breast lesions may be detected by visual changes in the breast tissue, self-examination, physical examination, and mammography. Radiography of the breast has been enhanced by advances that have greatly reduced the radiation hazards.

Fibroadenoma

General Information. Fibroadenoma develops as a result of increased sensitivity of a focal area of the breast to estrogens. The lesions are usually *solitary* but can be multiple. The lesion is movable and averages 2 to 4 cm in diameter or larger. There usually are no changes in the overlying tissue, nor are there any changes within the axillary lymph nodes. This lesion is entirely benign.

Diagnosis. This lesion is readily palpable and is usually discovered by the patient during routine self-examination or during a physical examination. There is no pain associated with this mass, and without self- or physical examination the lesion may go undetected. The lesion is identified on mammography (Fig. 8–30).

Treatment. Following analysis of the biopsied specimen and confirmation of the benign nature of the adenoma, the remainder of the lesion is excised. This surgical procedure usually renders a total cure.

Fibrocystic Disease/Mammary Dysplasia

General Information. Fibrocystic disease is a common female disorder associated with an estrogenic hormone imbalance and does not become clinically significant until ovarian function is fully evolved. It

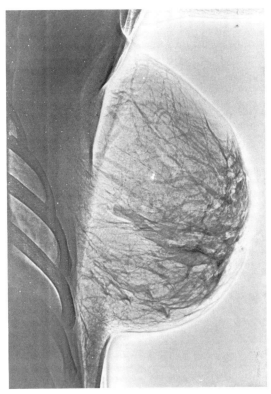

Figure 8–31. Benign fibrocystic disease of the right breast in a 45-year-old woman.

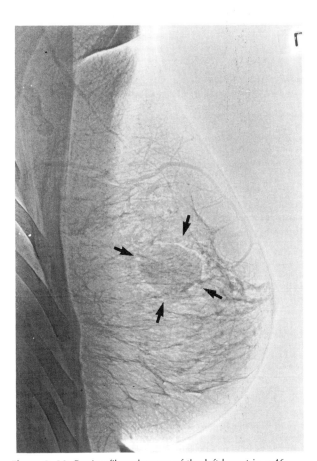

Figure 8–30. Benign fibroadenoma of the left breast in a 46-year-old woman.

is estimated that about 10% of adult women in the United States have symptoms of proliferative fibrocystic disease. Women with this disease have as great as four times the average risk of developing breast cancer. Cysts that are larger than 3 mm in diameter are considered a higher risk for breast cancer. The cystic lesions are frequently *multiple* and occur *bilaterally.* The upper outer quadrant is the part of the breast most often involved.

Diagnosis. The patient usually complains of a dull, heavy pain and tenderness on palpation. Routine mammography demonstrates this lesion (Fig. 8–31).

Treatment. Although the treatment methods vary, the cysts are often aspirated. This procedure assures that the lesions are cystic and not solid.

Carcinoma of the Breast

General Information. Adenocarcinoma of the breast is second only to lung cancer as the leading fatal cancer of women. It is estimated that 41,000 women died of breast cancer in 1987 and 1 of 10 women will develop breast cancer during their lifetime. The greatest risk of breast cancer involves women older than 50 who have a family history of breast cancer, women who have never had children, and women who bore their first child after age 30.

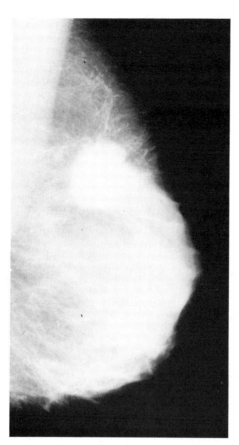

Figure 8–32. An obvious 2.5-cm lesion of the upper central left breast in a 47-year-old woman. The hallmarks of infiltrating margins with skin retraction are present. These findings are consistent with carcinoma.

The ingestion of dietary fat is one of the leading environmental factors that is believed to predispose to the development of breast cancer. Women with large breasts are more prone to develop breast cancer. The majority (50%) of lesions are found on the **upper outer** breast quadrant. Twenty percent are centrally located, 20% are located in the medial quadrant, and 10% are found in the lower anterior portion. The BCDDP, initiated in 1973, included 28 centers and involved 273,108 women who were screened for 5 consecutive years. In controlled surveillance of asymptomatic patients, the BCDDP study found that 80% of detected lesions were localized. Other studies report that 45% of lesions are found prior to regional spread.

Diagnosis. Breast cancer is usually found during a routine self-examination. Although many lesions are not palpable, many are represented as painless lumps or masses. Later signs include nipple retraction, bleeding from the nipple, ulceration, reddening of the skin, pain, and enlarged axillary nodes.

The advantage of mammography as a diagnostic tool is that it is able to demonstrate lesions that are not perceptible by palpation. Although the efficacy and frequency of mammography versus the risks have been debated by physicians for years, modern mammographic equipment results in a much lower radiation dose than that previously administered. Because early detection is so important, the benefits provided by mammography outweigh the radiation risks. For asymptomatic women between the ages of 40 and 49 years, the American College of Radiology recommends a baseline mammogram at age 40, a physical examination with breast examination annually, and mammography at intervals of 1 to 2 years. Women with a direct family history (mother, grandmother, or sister) of breast carcinoma are urged to have an annual mammogram. In baseline mammographic screening of asymptomatic patients, more than 95% of the cancers detected by mammography alone were localized lesions. Mammography has an accuracy rate of 85 to 92%. The 10-year survival rate of patients diagnosed via mammography is 95%. Currently, mammography is performed with specialized equipment using a film-screen combination or xeroradiographic technique. Thermography has been used as a diagnostic tool, but the results have been too nonspecific to be of much value. Both false-negative as well as false-positive rates are very high. Ultrasonography currently is unable to perceive a lesion that is less than 1 cm in diameter.

Once a lesion is demonstrated on mammography, an excisional biopsy with or without a mastectomy is completed. A staging workup includes a chest x-ray, complete blood count, and liver chemistry studies for all patients. Radionuclide bone scans can identify areas of metastasis even before the patient has pain. However, the bone scan also reveals other areas of increased isotope activity, which may be produced by any number of inflammatory disorders. CT and ultrasonography as well as nuclear medicine are able to demonstrate late-stage liver metastases. Estrogen and progesterone receptor analysis is performed on the surgical specimens. Estrogen receptors are found in about 60% of lesions in women younger than 50 years and in about 75% of women older than 50. These receptors are cytoplasmic proteins that form complexes with the respective hormones. They are subsequently translocated into the cell nuclei, where binding to chromatin leads to alterations of protein synthesis characteristic of a response to the hormone. Generally, breast carcinoma metastasizes to the **lungs** and **bone** first and to the **brain** and **liver** later (Fig. 8–32).

Treatment. Following confirmation by biopsy, the axillary lymph nodes are resected for staging purposes. If the lesion is localized, a modified radical mastectomy is performed. This is the treatment of choice of most surgeons. The entire breast is removed, with preservation of the pectoralis muscles. Currently, a significant number of surgeons are performing surgical lumpectomy, a simple removal of the lesion. The remainder of the breast is preserved, and there is little breast deformity. This of course is performed only on localized lesions. Some studies report that lumpectomy, when combined with chemotherapy or radiation therapy, is as successful as the modified radical or simple mastectomy. When regional metastases are noted, a radical mastectomy is performed. This procedure involves the removal of the entire breast, pectoral muscles, and axillary lymph nodes. Radiation therapy is employed for many localized lesions following surgery. Radiation is administered to the lymph nodes in the chest, since the early metastases settle in the lungs. Cancers that are not resectable are treated with combined radiation therapy and chemotherapy. Without chemotherapy, 75% of patients will develop further metastases within 10 years. In the presence of distant metastastes, total cure is rare and remission is uncommon. With distant metastases, the goal is to maximize the quality of life. Typically there is a 1- to 3-year survival period following therapeutic treatment. If the lesion is detected early and is localized, it is not uncommon for 90% of patients to survive at least 5 years. Once the cancer has spread, the 5-year survival rate decreases to 60%. Breast carcinoma in men has a poorer prognosis than in women. Endocrine therapy is more successful than chemotherapy.

Central Nervous System Tumors

Primary tumors of the central nervous system account for 9 to 10% of all cancer deaths. Approximately 10% of all nervous system disorders are neoplasms. It is estimated that 14,700 new cases of primary central nervous system tumors and 10,200 deaths occurred in 1987. Gliomas account for about 50% of all primary brain tumors, and glioblastomas account for 50% of all gliomas. Other forms of glioma include astrocytoma, oligodendroglioma, and ependymoma.

Brain tumors can occur in any age-group. The majority of tumors in adults are found in the *cerebrum*, and they most frequently affect persons 40 to 60 years of age. Meningiomas are the most frequently occurring nonglial tumors, primarily affecting adults around the age of 50. Meningiomas are typically nonaggressive tumors. Pituitary adenomas are responsible for 12 to 18% of intracranial neoplasms. Adenomas are almost always benign. Neurilemoma or schwannoma is chiefly a benign tumor affecting adults. In children, 20% of all tumors are brain tumors, and 60 to 70% of these are located in the *cerebellum* or *posterior fossa*. *Medulloblastomas* account for 30% of primary pediatric brain tumors. Ependymomas are the most frequently occurring tumors of the fourth ventricle. Optic pathway tumors account for 5% of intracranial tumors in children. The most prevalent brain tumors in adults are astrocytomas, glioblastomas, metastatic tumors, and meningiomas. In children, the most prevalent brain tumors are astrocytomas, medulloblastomas, ependymomas, and craniopharyngiomas. All types of brain tumor have a greater incidence in males. Brain tumors often interfere with the circulation of cerebrospinal fluid, producing internal hydrocephalus.

Brain tumors are divided into two groups, glial and nonglial. The glial tumors tend to grow through infiltration. This infiltrative quality coupled with the sponge-like quality of the brain makes these tumors biologically malignant and almost impossible to resect. Nonglial tumors typically grow by expansion and therefore are more accessible to the surgeon. Brain tumors do not usually metastasize outside of the central nervous system.

Tumors of the brain produce symptoms that interfere with normal neurological function. Edema fluid is perhaps the most important cause of the symptoms of brain tumors and is the supreme determinant of the level of neurological function that can be expected in the presence of the tumor. Some of the common symptoms of brain tumors include headache, nausea and vomiting, lethargy, seizures, paralysis, aphasia, blindness, deafness, and abnormal changes in personality and behavior. Herniation and hemorrhage are a major consequence of brain swelling affecting the midbrain and pons. Eventually there is destruction of the brain stem, resulting in loss of consciousness, respiratory failure, and death.

Gliomas account for 23% of spinal cord tumors, with two-thirds of them being ependymomas arising in the filum terminale and conus medullaris. Meningiomas and schwannomas account for about 56% of spinal cord tumors and are most often located in the thoracic spine.

Astrocytoma

General Information. Astrocytomas account for about 30% of all gliomas in both adult and pediatric patients. Pediatric astrocytomas almost always affect those younger than 20 years of age. In terms of histological differentiation, patients with grades I and II will survive from a few to several years. Those with grades III and IV usually will not survive more than 12 to 18 months. An astrocytoma that has more of an aggressive tendency and is highly malignant is referred to as *glioblastoma multiforme*. Typically, glioblastoma multiforme is actually a grade III or IV astrocytoma. *Oligodendrogliomas* are tumors of astrocytic origin that often may appear as calcified lesions on plain skull radiographs. They account for between 5 and 8% of all intracranial tumors found in the cerebrum. When surgery is possible, approximately 50% of patients will survive 5 years.

Diagnosis. CT scanning and MR imaging can graphically illustrate the extent of the brain tumor. Except for when a contrast agent is injected intravenously for tumor enhancement, both CT and MR are essentially noninvasive. They are most useful for determining the tumor response to radiation as well as for evaluating the level of recurrence following

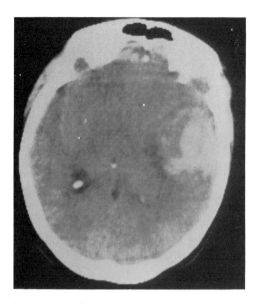

Figure 8–33. CT scan demonstrating a 5-cm blood-containing circumscribed mass in the left temporal fossa, displacing midline structures to the right. These findings are consistent with glioblastoma. The patient is a 45-year-old woman.

surgical resection (Figs. 8–33 and 8–34). When necessary, the cerebral angiogram will reveal *displacement* of vascular structures and is especially accurate in locating tumors of the anterior two-thirds of the cerebrum. These findings are of special importance to the surgeon who will be removing the lesion (Fig. 8–35). An analysis of spinal fluid is valuable, because when protein is elevated, a lesion is almost certain to be evident in the brain or spinal cord. MR imaging offers a new capability in three-dimensional tumor imaging.

Treatment. Surgical excision is the primary treatment for intracranial neoplasms. Malignant brain

tumors are usually responsive to radiation, and these treatments are very important following surgery. The patient usually tolerates the radiation well. Chemotherapy is employed when metastatic lesions are present. The data thus far on numerous combinations of chemicals have been inconclusive.

Ependymoma

General Information. Ependymomas are derived from the lining cells of the ventricles and central canal of the spinal cord. These account for fewer than

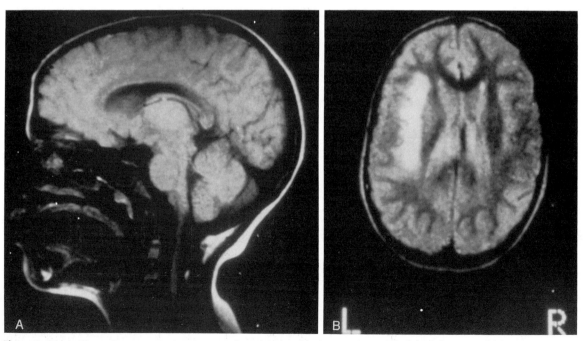

Figure 8–34. *A,* Magnetic resonance imaging reveals an intense signal occupying most of the left temporal lobe. *B,* The mass effect is noted on the left lateral ventricle. These findings indicate the presence of a primary glioma or astrocytoma in this 34-year-old woman.

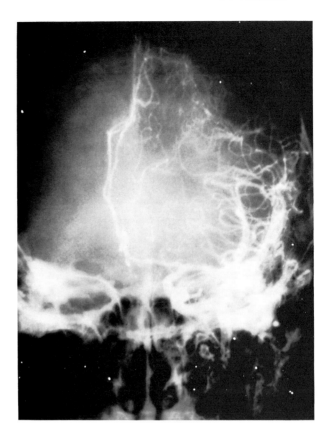

Figure 8–35. Cerebral angiogram, axial view, reveals a large mass in the upper right cerebral hemisphere, described as a subdural hematoma. There is a significant shift of the anterior cerebral artery and midline structures to the left in this 58-year-old man.

2% of all brain tumors. Fifty percent are located above the tentorium, and 40% are located below the tentorium. Some can be found in the filum terminale. Although this tumor can afflict almost any age-group, it predominates in 3- to 4-year-old children.

Diagnosis. This tumor is diagnosed in a similar manner to that of other astrocytomas (Fig. 8–36).

Treatment. Ependymoma is a slow-growing tumor that is known to recur very late, and the primary treatment is determined by the grade of the tumor. Grades I and II have a better prognosis. Radiation

combined with surgery may yield a survival rate as high as 80% over a 5-year period. This rate of survival decreases to 30% over a 10-year period.

Medulloblastoma

General Information. Medulloblastomas typically are highly malignant tumors that occur at a mean age of 14 years. The *cerebellum* is the usual site of the tumor, and 50 to 80% arise posteriorly in the mid-

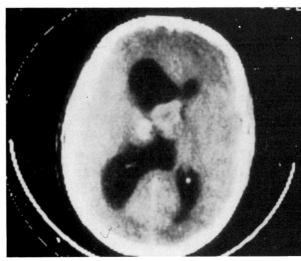

Figure 8–36. A 3 × 4.5-cm biloculated mass of the third ventricle and thalamus superiorly, lying within the bodies of both lateral ventricles. There is some irregularity of the tumor margins, with partial calcification. The patient is a 23-year-old man.

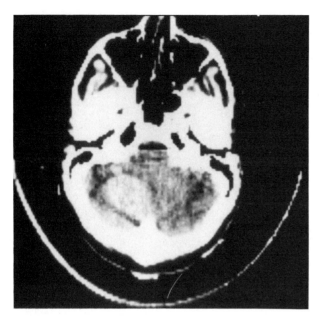

Figure 8–37. Medulloblastoma of the cerebellum with secondary internal hydrocephalus in a 20-year-old man.

sagittal plane from the roof of the fourth ventricle. They often inhibit the flow of cerebrospinal fluid along its pathways, thus they are often associated with hydrocephalus.

Diagnosis. CT, MR imaging, and vertebral angiography provide the best means of identifying the location and extent of the tumor (Fig. 8–37).

Treatment. Medulloblastoma is seldom ever cured by surgery alone. There is direct extension of this lesion into the spinal canal. The use of radiation to

the craniovertebral region has improved the survival rate to between 40 and 50% over a 5-year period. Unfortunately, the rate of recurrence (50 to 60%) is quite high. Chemotherapy has been somewhat successful in increasing the survival rate to about 71%.

Meningioma

General Information. Meningiomas account for approximately 15 to 20% of all adult intracranial tumors. They are usually benign and are the most frequently occurring nonglial tumors. They occur more frequently in females than in males and are rare in children. The lesion evolves slowly, and the neurological deficits appear gradually. Approximately 50% of these lesions are located *parasagittally* on the *vertex* of the cranium. Meningiomas are also known to develop within the spinal canal, but this site is far less common than the brain.

Diagnosis. Because of the slow-growing nature of this tumor, *calcification* is common. This lesion, when calcified, produces an obvious appearance on routine radiographs of the skull. CT reveals this lesion as a well-enhanced lesion. Because of the increased density of the lesion, it is not necessary to infuse the patient with contrast media (Fig. 8–38).

Treatment. Because of their superficial approximation to adjacent tissue, meningiomas are usually easier for the surgeon to remove than are other intracranial lesions. Typically, the tumor is nonaggressive and usually does not have any malignant tendencies. The prognosis is excellent, with 73 to 78% of individuals surviving a 5- to 10-year period following surgery and irradiation.

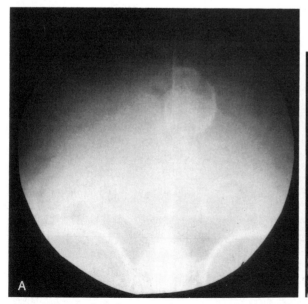
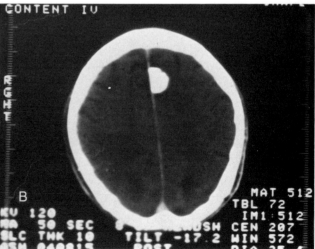

Figure 8–38. A calcified parasagittal meningioma as observed on *(A)* anterior view of the skull and *(B)* CT scan, to the right of the anterior falx. The patient is an 80-year-old man.

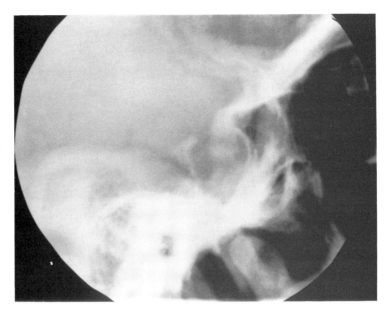

Figure 8–39. A symmetrical, ballooning, abnormally enlarged sella turcica in a 53-year-old man. These findings are consistent with chromophobe adenoma.

Pituitary Adenoma

General Information. Pituitory adenomas account for 12 to 18% of all intracranial neoplasms. These usually benign tumors have an extremely high rate of cure with surgery and irradiation and a low mortality rate and are usually slow growing and well *encapsulated*. The most common type of pituitary adenoma is the chromophobe adenoma.

Diagnosis. The symptoms of pituitary adenoma are the result of pressure on adjacent tissue due to the presence of the lesion. The neurological features include vision defects, headaches, seizures, and erosion and other changes that render the sella turcica *asymmetric* and that can best be seen on radiographically as a *ballooning* enlargement on the lateral view of the skull (Fig. 8–39). The lateral view of the cerebral angiogram is useful in demonstrating the carotid siphon as it courses along the sella turcica. Adenomas typically are located above or within the sella turcica and displace the carotid siphon. This lateral view also may reveal displacement of vessels involving the *sylvian triangle* (Fig. 8–40). CT scan

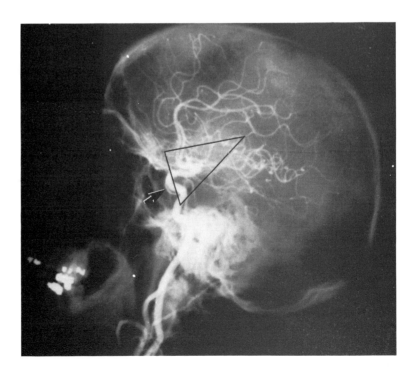

Figure 8–40. Normal appearance of the internal carotid artery and its branches. The carotid siphon (arrow) follows the course of the sella turcica. The vessels forming the sylvian triangle are noted (triangle).

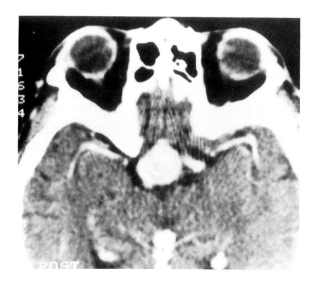

Figure 8–41. A contrast-enhancing infrasellar and suprasellar mass with an apparent cystic component near its apex on the left. This most likely represents a chromophobe adenoma in this 76-year-old man.

demonstrates the adenoma with the assistance of contrast enhancement (Fig. 8–41).

Treatment. Pituitary adenomas usually respond well to surgery and radiation, depending on the location of the lesion. When they are resectable, the rate of recurrence is only 5 to 10%. When an adenoma is not resectable, radiation therapy is used palliatively to shrink the size of the tumor.

Craniopharyngioma

General Information. Eighty percent of craniopharyngiomas occur before the age of 30, usually between the ages of 4 and 16. They are *cystic* tumors that are essentially benign. This congenital tumor arises from remnants of Rathke's pouch and may be suprasellar or intrasellar, in a location similar to that of a pituitary adenoma. As many as 80% of these tumors are calcified in children, but they are less likely to be calcified in adults. Erosion of the dorsum sellae is the most frequent finding.

Diagnosis. Radiographically, craniopharyngioma appears as a characteristic suprasellar calcification on the lateral skull film (Fig. 8–42). The cerebral angiogram may also disclose similarities to the pituitary adenoma, namely displacement of the carotid siphon and stretching and displacement of the vessels of the sylvian triangle. This tumor produces visual disturbances.

Treatment. Craniopharyngioma is treated surgically, but excision is often difficult because the

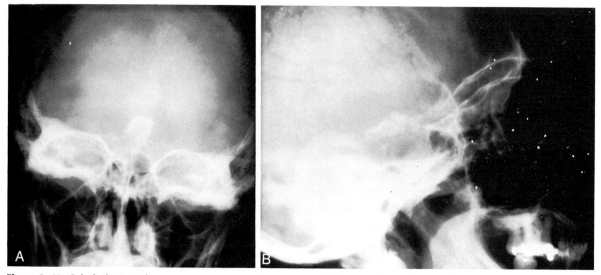

Figure 8–42. Calcified craniopharyngioma as seen on *(A)* anterior and *(B)* lateral views of the skull in a 16-year-old male.

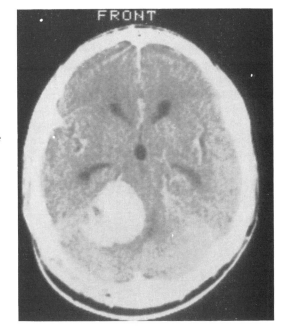

Figure 8–43. A contrast-enhanced mass in the cerebellar pontine angle, which has been revealed as an acoustic neuroma in this 25-year-old man. The mass is about 4.3 cm in diameter. There is a shift of the fourth ventricle to the left, and the right quadrigeminal cistern is effaced and displaced anteriorly.

lesion extends into the suprasellar region and involves the hypothalamus and third ventricle, the circle of Willis, and the optic nerve. There is an operative mortality of 30 to 40%, and the long-term results are poor, with only 20% surviving 10 years. With the addition of radiation therapy to surgery, the success rate approximates that of a grade I astrocytoma.

Acoustic Neurilemoma/Neuroma/ Schwannoma

General Information. Acoustic neurilemoma, neuroma, and schwannoma are tumors of the peripheral nerve sheath. They are found mostly in middle-aged adults and account for 8 to 10% of all intracranial tumors. The most common location is the *eighth* cranial nerve. They may be solid or cystic.

Diagnosis. Patients present with symptoms of hearing loss, tinnitus, vertigo, headaches, and ataxia. Plain skull films and CT scans demonstrate a funnel-like expansion of the internal auditory canal (Fig. 8–43).

Treatment. Surgical removal of as much of the tumor as possible is the primary treatment. If total resection is not achieved, the tumor often recurs. Overall, the prognosis is good.

Hemangioblastoma

General Information. Hemangioblastoma is a highly *vascular* lesion that consists of a conglomeration or tangle of capillary vessels.

Diagnosis. This common tumor may appear as a solitary dense nodule or a tangle of vessels. This lesion is best seen in the capillary and venous phases of a cerebral angiogram as a deep stain or blush. There usually is displacement of the fourth ventricle toward the opposite side, with possible obstruction (Fig. 8–44).

Treatment. Hemangioblastomas can almost always be successfully removed by the neurosurgeon.

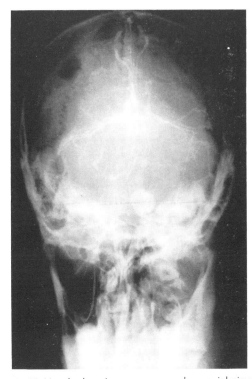

Figure 8–44. Vertebral angiogram, venous phase axial view, revealing a left hemangioblastoma.

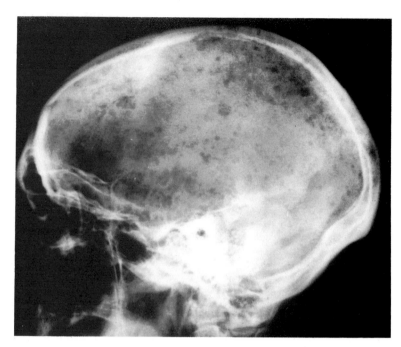

Figure 8–45. A right lateral view of the skull revealing numerous punched-out osteolytic lesions of the flat bones of the skull, consistent with multiple myeloma, in this 72-year-old woman.

Metastatic Tumors

General Information. Twenty to 25% of all brain tumors are metastatic. Primary lung carcinoma is the leading contributor to brain metastases. Forty to 50% of patients who die from this disease show brain involvement. Both solitary and multiple lesions are possible, but a solitary metastatic lesion is usually present. Other primary sites sending metastases to the brain include the colon, kidney, breast, and bone marrow. Fifty percent of patients with malignant melanoma have brain metastases.

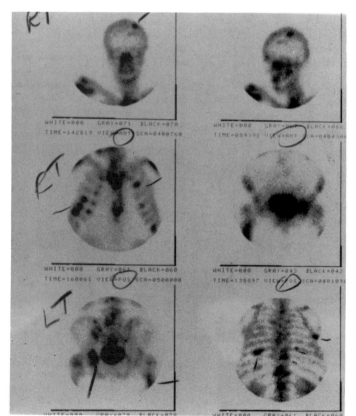

Figure 8–46. Increased isotope activity of the skull consistent with metastases.

Diagnosis. The symptoms and signs of metastatic brain carcinoma are typical of other brain tumors. Symptoms of metastases may occur before the primary lesion is discovered. Displacement of normal structures and a calcified pineal gland are common. Metastatic lesions may be observed on plain skull films, CT, MR and radioisotope scans (Figs. 8–45, 8–46, and 8–47). Chest x-rays of patients with brain tumor often reveal a silent bronchogenic carcinoma.

Treatment. The only treatment for malignant disease is chemotherapy. The prognosis is usually poor. Corticosteroids appear to be the drugs of choice at this time, although many investigational drugs may be administered on an experimental and controlled basis.

Spinal Cord Tumors

General Information. Spinal cord tumors are categorized into three distinct groups: intramedullary, extramedullary intradural, or extradural. The identification is important because of the various surgical approaches undertaken. Most of the primary tumors found in the brain can also be found in the spinal cord. Metastatic neoplasms can cause compression of the spinal cord, disabling the patient and causing a great deal of pain. Gliomas account for 23% of spinal cord tumors. Two-thirds of these are ependymomas. The majority of gliomas are well-differentiated astrocytomas. Meningiomas and schwannomas account for 56% of spinal cord tumors. The gliomas most often

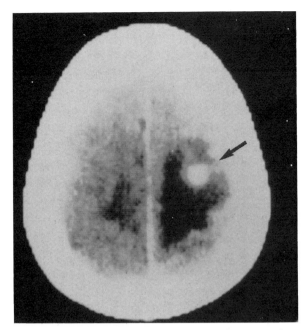

Figure 8–47. Multiple metastatic lesions with a large area of surrounding edema in a 45-year-old man.

arise in the filum terminale and conus medullaris. Meningiomas and schwannomas are most often found in the thoracic spine.

Diagnosis. Myeolography is able to differentiate between the three types of masses that may be located within the spinal canal (Figs. 8–48, 8–49, and 8–50).

Figure 8–48. Thoracic myelogram revealing intramedullary widening of the spinal cord at T-2, T-3, and T-4 in a 26-year-old man. These findings are consistent with an ependymoma or astrocytoma of the spinal cord.

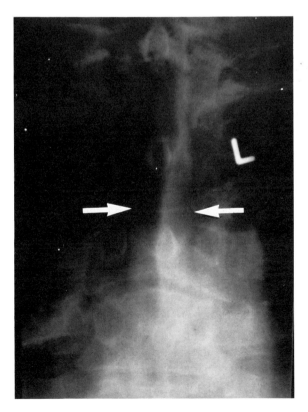

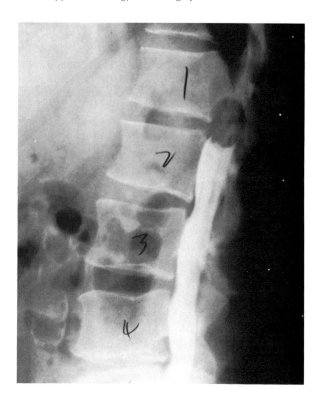

Figure 8–49. Lumbar myelogram revealing a complete block at the L1-2 level, with a sharp concave filling defect. This lesion is most likely an ependymoma or astrocytoma.

Treatment. The prognosis depends on the type, location, and extent of the tumor. Many of these tumors are not resectable, and radiation and chemotherapy often are the primary modes of treatment.

Lymphatic System Cancer

Malignant lymphomas are solid neoplasms afflicting the lymph nodes, spleen, bone marrow, thymus, liver, and submucosa of the respiratory and digestive tracts. They usually present as a firm, painless enlargment of the lymph nodes. Diffuse lymphomas are more aggressive than nodular lymphomas. Lymphoma has no benign counterpart. Classification of neoplasms of the lymphatic system is based on the cell of origin. The exact etiology of lymphoma is unknown, but there is evidence linking lymphoma with acquired immunological disorders such as Sjögren's syndrome, systemic lupus erythematosus,

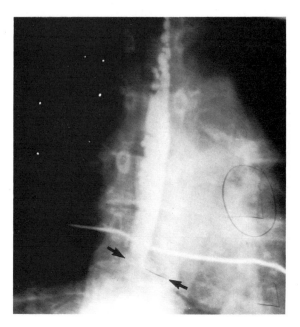

Figure 8–50. Thoracic myelogram revealing an extramedullary extradural mass in the spinal canal extending through most of the T-7 level and much of the T-8 level along the left later anterior aspect of the canal, displacing the cord to the right. The patient is a 48-year-old woman.

rheumatoid disease, and Hashimoto's disease. The presence of any of these disorders increases the probability of lymphoma 50 times.

Hodgkin's Disease

General Information. Hodgkin's disease was named for Thomas Hodgkin, who performed research on the lymphatic system in 1832 and is credited with identifying the characteristics of this disease.

Hodgkin's disease accounts for 40 to 45% of all lymphomas and is the most common and curable form of lymphoma. In 1987, 7300 new cases and 24,900 related deaths were anticipated. Approximately 50% of the cases involved persons between the ages of 20 and 40 years. Fewer than 10% of cases have their onset after age 60, and 10% before the age of 10 years. Males have a higher incidence and poorer prognosis than females.

This disease directly affects the lymph nodes and later involves the liver, spleen, bone marrow, and lungs. The cells that undergo proliferation are mononuclear **Reed-Sternberg** cells. Patients with Hodgkin's disease are susceptible to viral, mycobacterial, and fungal infections.

Diagnosis. Many radiographic procedures are used in diagnosing Hodgkin's disease. PA chest radiographs often reveal enlargement and widening of the superior mediastinum (Fig. 8–51). IVP can rule out asymptomatic kidney involvement. Bipedal lymphangiography can demonstrate the *classic foamy* appearance of the lymph nodes, which may be indicative of Hodgkin's disease and other types of lymphoma (Figs. 8–52, 8–53, and 8–54). Nuclear medicine gallium scanning is an excellent way of detecting abnormal

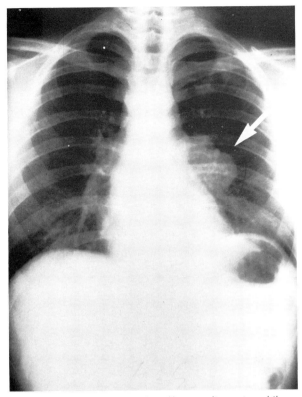

Figure 8–51. Posteroanterior chest film revealing a 4-cm hilar mass, consistent with Hodgkin's disease, in a 23-year-old man.

lymph nodes throughout the body. Hodgkin's disease affects bone more frequently than does non-Hodgkin's lymphoma. Osteolytic and osteoblastic metastases may appear individually or together on bone. CT is useful in staging all forms of lymphoma.

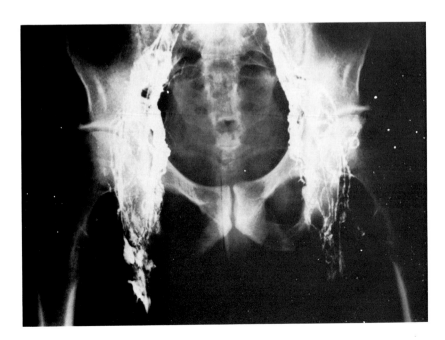

Figure 8–52. A normal-appearing bipedal lymphangiogram in a 35-year-old man.

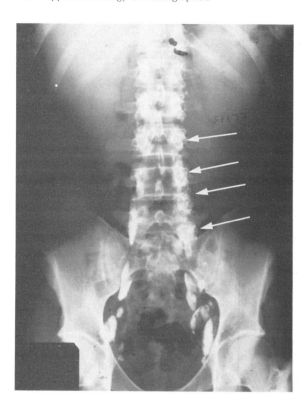

Figure 8–53. Bipedal lymphangiogram revealing multiple abnormal lymph nodes that have a classic foamy, soapsuds appearance involving the left paraaortic, iliac, and inguinal nodes with multiple small filling defects and some abnormal displacement. The patient is a 23-year-old man.

Treatment. The primary role of surgery is to obtain a tissue diagnosis through biopsy. Abdominal exploration with biopsies of the lymph nodes, bone marrow, and removal of the spleen are performed to rule out visceral involvement. Radiation therapy is the primary treatment for stages 1 and 2. Chemotherapy is technically designed to treat stages 3 and 4 but can be employed for stages 1 and 2 when the patient cannot tolerate radiation treatments. There is an excellent chance of a total cure following surgery and radiation treatments. Sixty to 90% of patients will survive for 10 or more years after treatment.

Leukemia

General Information. Leukemia is a blood neoplasia that is characterized by an abnormal proliferation and incomplete maturation of leukocytes and lymphocytes. The primary clinical manifestation is an abnormal decrease of red cells, granulocytes, and platelets. It can be classed as either *myelocytic* or *lymphocytic*. Leukemia originates in the marrow and has the ability to infiltrate other structures such as the lymph nodes, liver, spleen, and other tissues. Leukemia can occur as an acute or chronic disease in

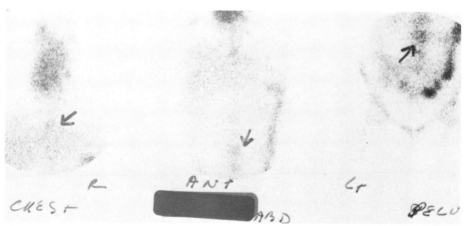

Figure 8–54. Increased uptake in the mediastinal and supraclavicular lymph nodes and at the level of the diaphragm in the posterior mediastinum and possibly the body of L-3 on 120-hour gallium scan. The patient is a 26-year-old woman.

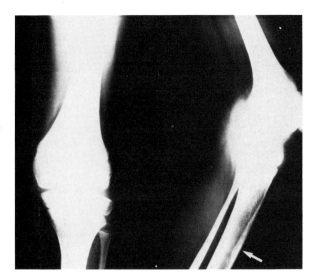

Figure 8–55. Patchy areas of destruction of the metaphyses of the knee joint in a 12-year-old girl. These findings are compatible with leukemia.

adults and children. The incidence rates vary according to the type of involved cell. The exact cause of leukemia is unknown. Evidence from epidemiological studies suggests that enviromental and genetic factors may be causes of leukemia, although there is limited evidence. *Acute* lymphocytic leukemia is typically a disease affecting *children*. *Chronic* lymphocytic leukemia most often affects the *elderly*. Acute myelocytic leukemia can occur in any age-group. Chronic myelocytic leukemia occurs in middle-aged adults. All forms of leukemia have a slight male predominance, except for chronic lymphocytic leukemia, which has a more striking male predominance. In 1987, 26,400 new cases and 17,800 related deaths were anticipated. The incidences of acute and chronic leukemia are about equal.

Diagnosis. Symptoms of leukemia usually occur suddenly in children and gradually in adults. The afflicted child is often listless and pale, suffers from repeated infections, experiences unexplained weight loss, bruises easy, and often has nosebleeds and subcutaneous skin hemorrhages. The symptoms of chronic leukemia are often very vague rather than overt. Diagnosis can be made through hematological tests and bone marrow biopsy. Generally, radiographic abnormalities are more common in children. A *lucent* metaphyseal *band* appearing in the knees and wrists is an important radiographic sign of leukemia in children. Fine, patchy areas of bone destruction are also common in the metaphyses. Changes may also be observed in the skull, where the sutures may be separated, patchy bone destruction is apparent, and occasional vertical bony spicules are frequently observed in the margin of the skull table (Fig. 8–55).

Treatment. According to the American Cancer Society, chemotherapy is the most effective method of treating leukemia. Drugs are used independently or in combination. In some instances, bone marrow

transplants are successful in the treatment of certain leukemias. Transfusion of blood components and antibiotics are used as supportive treatments, because when leukemia occurs, millions of abnormal, immature white blood cells are released. The rate of survival for children has improved significantly. Because of continued research, some cancer centers are reporting as much as a 75% 5-year survival rate. The overall survival rate for whites is 33% and for blacks is 28%.

Bone Tumors

Primary bone sarcoma is accountable for fewer than 0.5% of total deaths due to cancer. Bone tumors account for about 1% of all malignancies. Cancer of bone is most often secondary rather than primary. Bone cancer is most prevalent in adolescence, with a rate of 3 per 100,000. Despite this significant rate at this age, bone tumors account for only 3.2% of childhood malignancies occurring before the age of 15. Males appear to have a slightly higher incidence than females.

Primary cancers of the breast, prostate gland, lungs, kidney, and thyroid commonly metastasize to bone, and 65% of these spread to the spine and pelvis. Bones closest to the trunk are the most common recipients of metastasis.

The most common symptom of bone cancer is persistent pain, which typically worsens at night. In children, these complaints are often dismissed as the results of normal activity in this age-group or as growing pains. As a rule of thumb, any pain that persists for more than a few days requires a medical opinion. Generally, radiographs reveal most bone lesions. Radiographs demonstrate the gross anatomy of the lesion and the ability of the surrounding tissue to confine the developing neoplasm. There are three

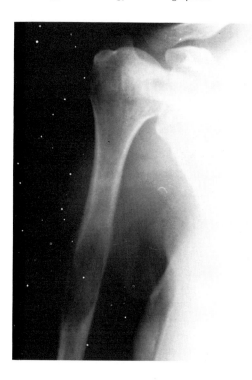

Figure 8–56. A slowly evolving destructive lesion of the right humeral shaft in a 41-year-old woman. The edge of the destroyed bone represents the true edge of the tumor and is characteristic of the geographic pattern of bone disease.

primary destructive patterns of primary bone neoplasms. These patterns vary according to the pathological aggressiveness. A *geographic* pattern denotes a slow rate of growth. The edge of destroyed bone represents the true edge of the tumor. A *moth-eaten* pattern forms where there is an intermediate rate of growth and the tumor has extended beyond the radiographic lesion. The *permeated* pattern indicates rapid growth, with the tumor penetrating the cortex and extending longitudinally within the bone. The

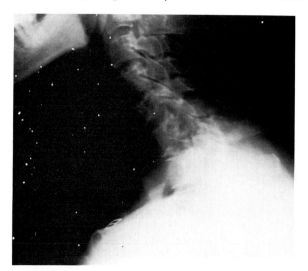

Figure 8–57. Lateral view of the cervical spine revealing an osteolytic moth-eaten appearance of C5-6 and localized kyphosis of the lower cervical spine in a 62-year-old woman.

visible lesion on the radiograph also indicates the desired location for needle biopsy (Figs. 8–56, 8–57, and 8–58).

Many types of bone tumors are most often located in the growth centers of the bone. There is a high degree of correlation between this location and the rapid growth taking place. Although the etiology of bone tumors is unknown, it is postulated that prolonged growth or overstimulated metabolism may be related to the development of a primary bone neoplasm. These conditions may occur in adult patients with Paget's disease, hyperparathyroidism, chronic osteomyelitis, old bone infarcts, and fracture callus. There are some forms of hereditary exostoses (chondromatosis) that have the ability to develop into chondrosarcomas. There has been some evidence linking x-ray and radioisotope treatments with the formation of osteogenic sarcoma, chondrosarcoma, and fibrosarcoma. Most recently it has been suggested that viruses cause osteosarcoma. The role of cancer-causing infectious agents is currently being researched in the laboratory using mice, chickens, and hamsters. In addition to radiography, CT can provide excellent detail of bone and soft tissues for diagnosis as well as for selecting the best site for biopsy. Radioisotope bone scans are useful in determining the degree of bone involvement and metastasis.

Most bone sarcomas are described as osteogenic. Other connective tissue sarcomas are named for their tissue origin. Osteogenic sarcoma accounts for 28%

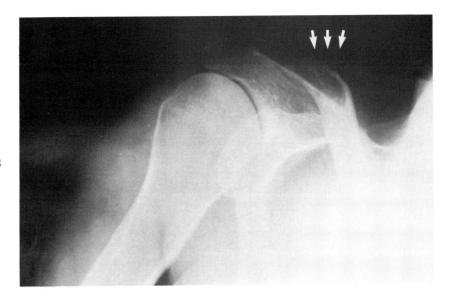

Figure 8–58. Permeated metastases of the right distal clavicle in a 57-year-old man. Note that the metastases have penetrated the cortex and are advancing longitudinally.

of malignant bone lesions, chondrosarcoma for 13%, fibrosarcoma for 4%, and others are even less common. Other forms of disease, such as a wide variety of benign tumors and cysts, fibrous dysplasias, and congenital disorders, must be differentiated from early osteogenic malignancy. There are also specific disorders of bone marrow and of the plasma cells of bone marrow.

A bone lesion can be described in several ways: (1) An osteoblastic lesion is a bone-forming sclerotic growth or tumor in which there is an **increase** in bone density (Fig. 8–59). (2) An osteolytic lesion is a bone-***destroying*** growth or tumor that results in decreased bone density in the affected area. Osteolytic disease has to be differentiated from osteomalacia and osteoporosis (Fig. 8–60). (3) A periosteal reaction

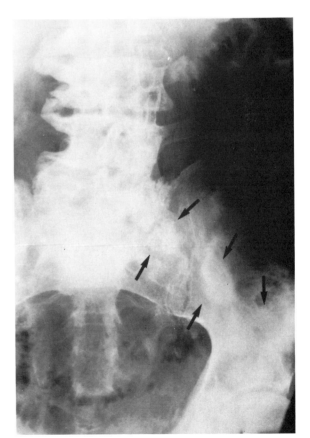

Figure 8–59. Marked osteoblastic metastases of the left hemipelvis and sacrum in an 85-year-old man.

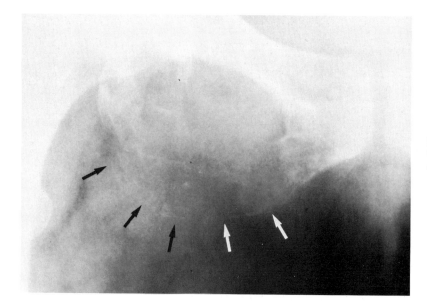

Figure 8–60. Metastatic osteolytic lesions of the right ischium, secondary to primary breast carcinoma, in a 62-year-old woman.

is excess bone produced by the periosteum. This type of lesion can be a simple osteomyelitis or an early osteosarcoma (Fig. 8–61). (4) Cortical thickening occurs when new bone is laid down by the periosteum. Unlike a periosteal reaction, cortical thickening resembles the normal cortex and usually involves a long-term healing process (Fig. 8–62). (5) Alteration in trabecular pattern usually results in a **decrease** in the number of trabeculae and a **thickening** of the remaining trabeculae (Fig. 8–63). (6) Alteration in the bone shape is important in assessing a congenital bone dysplasia or an acquired disorder such as acromegaly (Fig. 8–64). For diagnostic purposes, bone lesions can be categorized as solitary lesions, multiple lesions in one or more bones, and generalized lesions in which all bones are diffusely affected.

In terms of treatment, benign tumors are best removed surgically. Defects in bone can be replaced and filled in with bone grafts. Malignant tumors are best treated with surgery, radiation therapy, and chemotherapy in combination. Treatment depends on the relative sensitivity or resistance to radiation. Osteosarcoma is the most radioresistant tumor, and thus amputation is often necessary.

Cystic Bone Lesions

General Information. It is not known how or why bone cysts appear. There is thought to be some

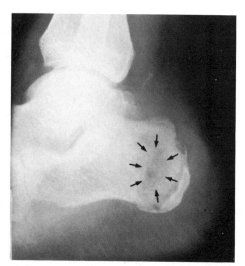

Figure 8–61. Periosteal reaction (arrows) occurring 2 weeks after a minor heel injury in an adolescent male. Osteomyelitis was indicated as the diagnosis.

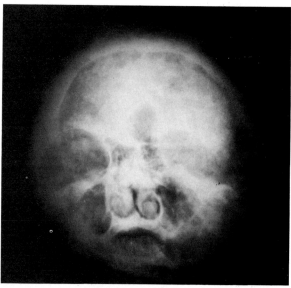

Figure 8–62. Paget's disease of the skull in an 85-year-old woman. There is significant thickening of the bony cortex.

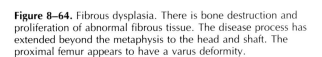

Figure 8–63. *A,* Traumatic comminuted fracture involving both bones of the lower leg, above the ankle. *B,* Re-forming of the trabecular bone, which represents the final stage of healing. The trabecular pattern appears thickened as a result of callus formation. This film of a 34-year-old man was taken 26 months after injury.

relationship to trauma or a hemorrhagic disorder. Typically, the patient is a fairly young child or adolescent. Bone cyst formation is three times more common in males and usually involves the metaphysis into the diaphysis. The femur and humerus are the sites of approximately 75% of bone cysts, which are commonly found at the distal locations in the femur and at proximal areas of the tibia and humerus. The earliest symptom is usually pain, most often associated with fracture. There is often no correlation with a traumatic event. The incidence in males is twice that in females.

Diagnosis. Cysts are radiographically apparent as a *lytic* lucency in the central part of the long bone with *thinning* of the cortex, accompanied by symmetrical *expansion*. A bone cyst usually has a wall of

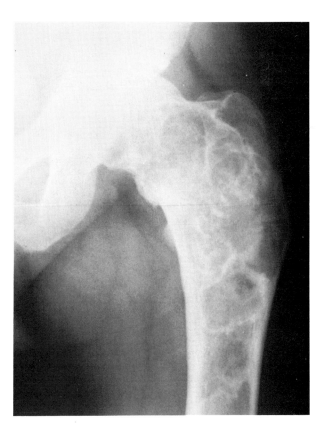

Figure 8–64. Fibrous dysplasia. There is bone destruction and proliferation of abnormal fibrous tissue. The disease process has extended beyond the metaphysis to the head and shaft. The proximal femur appears to have a varus deformity.

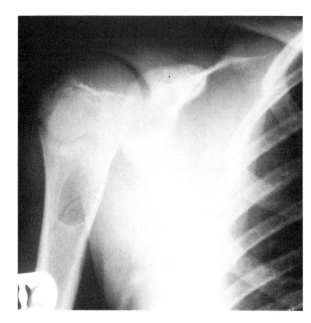

Figure 8–65. Pathological fracture of the proximal shaft of the right humerus in an 11-year-old boy. There is a 2.5 × 1.5–cm unicameral bone cyst.

fibrous tissue and is filled with fluid. Many cysts are of the *unicameral* type, meaning that they contain a solitary cavity (Fig. 8–65). Unicameral bone cysts are often associated with fracture. Fractures associated with disease are referred to as pathological, trophic, or spontaneous fractures. Pathological fractures occur in about 60% of unicameral cysts. As the cyst develops, it descends beneath the epiphyseal plate and

spreads downward toward the shaft and transversely travels toward the periosteal margins. When the margin is penetrated, a fracture occurs. *Multicameral* or *multilocular* bone cysts usually contain numerous cavities (Fig. 8–66). *Aneurysmal* bone cysts are thought possibly to be formed secondary to injury. This lesion has been found in some patients having giant cell tumor. Aneurysmal bone cysts are often

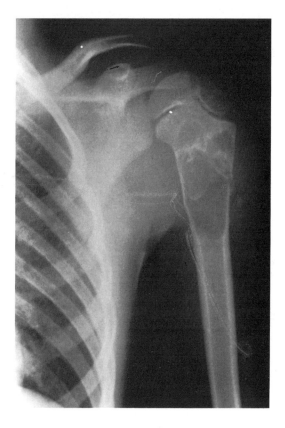

Figure 8–66. Pathological fracture of the upper one-third of the left humeral shaft, with a multicameral cyst that extends well into the metaphysis. The patient is a 6-year-old boy.

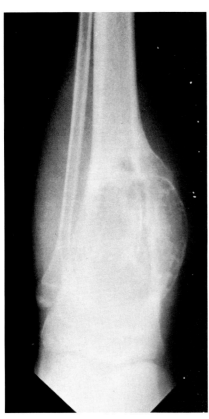

Figure 8–67. Large oval osteolytic lesion with the septa in the proximal tibia. Because of this 17-year-old male's history of prior trauma, the radiographic appearance is consistent with that of an aneurysmal bone cyst of the tibia.

within the bone. When it is located within bone, it is referred to as *enchondroma*. The site of this lesion is usually the small bones of the hands and feet. Adults between the ages of 20 and 30 are most often affected, and both sexes are affected equally often. Enchondroma is significantly more common than periosteal chondroma. In the early stage of the disease, this lesion must be differentiated from chondrosarcoma. A surgical bone biopsy is used to distinguish between the benign and malignant processes. Radiographically, the lesion is revealed as a *localized*, radiolucent, cystic defect with distortion of the contour of bone. Centralized areas of calcification may be apparent. This lesion may also be found in the ribs, sternum, and spine (Fig. 8–68).

Osteochondroma is the most common benign tumor of bone affecting patients younger than 21 years. It is often referred to as an *exostosis*, which is an osteoblastic lesion that may be solitary or multiple and usually appears as an outgrowth from the surface at the metaphysis of long bones. This tumor emanates from bone and cartilage and may also be found on flat bones, especially of the scapula and pelvis. It is not uncommon for this lesion to appear simultaneously in several locations. When this occurs, it is referred to as hereditary multiple exostoses. Osteo-

unicameral and can become very large. They usually assume an asymmetric appearance in the metaphysis (Fig. 8–67).

Treatment. Bone cysts are treated with curettage and implantation of new bone cells into the cystic cavity. The lesion usually heals completely, but despite this treatment, 30% of these will recur. Fifteen percent will heal following fracture. Radiation treatments in addition to surgery have reduced the rate of recurrence. Although the prognosis is favorable, there is documentation of sarcoma following irradiation of aneurysmal bone cysts.

Benign Tumors

General Information. Typically, benign tumors of bone and adjacent tissue are small, have sclerotic margins, and rarely involve cortical destruction. The large majority are osteoblastic. Others originate as cartilaginous tumors.

Diagnosis. Practically all bone tumors can be differentiated radiographically. Chondroma/enchondroma is a cartilaginous tumor. It can be a solitary or multiple lesion, which may be either periosteal or

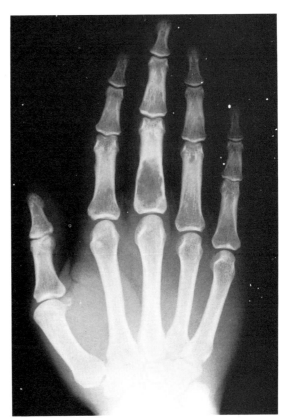

Figure 8–68. Osteolytic lesion of the proximal and middle portion of the proximal phalanx of the right middle finger in a 32-year-old man. The findings are compatible with enchondroma.

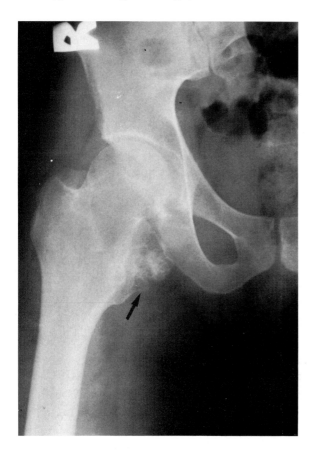

Figure 8–69. Osteoblastic lesion situated adjacent to the lesser trochanter of the right femur. This finding is consistent with benign osteochondroma or hereditary exostosis.

chondroma presents a characteristic mushroom or cauliflower-like radiopaque appearance (Fig. 8–69).

Osteomas are uncommon lesions found almost exclusively in the skull and facial bones, with the frontal sinus being the most common site. This lesion afflicts males more often than females, and it can occur at virtually any age. The lesion is usually asymptomatic. It occurs mostly as a solitary lesion and is composed of compact bone (Fig. 8–70).

Osteoid osteomas are usually small solitary osteo-

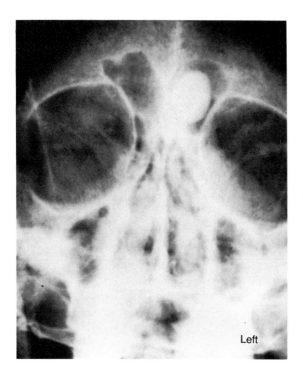

Figure 8–70. Posteroanterior skull view revealing an osteoma in the left frontal sinus cavity.

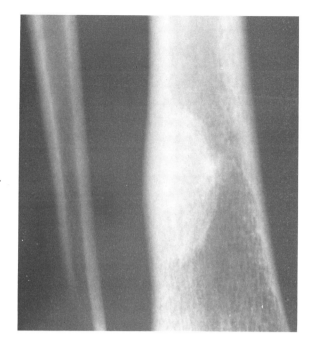

Figure 8–71. Sclerotic density along the distal lateral tibia, consistent with an osteoid osteoma, in a 26-year-old woman.

blastic lesions found in most any bone, but almost always in the femur and tibia. The distal tibia just superior of the epiphysis is a common site. This condition afflicts mostly males and becomes obvious at night, when the pain tends to be more severe. Radiographs reveal a centralized area of radiolucency surrounded by dense sclerotic bone (Fig. 8–71)

Treatment. Curettage is a surgical procedure in which diseased tissue is scraped from a surface. It is the treatment of choice for most benign bone tumors. Chondroma/enchondroma has a tendency to recur after surgical excision. Osteochondromas are surgically removed when the patient complains of pain, and pain is most common when the lesions are multiple. Osteochondroma has been known to transform into a chondrosarcoma. This malignancy is most common in the presence of multiple exostoses. Patients having an osteoma of the frontal or maxillary sinus do not usually require any treatment, unless the lesion is interfering with the drainage of the passageway. In many cases, an osteoma in the sinuses is an incidental finding. In treating an osteoid osteoma, it is necessary to excise all elements of the lesion including some of the surrounding sclerotic bone.

Malignant Tumors

General Information. Malignant tumors are usually larger than their benign counterparts. These lesions usually include a periosteal reaction and no respect whatsoever for tissue margins. Cortical destruction and a loss of bony trabeculation are common. Primary bone lesions usually assume one of three destructive patterns, which are indicative of the degree of aggressiveness of the tumor.

According to the American Cancer Society, multiple myeloma, a nonosseous malignant tumor emanating from the plasma cells of bone marrow, should be considered a bone tumor, and in that context it is the most common malignant bone tumor. In 1978, it was reported that multiple myeloma accounted for 35 to 43% of all malignant bone tumors. Osteosarcoma is the most frequently occurring primary osseous malignant bone tumor, followed by chondrosarcoma, fibrosarcoma, Ewing's sarcoma, and giant cell tumor. Approximately 60 to 65% of malignant bone lesions are metastatic from elsewhere in the body. It is not uncommon for osteolytic bone metastases to be noted on radiographic studies, with the primary tumor site unknown and the patient totally asymptomatic. Metastatic carcinoma of bone is most often found in structures of the axial skeleton, such as the spine, pelvis, and skull. It has been suggested that metastases are less frequent in anatomical sites away from the midsagittal plane. Following confirmation of a primary malignancy, nuclear medicine bone scans are performed to rule out bone metastases. Areas of increased uptake of the radioisotope are revealed as areas of *increased* density, or *hot spots.*

Diagnosis. Multiple myeloma or plasma cell myeloma most frequently afflicts men between the ages of 60 and 80. This condition is characterized by the proliferation of the plasma cells in the medullary cavity. Multiple myeloma is a *multicentric* disease, meaning that it is found in several sites at the time of diagnosis. Patients often complain of pain in the upper and lower back, thorax, and head. An abnormal protein (Bence Jones protein) is found in the urine. As is the case with most malignancies, the cause is unknown. Radiographically noted are multiple *punched-out osteolytic* lesions, especially apparent

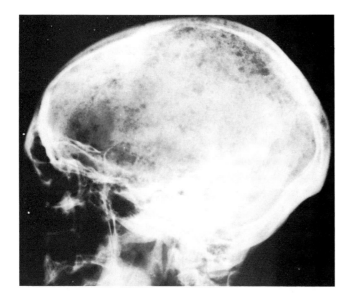

Figure 8–72. Multiple punched-out lesions of the lateral skull, compatible with multiple myeloma, in a 72-year-old woman.

on the flat bones of the skull. This punched-out appearance gives rise to the name *sieve skull* (Fig. 8–72). Compression fractures of the spine are difficult to distinguish from those caused by osteoporosis. According to manufacturers of iodinated contrast media, IVP is contraindicated in patients with a history of multiple myeloma, especially if the patient has been dehydrated. Dehydration may promote precip-

itation of casts and cells in the renal tubules and can cause renal failure.

Osteosarcoma is found to affect persons in the age-group from 10 to 25 years, with a higher incidence in males. It is also common in older adults as a malignant change in Paget's disease. The **metaphyseal** regions of the distal femur and proximal humerus are most frequently involved with osteosarcoma. Sev-

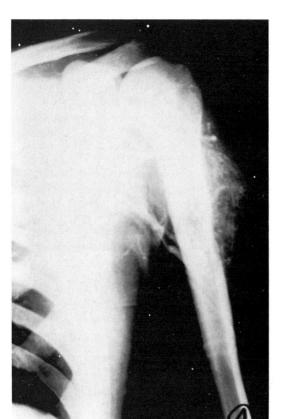

Figure 8–73. Soft tissue mass lesion with osteoblastic activity involving the proximal humerus in a 17-year-old. These findings are consistent with primary osteogenic sarcoma.

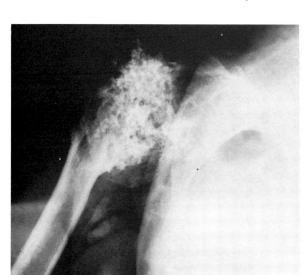

Figure 8–74. A large, soft tissue mass lesion that encompasses the entire right humeral head, neck, and metaphyses. This moth-eaten appearance is compatible with chondrosarcoma. The patient is a 55-year-old woman.

enty-five percent are found in the distal femur at the knee. This tumor can occur without explanation, but many patients have a hisotry of trauma, with pain in the knee lasting for 3 to 4 months before the lesion is detected. Radiographically, osteosarcoma can be described as a most destructive, often large soft tissue mass, with new *osteoblastic* activity (spicules) within the soft tissue mass. The formation of the bone spicules is sometimes referred to as the *sun-ray* appearance. In addition, the periosteum may lift up, forming a cuff. This is common with osteosarcoma and with other aggressive bone conditions. Thus, osteosarcoma must be included in the differential diagnosis of any abnormal bone condition (Fig. 8–73).

Chondrosarcoma is an *expanding* osteolytic lesion that may form from a benign chondroma. This condition occurs mostly in men from 30 to 60 years old and accounts for between 7 and 15% of all bony neoplasms. This tumor usually invades the soft tissues following the initial bone destruction. The average age of onset is 45 years, and the pelvis, ribs, scapulae, humeri, and proximal femora are the most common locations. Radiographically, this is a slow-growing, large *soft tissue mass,* with or without flecks of calcification. This lesion is most destructive to underlying bone (Fig. 8–74).

Fibrosarcoma is a malignant tumor of the metaphyses of long bones, flat bones, and soft tissues. The bones of the knee and pelvis are most commonly involved. It primarily affects adults from 45 to 60 years old. This is characteristically a *lytic* lesion with a *moth-eaten* appearance, which may vary in severity from erosion to total destruction and is often associated with a soft tissue mass. The peak age of onset is in the mid-30s. This tumor is known to develop into Paget's disease. Fibrosarcoma may also be difficult to differentiate from metastatic bone disease (Fig. 8–75).

Ewing's sarcoma is a rare primary bone lesion affecting a typically young age-group between the ages of 10 and 30, with 80% occurring before the age of 20. Sixty percent of cases involve the *shafts* of long bones and some flat bones. Early symptoms of Ewing's sarcoma include severe pain, fever, and leukocytosis. These symptoms also mimic osteomyelitis, therefore differentiation is necessary. Ewing's sar-

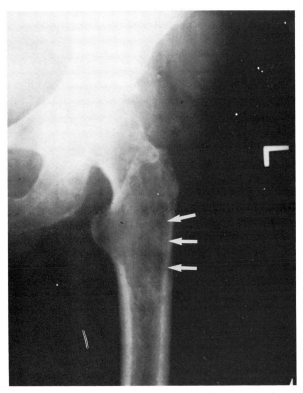

Figure 8–75. Lytic, moth-eaten appearance of the proximal femur in a 60-year-old man. This is consistent with fibrosarcoma.

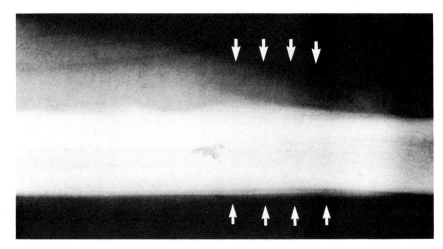

Figure 8–76. Laminated periosteal reaction of the midshaft of the femur in a 15-year-old male. This laminated onionskin appearance is consistent with Ewing's sarcoma.

coma is a destructive lesion that originates in the medullary cavity, expands, and eventually breaks through the cortex and elevates the periosteum so that it appears radiographically as a reactive, *laminated* formation on the periosteum of the bony shaft, resembling a layered *onionskin* pattern (Fig. 8–76).

Giant cell tumor or osteoclastoma is an uncommon malignant tumor characterized by a multicameral cystic or *bubble-like* appearance. It occurs predominantly in women after the age of 19. This lesion is almost always localized in the distal portion of the femur or humerus, with about 50% involving the knee joint. X-rays reveal the multilocular or multicameral area of radiolucency with no reactive sclerosis in the bone margins. Giant cell tumor has the same characteristics as benign chondroblastoma. Histologically, the potential toward malignancy cannot be determined. This lesion can occur as a benign tumor as well as one that is malignant. Fifty percent of benign giant cell tumors will recur, and some may have the ability to metastasize. It has been found that some giant cell tumors that were malignant contained some osteoid tissue, which may appear to have some connection with osteosarcoma (Figs. 8–77, 8–78, and 8–79).

Metastatic bone tumors are the most common form of bone malignancy in adults. Those that frequently metastasize are carcinomas of the kidney, prostate gland, lung, ovary, breast, testis, thyroid gland,

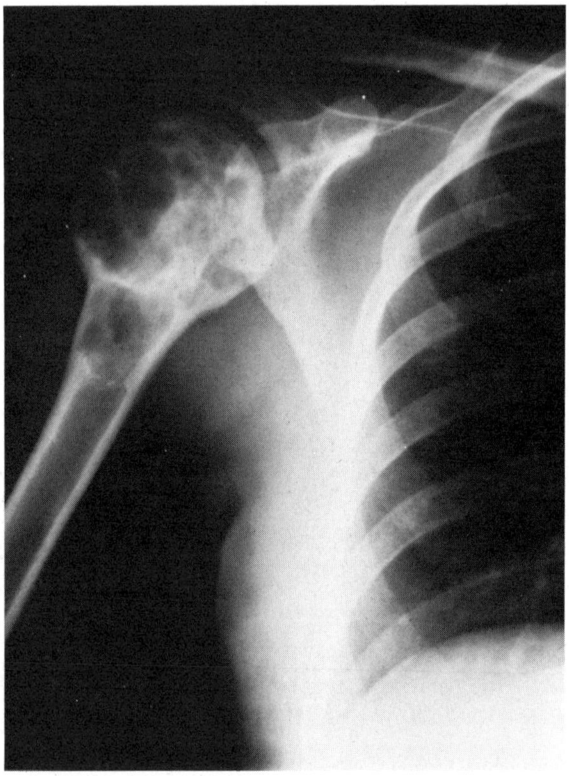

Figure 8–77. Multicameral bubble-like cystic lesion of the right proximal humerus, consistent with giant cell tumor.

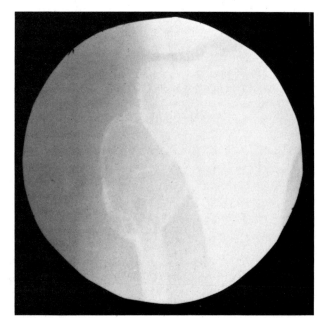

Figure 8–78. Large, cystic lucency of the proximal fibula, consistent with giant cell tumor. The patient is a 20-year-old woman.

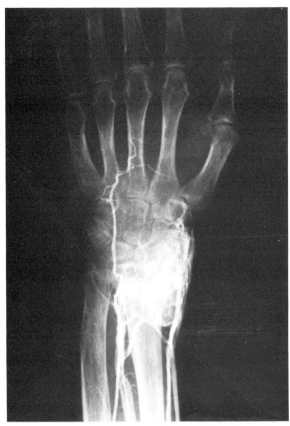

Figure 8–79. Vascularized giant cell tumor of the distal radius in a 73-year-old man. This is consistent with giant cell tumor.

such as arthritis and osteomyelitis. Clinical correlation is necessary (Fig. 8–80).

All radiographers (students and graduates) must be aware of the patient's clinical history at all times, but especially when mobile radiographs are taken in the patient's room. Primary malignancies of the lung and kidney can spread to the long bones. This secondary disease serves to weaken the bone substantially. The major point of weakness occurs in the *midshaft* of long bones, especially the femur and humerus. Pathological fractures can occur with the slightest trauma. The radiographer must exercise great care when performing radiographic procedures at the patient's bedside. The student should be made aware of the proper way to handle patients with terminal cancer so that fractures of diseased limbs do not occur. A pathological fracture creates an additional complication to an already serious condition. Buckling fractures occur with osteoporosis, such as in osteogenesis imperfecta. Transverse fractures extend at right angles to the longitudinal axis of the bone. The bone

stomach, and intestine. Both osteolytic as well as osteoblastic metastasis are possible. Typically, lytic metastases are received from the lung, kidney, intestine, breast, and thyroid. Blastic or sclerotic metastases in the male emanate from the prostate but may be disseminated from bladder carcinoma that has invaded the prostate or from a male breast carcinoma. Typically, the bones containing red marrow are the ones most likely to be affected. The spine, skull, ribs, pelvis, humeri, and femora are the bones most commonly involved with metastases. Pediatric patients most often are afflicted with metastases via neuroblastoma and leukemia. Mixed lytic and blastic metastases are common with breast carcinoma. It is thought that metastatic bone disease represents the first sign of malignancy elsewhere in the body. Following diagnosis of a primary tumor, a nuclear medicine bone scan is performed to help stage the disease. When results are positive, the bones demonstrate areas of increased radionuclide uptake. These areas of increased activity are of increased density and are often referred to as hot spots. They designate the areas of bone in which tumor cells are seeded and are growing. Bone scans also reveal an increased uptake with other inflammatory conditions

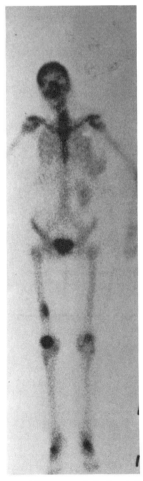

Figure 8–80. Abnormal isotope activity involving the right femur. This metastatic lesion is compatible with this 70-year-old woman's history of renal carcinoma.

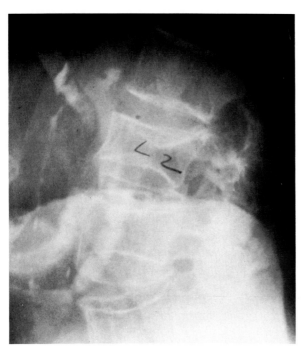

Figure 8–81. Osteoporotic compression and a buckling fracture of the body of L-2 in an 84-year-old woman.

ends are irregular or fragmented (Figs. 8–81 and 8–82).

Treatment. Bone malignancies are most effectively treated with combinations of surgery, radiation, and chemotherapy. The radiosensitivity of certain bone malignancies varies. In the absence of regional spread, surgical amputation is the treatment of choice for osteosarcoma, which is also radioresistant. Many patients with primary bone cancer are now being treated successfully by removing and replacing a section of bone rather than by amputation. The level of amputation should include the joint immediately above the primary sarcoma. Other radioresistant bone malignancies include chondrosarcoma and fibrosarcoma. The extent of their radioresistance depends on their histological characteristics and cellular differentiation. Radiosensitive tumors include Ewing's sarcoma and multiple myeloma. Metastasis is the primary complication of osteosarcoma, and chemotherapy is the primary treatment of choice. The most recent survival data are not encouraging. Only 20 to 25% of patients will survive 3 years after surgical amputation. The common cause of death is pulmonary metastatic disease. Ewing's sarcoma typically has a very poor prognosis, with a 5-year survival rate of approximately 15% even after surgery and radiation therapy. More than 75% of patients will develop metastases within 2 years. Ewing's sarcoma that has not yet metastasized usually responds favorably to chemotherapy. Complete remission with prolonged

survival has been noted in some patients who have received a combination of radiation therapy and chemotherapy. Chondrosarcoma is typically a slow-growing tumor that is very difficult to eradicate with radiation. Radiation often only serves to slow the metastatic spread. Surgical amputation of soft tissue and possibly the limb is the treatment of choice for chondrosarcoma. Multiple myeloma, when a solitary lesion, can be treated with radiation. However, it most often presents as numerous lesions located over several locations in the skeleton. Survival time is 1½ to 3 years after diagnosis. Giant cell tumor can occur in both benign and malignant forms, and there is a definite risk of malignant transformation when a recurring benign giant cell tumor is irradiated.

Immunotherapy currently is a most controversial but promising method of treatment. Data regarding its effectiveness are so far inconclusive.

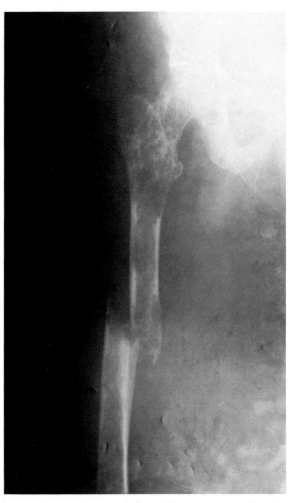

Figure 8–82. Transverse pathological fracture 11 cm in length, middle one-third of the left femur. There are metastatic bone changes noted in the proximal left femur, inferior pubic ramus, and ischium in this 67-year-old woman.

Self-Assessment Quiz

For each of the following questions, select the one best response and circle the letter that precedes it.

1. It is estimated that over the next several years cancer will strike how many American families?
   a. one of two
   b. one of three
   c. two of five
   d. three of four

2. The rising incidence of cancer in the United States is primarily due to an increase in cancers of the
   a. colon
   b. breast
   c. lung
   d. prostate

3. Which of the following groups has the highest cancer risk factors?
   a. white males
   b. black males
   c. white females
   d. black females

4. The highest mortality rate is associated with cancer of the
   a. pancreas
   b. ovary
   c. breast
   d. lung

5. The key to cancer cure is
   a. early detection
   b. surgery
   c. chemotherapy
   d. radiation therapy

6. Which of the following are probable causes of cancer?
   a. food
   b. cosmetics
   c. plastics
   d. radiation
   e. all of the above

7. Which of the following are probable causes of cancer?
   a. cigarettes
   b. pollution
   c. stress
   d. chemicals
   e. all of the above

8. The TNM system is a method for cancer
   a. grading
   b. staging

9. An in situ lesion can be best described as one that is
   a. benign
   b. a spreading cancer
   c. confined to the basement membrane
   d. multiple

10. Which route of metastasis is typical for most carcinomas?
    a. transcoelomic
    b. lymphatic
    c. hematogenous
    d. through body spaces

11. Which of the following are common sites of metastasis?
    a. lungs
    b. bone
    c. liver
    d. lymph nodes
    e. all of the above

12. Primary breast carcinoma can metastasize to almost any site.
    a. true
    b. false

13. Pain is typically an early symptom of cancer.
    a. true
    b. false

14. Bleeding is typically an early sign of cancer
    a. true
    b. false

15. Cachexia is defined as
    a. a form of metastasis that is fatal to Caucasians
    b. an early complication of cancer of the colon
    c. a type of bone cyst that causes pathological fractures
    d. an emaciated and debilitated state present with advanced cancer

16. The passage of black tarry stool describes
    a. melena
    b. hematochezia
    c. hematemesis
    d. hemoptysis

17. Breast cancer, once the most common cancer in women, has recently been surpassed by cancer of the
    a. ovary
    b. endometrium
    c. bladder
    d. lung

18. The most common tumor of the lung is
    a. lipoma
    b. squamous cell
    c. oat cell
    d. bronchogenic

19. Which of the following has the highest rate of metastasis?
    a. bronchogenic carcinoma
    b. squamous cell carcinoma
    c. basal cell carcinoma
    d. osteogenic sarcoma

20. The high mortality rate of lung cancer is mainly due to the lack of symptoms in the early stages of the disease.
    a. true
    b. false

21. Metastases to the lungs are most often disseminated by cancers of the
    a. breast and prostate gland
    b. breast and ovaries
    c. prostate and bone
    d. bone and breast

22. The highest incidence of esophageal cancer is found in
    a. the United States
    b. Norway and Sweden
    c. Russia
    d. the Orient

23. The earliest and most common symptom or sign of esophageal cancer is
    a. dyspnea
    b. hemorrhage
    c. dysphagia
    d. aphasia

24. The most obvious symptom of gastric carcinoma is
    a. pain
    b. hemorrhage
    c. achalasia
    d. diarrhea

25. Fifty percent of stomach cancers are located in or at the
    a. pylorus
    b. fundus
    c. lesser curvature
    d. greater curvature

26. Factors that predispose one to gastric carcinoma include all of the following EXCEPT
    a. type A blood
    b. history of gastric ulcer
    c. type O blood
    d. presence of gastric atrophy

27. As a rule, radiation therapy is not effective in the treatment of gastric carcinoma.
    a. true
    b. false

28. The majority (62%) of colon cancers are found in the
    a. rectum
    b. anus
    c. rectum and sigmoid colon
    d. sigmoid colon

29. A colon polyp that has a stalk is referred to as
    a. pedunculated
    b. sessile
    c. stratified
    d. villous

30. Which of the following has greater malignant potential?
    a. simple polyp
    b. villous adenoma

31. Which of the following are among the earliest symptoms of colon cancer?
    a. hemorrhage
    b. pain
    c. altered bowel habits
    d. hemorrhage and altered bowel habits
    e. all of the above

32. Primary carcinoma of the liver is
    a. uncommon
    b. very common
    c. moderately common
    d. treated with radiation

33. The liver is the main site of metastasis from many other organs.
    a. true
    b. false

34. The earliest sign of extrahepatic biliary cancer is
    a. hemorrhage
    b. nausea
    c. jaundice
    d. ascites

35. Hepatic and biliary cancer are characterized by elevated serum levels of
    a. bilirubin and alkaline phosphatase
    b. creatinine and blood urea nitrogen
    c. uric acid and amylase
    d. creatine and uric acid

36. Cancer of the pancreas is known as the silent disease because symptoms are not apparent until the cancer has significantly advanced.
    a. true
    b. false

37. The portion of the pancreas that lies within the loop of the duodenum is the
    a. head
    b. head and body
    c. body
    d. tail

38. The most important laboratory test for evaluating diseases of the urinary tract is
    a. blood urea nitrogen analysis
    b. serum uric acid analysis
    c. serum creatinine analysis
    d. complete urinalysis

39. Which of the following is the most common malignant lesion of the kidney?
    a. cyst
    b. leiomyoma
    c. hypernephroma
    d. lipoma

40. Renal cell carcinoma most frequently afflicts
    a. women
    b. children
    c. men
    d. adolescents

41. Hypernephromas are highly vascularized lesions.
    a. true
    b. false

42. Wilms' tumor of the kidney primarily affects
    a. children
    b. adolescents
    c. young adults
    d. the elderly

43. The most significant risk factor for bladder cancer is
    a. exposure to aniline dies
    b. working in the leather industry
    c. working in the rubber industry
    d. long-term use of artificial sweeteners
    e. smoking

44. Transitional carcinoma of the bladder is best described as
    a. an area of increased vascularity
    b. increased trabeculation
    c. the presence of diverticula
    d. the presence of a filling defect

45. The most common gynecological cancer involves the
    a. endometrium
    b. cervix
    c. ovary
    d. fallopian tubes

46. Leiomyomas of the uterus and cysts of the ovary are correctly described as
    a. benign tumors
    b. forms of cancer

47. The common fibroid tumor is closely associated with
    a. diet
    b. smoking
    c. environment
    d. pregnancy

48. Prostate cancer mainly afflicts men of what age-group?
    a. 17 to 25 years
    b. 26 to 50 years
    c. 51 to 65 years
    d. over 65 years

49. Prostate cancer is usually revealed as an outlet obstruction due to prostate enlargement.
    a. true
    b. false

50. The earliest site of metastasis of prostate cancer involves the
    a. bone
    b. lungs
    c. liver
    d. brain

51. Fibrocystic disease is also referred to as
    a. adenocarcinoma
    b. polycystic disease
    c. fibroadenoma
    d. mammary dysplasia

52. The highest mortality rate of breast cancer occurs in which age-group?
    a. 15 to 30 years
    b. 30 to 45 years
    c. 45 to 60 years
    d. 55 to 74 years

53. The typical fibroadenoma of the breast is
    a. cystic
    b. nonmovable
    c. accompanied by nipple retraction
    d. solitary and movable

54. The majority of cancerous breast lesions are found
    a. near the nipple
    b. in the lower outer quadrant
    c. in the upper inner quadrant
    d. in the upper outer quadrant

55. Currently, which method of breast cancer detection is *most* recommended?
    a. self-examination
    b. mammography

56. The primary disadvantage of thermography as a diagnostic tool is
    a. its high false-negative and false-positive rates
    b. the risk of radiation exposure
    c. the risk of burns
    d. that it is a painful procedure

57. Ultrasonography is able to detect a lesion that is less than 1 cm in diameter.
    a. true
    b. false

58. What are the earliest and latest sites of metastasis of breast carcinoma?
    a. lungs and bone; brain and liver
    b. lungs and brain; bone and liver
    c. lungs and liver; bone and brain

59. In adults, the majority of brain tumors are found in the
    a. cerebrum
    b. cerebellum
    c. pons
    d. brain stem

60. In children, the majority of brain tumors are found in the
    a. cerebrum
    b. cerebellum
    c. pons
    d. cerebrum and pons

61. Which tumor has a more favorable prognosis?
    a. pituitary adenoma
    b. parasagittal meningioma

62. Medulloblastomas most frequently afflict
    a. children
    b. adolescents
    c. adults

63. Astrocytomas most frequently afflict
    a. children
    b. adults
    c. adolescents

64. All of the following are frequent symptoms of brain tumors EXCEPT
    a. headache
    b. vomiting
    c. hemorrhage
    d. nausea
    e. seizures

65. The primary treatment for all intracranial neoplasms is
    a. surgery
    b. radiation
    c. chemotherapy
    d. hormonal therapy

66. All of the anatomical structures listed below are identified when viewing a lateral cerebral angiogram EXCEPT the
    a. carotid siphon
    b. sylvian triangle
    c. basilar artery
    d. middle cerebral artery
    e. anterior cerebral artery

67. What percent of brain tumors are metastatic?
    a. 10%
    b. 20 to 25%
    c. 50%
    d. 75%

68. Which of the following primary cancers commonly does NOT metastasize to the brain?
    a. Colon
    b. Kidney
    c. Breast
    d. Liver
    e. Leukemia

69. Lymphoma has no benign form.
    a. true
    b. false

70. The most common and curable form of lymphatic cancer is
    a. Hodgkin's lymphoma
    b. non-Hodgkin's lymphoma
    c. multiple myeloma
    d. lymphocytic leukemia

71. Lymph nodes that appear foamy are indicative of lymphatic cancer.
    a. true
    b. false

72. Acute lymphocytic leukemia typically affects
    a. children
    b. adolescents
    c. adults

73. Chronic lymphocytic leukemia typically affects
    a. the elderly
    b. young adults
    c. children
    d. only women

74. Radiological indications of leukemia include all of the following EXCEPT
    a. trumpeting of the metacarpals
    b. lucent metaphyseal bands in the knees and wrists
    c. patchy areas of bone destruction in the metaphyses
    d. separation of cranial sutures
    e. bony spicules at the margin of skull tables

75. Bone cancer is most often secondary rather than primary.
    a. true
    b. false

76. Primary cancers that metastasize to bone include all of the following EXCEPT those of the
    a. breast
    b. prostate gland
    c. liver
    d. lungs

77. The bones that are most susceptible to metastases are those
    a. of the extremities
    b. closest to the trunk
    c. farthest from the midline
    d. of the extremities and those farthest from the midline

78. The terms *geographic, moth-eaten,* and *permeated* pertain to destructive patterns of primary bone neoplasms.
    a. true
    b. false

79. Excluding multiple myeloma, the most common bone cancer is
    a. Ewing's sarcoma
    b. aneurysmal bone cyst
    c. osteosarcoma
    d. Paget's disease

80. A bone-forming sclerotic growth is described as
    a. osteoblastic
    b. osteolytic

81. A bone-destroying lesion is described as
    a. osteoblastic
    b. osteolytic

82. Bone cysts are most frequently found in which joint?
    a. wrist
    b. ankle
    c. knee
    d. shoulder

83. A solitary bone cyst may be described as
    a. multicameral
    b. osteoblastic
    c. osteolytic
    d. unicameral
    e. osteolytic and unicameral

84. Bone cysts are often associated with what type of fracture?
    a. traumatic
    b. pseudofracture
    c. pathological
    d. traumatic

85. Which type of bone cysts are common following trauma?
    a. anceurysmal
    b. traumatic

86. Another name for osteochondroma is
    a. enchondroma
    b. exostosis
    c. multicameral bone cyst
    d. aneurysmal bone cyst

87. Which of the following terms correctly describes osteoid osteomas?
    a. cystic
    b. osteolytic
    c. osteoblastic
    d. sclerotic
    e. osteoblastic and sclerotic

88. Areas of increased uptake of a radioisotope as revealed on a bone scan may indicate metastases and are referred to as hot spots.
    a. true
    b. false

89. Multiple punched-out lesions noted on a lateral view of the skull indicative of
    a. Ewing's sarcoma
    b. osteosarcoma
    c. multiple myeloma
    d. lymphoma

90. The presence of Bence Jones protein in the urine usually is indicative of
    a. Ewing's sarcoma
    b. osteosarcoma
    c. multiple myeloma
    d. lymphoma

91. Giant cell tumor is most accurately described as
    a. a multicameral lesion
    b. an osteoblastic lesion
    c. either benign or malignant
    d. a benign or malignant multicameral lesion

Study Questions

1. List and describe the two primary components of a neoplasm.

2. Explain the behavior differences between a benign and malignant lesion.

3. List the four types of cancers.

4. Explain the differences between grading and staging.

5. Explain the significance of the TNM system.

6. List several sites of early and late metastases.

7. What are some of the manifestations of a malignant neoplasm?

8. Define the term lesion.

9. Describe the action of cancer on the host cell.

10. What are some of the advantages of linear tomography and computed tomography in the diagnosis of lung cancer?

11. What types of bone tumors are most common? Describe the radiographic appearance of each.

Glossary

In order to minimize diacritical marks, a simplified method (the same as that in *Dorland's Illustrated Medical Dictionary*) is used. Essentially, an unmarked vowel ending a syllable is long, and an unmarked vowel in a syllable ending with a consonant is short. Otherwise, a macron or breve is used to indicate vowel length.

A

abate (ah-bāt′)   To lessen or decrease.

abduction (ab-duk′shun)   The drawing way from the midline.

abscess (ab′ses)   A localized spherical collection of pus.

achalasia (ak″ah-la′ze-ah)   Cardiospasm.

achondroplasia (ah-kon″dro-pla′ze-ah)   A congenital cartilaginous disturbance; the leading cause of dwarfism.

achlorhydria (ah″klor-hi′dre-ah)   An absence of hydrochloric acid in gastric juice.

acidosis (as″ĭ-do′sis)   An increase in the hydrogen ion concentration in body fluids.

acromegaly (ak″ro-meg′ah-le)   Abnormal enlargement of facial features and hands due to excess production of the growth hormone.

acute (ah-kūt′)   Having a sudden onset of symptoms, which may be severe and last only a short time.

adduction (ah-duk′shun)   The drawing toward the midline.

adeno- (ad′ĕ-no)   Pertaining to a gland.

adenoids (ad′ĕ-noidz)   Pharyngeal tonsils.

adenoma (ad″ĕ-no′mah)   A benign glandular tumor.

adenomatous (ad″ĕ-nom′ah-tus)   Pertaining to an adenoma.

adjuvant (ad′ju-vant)   Something that aids or assists.

adynamic ileus (ad″i-nam′ik il′e-us)   Intestinal obstruction resulting from lack of mobility or peristalsis.

aerated (a′er-āt″ed)   Filled with air.

aerosol (a′er-o-sol″)   A stable suspension of liquid that is dispersed in a fine mist.

aganglionic (a-gang″gle-on′ik)   Lacking ganglion cells.

agenesis (ah-jen′ĕ-sis)   Absence of an organ or structure.

Agent Orange (a′jent or′anj)   A chemical defoliant used in the Vietnam War.

aggressive (ah-gres′iv)   Marked by destructive behavior, such as tumor.

AIDS   Acquired immunodeficiency syndrome.

Albers-Schönberg disease (al′berz shān′berg dĭ-zēz′)   Eponym for osteopetrosis.

alkaline phosphatase (al′kah-līn fos′fah-tās)   An enzyme that is found in most body fluids and cells.

allergen (al′er-jen)   Anything that produces an allergic reaction.

alveolus (al-ve′o-lus)   A small sac-like dilatation, as of the lungs.

ambulation (am″bu-la′shun)   The act of walking.

ameba (ah-me′bah)   A minute one-celled protozoon.

amide (am′īd)   A compound derived from ammonia by substitution of an acid radical for oxygen.

amine (ah-mēn′)   An organic compound containing nitrogen.

ampulla of Vater (am-pul′lah ov fah′ter)   The junction where the common bile duct and pancreatic ducts meet.

amylase (am′ĭ-lās)   An enzyme that catalyzes the hydrolysis of starch into simpler compounds.

analgesic (an″al-je′zik)   Pain-relieving medication.

anaplasia (an″ah-pla′ze-ah)   Loss of differentiation of cells, an irreversible alteration in adult cells toward more primitive cell types; a characteristic of tumor cells.

anaplastic (an″ah-plas′tik)   Characterized by anaplasia.

anasarca (an″ah-sar′kah)   A widespread accumulation of fluid throughout the body.

anastomosis (ah-nas″to-mo′sis)   A communication between two tube-like structures or organs.

anemia (ah-ne′me-ah)   A decrease in the number of circulating red blood cells; reduction of hemoglobin.

aneurysm (an′u-rizm)   A dilatation or ballooning out of an artery.

aneurysmal (an″u-riz′mal)   Pertaining to an aneurysm.

angina (an-ji′nah)   Any condition marked by suffocative spasms; may occur in the pectoral region.

angiogram (an′je-o-gram″)   A radiographic demonstration of blood vessels on x-ray film using a contrast medium.

angiography (an″je-og′rah-fe)   The radiological visualization of blood vessels.

aniline dye (an′ĭ-lin di)   A carcinogenic dye used in the manufacture of rubber and cable.

ankylosis (ang″kĭ-lo′sis)   A bent, deformed, and sometimes fused joint.

anomaly (ah-nom′ah-le)   Marked deviation from the normal.

anorexia (an″o-rek′se-ah)   Loss of appetite.

anoxia (ah-nok′se-ah)   Lack of oxygen supply to tissue.

antegrade (an′te-grād)   With the direction of flow.

antibiotic (an″tĭ-bi-ot′ik)   Medication that kills bacteria.

antibody (an′tĭ-bod″e)   An immune molecule produced by the body to counteract an antigen.

antigen (an′tĭ-jen)   An external agent that attacks the body.

antihypertensive (an″tĭ-hi″per-ten′siv) An agent that reduces high blood pressure.

antimicrobial (an″tĭ-mi-kro′be-al) An agent that kills microorganisms.

anulus fibrosis (an′u-lus fi-bro′sis) The peripheral part of an intervertebral disk.

aphasia (ah-fa′ze-ah) Defect or loss of the power of speech.

apophyseal (ap″o-fiz′e-al) Pertaining to a bony outgrowth forming a process, as in the vertebral column.

apoplexy (ap′o-plek″se) Cerebral hemorrhage.

appendicitis (ah-pen″dĭ-si′tis) Inflammation of the appendix.

aqueduct of Sylvius (ak′we-dukt″ ov sil′ve-us) The intraventricular channel that connects the third and fourth ventricles of the brain.

arachnodactyly (ah-rak″no-dak′tĭ-le) A condition characterized by extremely long and slender fingers and toes; Marfan's syndrome.

arrhythmia (ah-rith′me-ah) An abnormal heart rhythm.

arteriosclerosis (ar-te″re-o-sklĕ-ro′sis) Hardening or calcification of all three arterial layers.

arthritis (ar-thri′tis) An inflammation of one or more joints.

arthrodesis (ar″thro-de′sis) The surgical fusion of a joint.

arthrogram (ar′thro-gram) A radiographic examination of a joint following the injection of a contrast medium.

arthroplasty (ar′thro-plas″te) Repair of a joint; repair or reconstruction.

asbestosis (as″bĕ-sto′sis) A lung condition caused by the inhalation of asbestos dust fibers.

ascites (ah-si′tēz) An abnormal accumulation of serous fluid in the abdomen.

ascorbic acid (ah-skōr′bik a′sid) Vitamin C.

aseptic necrosis (a-sep′tik nĕ-kro′sis) Death of tissue in the absence of an infection.

aspiration (as″pĭ-ra′shun) The intake of foreign material into the lungs during respiration.

aspirin (as′pĭ-rin) Acetylsalicylic acid; an analgesic or pain killer.

asthma (az′mah) A functional or allergic reaction causing bronchoconstriction.

astrocyte (as′tro-sīt) A neuroglial cell of ectodermal origin.

astrocytic (as″tro-sit′ik) Pertaining to an astrocyte.

astrocytoma (as″tro-si-to′mah) A tumor composed of astrocytes.

asymmetric (a″sim-met′rik) Lacking symmetry; dissimilarity of corresponding parts.

asymptomatic (a″simp-to-mat′ik) Revealing no symptoms.

ataxia (ah-tak′se-ah) Loss of muscular coordination.

atelectasis (at″e-lek′tah-sis) Collapse of all or part of the lung.

atherosclerosis (ath″er-o″skle-ro′sis) Accumulation of fatty deposits in the intima, or inner layer, of an artery.

atresia (ah-tre′ze-ah) Absence of an opening or lumen.

atrophic (ah-trof′ik) Pertaining to a decrease in tissue mass.

atrophy (at′ro-fe) A wasting away of tissue; decrease in tissue size.

atropine (at′ro-pēn) A smooth muscle relaxant that is used as a premedication to prevent the buildup of secretions.

autoimmune (aw″to-im-mūn′) An attack against a body's own cells.

autolysis (aw-tol′ĭ-sis) The disintegration of cells or tissues by enzymes.

autopsy (aw′top-se)   Examination of the body after death.

autosomal (aw″to-so′mal)   Pertaining to a genetic trait that is not sex linked.

axial (ak′se-al)   Pertaining to or forming an axis.

azotomia (az″o-te′me-ah)   An excess of nitrogenous compounds in the blood.

B

Bouchard's nodes (boo-sharz′ nōdz)   Cartilaginous and bony processes that form in the proximal interphalangeal joints as a result of osteoarthritis.

Brodie's abscess (bro′dēz ab′ses)   A localized circumscribed hematogenous bone infection commonly found in the distal tibia as a result of persistent inflammation.

bronchiectasis (brong″ke-ek′tah-sis)   A permanent dilatation of terminal bronchi due to chronic inflammatory disease.

bronchiole (brong′ke-ōl)   The terminal end of a bronchus; the smallest bronchi.

bronchitis (brong-ki′tis)   Inflammation of the bronchi.

bronchogenic (brong-ko-jen′ik)   Originating in a bronchus.

bronchography (brong-kog′rah-fe)   Radiographic visualization of the bronchi with an oily, opaque contrast agent.

brucellosis (broo″sel-lo′sis)   A generalized infection involving the reticuloendothelial system.

bulla (bul′ah)   A blister, vesicle, or bleb.

BUN   Blood urea nitrogen; a blood chemistry test that measures renal function.

bursitis (ber-si′tis)   Inflammation of a bursa.

C

cachexia (kah-kek′se-ah)   A debilitated and emaciated state, as in a person suffering from the long-term effects of cancer.

calcaneus (kal-ka′ne-us)   The heel bone or os calcis.

calcification (kal″sǐ-fǐ-ka′shun)   Deposition of mineral salts in tissue.

calcified (kal′sǐ-fīd)   Hardness of a tissue due to deposition of calcium.

calcium (kal′se-um)   The most abundant mineral in the body, which, in combination with phosphorus, forms calcium phosphate in the major construction of bones.

calculi (kal′ku-li)   Plural of calculus.

calculus (kal′ku-lus)   An abnormal accumulation of mineral salts, forming a stone.

callus (kal′us)   New bone formation, as found in healing fractures.

calyx (ka′liks)   The cup-shaped structure of the renal pelvis.

cancellous bone (kan′sǔ-lus bōn)   A spongy bone consisting of a lattice-like bone matrix.

cancer (kan′ser)   A malignant neoplasm.

carcinogen (kar-sin′o-jen)   A cancer-causing substance.

carcinoma (kar″sǐ-no′mah)   Cancer of epithelial tissue.

cardiomyotomy (kar″de-o-mi-ot′ǒ-me)   A surgical cutting of the cardiac sphincter to relieve stenosis.

cardiospasm (kar′de-o-spazm″) Achalasia; failure of the esophagus to relax while swallowing.

cardiovascular (kar″de-o-vas′ku-lar) Pertaining to the heart and great vessels.

caries (ka′re-ēz) A disease of the teeth; tooth decay.

carotid siphon (kah-rot′id si′fun) The curving portion of the internal carotid that courses upward, tracing the path of the sella turcica.

cartilaginous (kar″tĭ-laj′ĭ-nus) Consisting of cartilage.

caseous (ka′se-us) Resembling cheese; a form of necrosis.

cataract (kat′ah-rakt) Opacification of the eye lens.

catheter (kath′ĕ-ter) A hollow tubular instrument passed through body channels for injection or removal of solids and fluids.

catheterization (kath″ĕ-ter-i-za′shun) The passage of a catheter into a body channel or cavity.

cavitation (kav″ĭ-ta′shun) The presence or formation of a cavity.

CBC Complete blood count.

celiac (se′le-ak) Pertaining to the abdomen.

cellulitis (sel″u-li′tis) A spreading inflammatory lesion within solid tissue.

centrilobar (sen″trĭ-lo′bar) Pertaining to the central portion of a lung lobe.

chalk bones (chawk′bōnz) Osteopetrosis.

chemotherapy (ke″mo-ther′ah-pe) Treatment of disease with chemical agents.

cholangiography (ko-lan″je-og′rah-fe) Radiographic examination of the bile ducts.

cholecystectomy (ko″le-sis-tek′to-me) Surgical removal of the gallbladder.

cholecystitis (ko″le-sis-ti′tis) Inflammation of the gallbladder.

cholecystogram (ko″le-sis′to-gram) X-ray study of the gallbladder.

choledocholithiasis (ko-led″ŏ-ko-lĭ-thi′ah-sis) A condition marked by gallstones in the common bile duct.

cholelithiasis (ko″le-lĭ-thi′ah-sis) The presence of gallstones.

cholesterol (ko-les′ter-ol) A steroid alcohol found in numerous body substances; one substance found in gallstones.

chondroblast (kon′dro-blast) An immature cartilage-producing cell.

chondroma (kon-dro′mah) A benign cartilaginous tumor.

chondromatosis (kon″dro-mah-to′sis) The formation of multiple chondromas.

chondrosarcoma (kon″dro-sar-ko′mah) A malignant cartilaginous tumor.

choroid plexus (kor′oid plek′sus) A network of veins that produce cerebrospinal fluid.

chronic (kron′ik) Persisting for a long time.

cirrhosis (sir-ro′sis) A chronic disease of the liver characterized by loss of liver cells and replacement with fibrous connective tissue, causing hepatomegaly.

clot (klot) A mass of coagulated blood, usually located outside a blood vessel.

clubfoot (klub′foot) Congenital downward and turning inward of the foot; talipes equinovarus deformity.

coagulate (ko-ag′u-lāt) To cause to clot, as in blood.

coccidioidomycosis (kok-sid″e-oi″do-mi-ko′sis) A lung disease characterized by a granulomatous fungal lung growth.

colitis (ko-li′tis) Inflammation of the colon.

collagen (kol′ah-jen) The fibrous structural protein found in connective tissue.

collateral (kŏ-lat′er-al) Secondary, accessory, or indirect side branches, as of blood vessels.

colonoscopy (ko"lon-os'ko-pe)   An endoscopic examination of the colon.

colostomy (ko-los'to-me)   Surgical creation of an artificial opening or stoma in the abdomen in which the colon is brought to the surface of the abdomen for the evacuation of feces.

coma (ko'mah)   A state of unconsciousness.

compensatory (kom-pen'sah-to"re)   Offsetting or counterbalancing a defect.

competence (kom'pě-tens)   Correct function of a body part.

compression (kom-presh'un)   The act of pressing upon or together.

concavity (kon-kav'ĭ-te)   A depression or hollowed-out area.

congenital (kon-jen'ĭ-tal)   Present at birth.

congestion (kon-jest'yun)   Engorgement of capillaries with blood; part of the inflammatory response.

connective tissue (kŏ-nek'tĭv tish'u)   A type of fibrous tissue.

consolidation (kon-sol"ĭ-da'shun)   Solidification into a mass, as with fluid.

constipation (kon"stĭ-pa'shun)   Infrequent and hard bowel movements.

contraindication (kon"trah-in"dĭ-ka'shun)   Any condition that renders a particular treatment undesirable.

contusion (kon-tu'zhun)   A bruise.

correlation (kor"ě-la'shun)   The degree of association.

cortex (kor'teks)   The outer layer of a structure; dense compact bone.

costovertebral (kos"to-ver'tě-bral)   Pertaining to the junction of the bony rib and vertebral body.

creatinine (kre-at'ĭ-nin)   A nitrogenous product of muscle breakdown.

crepitus (krep'ĭ-tus)   The grating sound of bone surfaces rubbing together.

cricothyroid (kri-ko-thi'roid)   Pertaining to or situated between the cricoid and thyroid cartilages.

Crohn's disease (knōnz dĭ-zēz')   Regional enteritis; inflammation of the terminal ileum.

croup (kroop)   Laryngitis with spasm producing a bark-like cough.

culture (kul'tūr)   Propagation of microorganisms in special media.

curettage (ku"rě-tahzh')   The scraping or cleaning of a diseased surface.

Cushing's syndrome (koosh'ingz sin'drōm)   A condition characterized by an increase in levels of cortisol from the adrenal cortex.

cyanosis (si"ah-no'sis)   A bluish discoloration of the skin indicating a lack of oxygen.

cylindrical (sĭ-lin'drĭ-k'l)   Shaped like a cylinder.

cyst (sist)   A closed, fluid-filled sac.

cystectomy (sis-tek'to-me)   Surgical removal of the urinary bladder.

cystic (sis'tik)   Pertaining to a cyst-like lesion.

cystitis (sis-ti'tis)   Inflammation of the urinary bladder.

cystoscopy (sis-tos'ko-pe)   An examination of the urinary bladder with a cystoscope.

cytology (si-tol'o-je)   The study of cells.

D

debridement (da-brēd'maw)   Excision of necrotic tissue and foreign matter from a wound.

decubitus (de-ku′bĭ-tus)   Lying down in a recumbent position. Associated with a horizontally projected x-ray beam.

defecation (def″e-ka′shun)   The elimination of feces.

deficit (def′ĭ-sĭt)   A lack or deficiency.

degeneration (de-jen″er-a′shun)   The deterioration of a cell following injury; nonlethal cell injury.

deglutition (deg″loo-tish′un)   The act of swallowing.

dehydration (de″hi-dra′shun)   The removal of water from the body or from a tissue.

demineralization (de-min″er-al-i-za′shun)   Excessive elimination of minerals from the body.

dentin (den′tin)   The chief substance of teeth.

DES   Diethylstilbestrol, a synthetic estrogen used to prevent spontaneous abortion, which has been linked to cancer of the vagina.

detachment (de-tach′ment)   The condition of being separated or disconnected.

diabetes (di″ah-be′tēz)   A disease characterized by the lack of insulin production needed for metabolism of glucose.

dialysis (di-al′ĭ-sis)   The removal of toxic wastes from the blood.

diaphysis (di-af′ĭ-sis)   The primary center of ossification; shaft or body of a long bone.

diarrhea (di″ah-re′ah)   The rapid movement of feces through the bowel resulting from poor absorption of water, producing abnormal frequency and liquid-like stools.

diastole (di-as′to-le)   The resting phase of the heart.

differentiation (dif′er-en″she-a′shun)   A histological process of distinguishing one type of cell from another; used in grading of cancer.

diffuse (dĭ-fūs′)   Not limited or localized.

digital (dij′ĭ-tal)   Pertaining to an examination of a body part or structure such as the rectum or prostate gland with the fingers.

digitalis (dij″ĭ-tal′is)   A medication used in treatment of congestive heart failure; causes increased strength of contraction of the heart.

dilatation (dil-ah-ta′shun)   The condition of being enlarged or stretched.

diphtheria (dif-the′re-ah)   A highly contagious disease affecting the throat.

disease (dĭ-zēz′)   A pathological process that produces a specific set of signs and symptoms.

dislocation (dis″lo-ka′shun)   The displacement of a bone from a joint space.

distal (dis′tal)   Farthest away from the point of reference.

disuse atrophy (dis-ūs′ at′ro-fe)   The result of inactivity of a body part.

diuretic (di″u-ret′ik)   A medication that promotes the excretion of urine.

diverticula (di″ver-tik′u-lah)   The plural of diverticulum.

diverticulitis (di″ver-tik-u-li′tis)   Inflammation of a diverticulum.

diverticulosis (di″ver-tik-u-lo′sis)   The presence of diverticula in the absence of inflammation.

diverticulum (di″ver-tik′u-lum)   An outpouching or sac in the mucous membrane of a hollow organ.

dominant (dom′ĭ-nant)   A genetic trait that is acquired from both parents.

dorsiflexion (dor″sĭ-flek′shun)   Backward flexion, as of the foot.

Down's syndrome (downz′ sin″drōm)   Mongolism; trisomy 21.

duck waddle (duk wad'l)   A peculiar walk pattern associated with congenital hip dysplasia.

duration (dūr-a′shun)   A period of time; life history of a disease.

dwarfism (dwarf′izm)   The state of being a dwarf or undersized individual.

dysfunction (dis-funk′shun)   A disturbance or impairment of an organ.

dyslexia (dis-lek′se-ah)   An inability to comprehend the written language.

dysphagia (dis-fa′je-ah)   Difficulty in swallowing.

dysplasia (dis-pla′se-ah)   The abnormal development of tissue.

dyspnea (disp′ne-ah)   Difficult, labored breathing.

dysuria (dis-u′re-ah)   Painful or difficult urination.

E

ecchymoses (ek″ĭ-mo′sēz)   Hemorrhagic spots that are larger than petechiae.

ectopia (ek-to′pe-ah)   Congenital displacement of an organ or structure.

edema (ĕ-de′mah)   An abnormal fluid collection within the intercellular spaces.

edematous (ĕ-dem′ah-tus)   Pertaining to edema.

effusion (ĕ-fu′zhun)   The collection of fluid in a body space or cavity.

electrolyte (e-lek′tro-līt)   A chemical substance that, when dissolved in water or melted, dissociates into electrically charged particles (ions) and thus is capable of conducting electric current.

embolism (em′bo-lizm)   Any foreign matter that may travel in blood, producing an obstruction of blood flow.

emboli (em′bo-li)   The plural of embolus.

embolization (em″bo-li-za′shun)   The process of becoming an embolus; the introduction of embolic material into a vessel for occlusive purposes.

embolus (em′bo-lus)   A blood clot that is often a part of a thrombus.

embryonal (em′bre-o-nal)   Pertaining to an embryo.

emesis (em′ĕ-sis)   The act of vomiting.

emphysema (em″fĭ-se′mah)   The swelling or overexpansion of alveoli.

empyema (em″pi-e′mah)   A collection of pus in a body cavity, as in the pleural cavity.

encapsulated (en-kap′su-lāt-ed)   Enclosed within a capsule.

encephalitis (en″sef-ah-li′tis)   Inflammation or infection of the whole brain.

encephalocele (en-sef′ah-lo-sēl″)   Protrusion or herniation of the brain.

encephalography (en-sef′ah-log′rah-fe)   Radiographic demonstration of the cerebral ventricles.

encephalopathy (en-sef′ah-lop′ah-the)   Any degenerative disease of the brain.

endobronchial (en″do-brong′ke-al)   Pertaining to the inner lining or inside of a bronchus.

endocarditis (en″do-kar-di′tis)   Inflammation of the inner heart lining.

endocrinology (en″do-krĭ-nol′o-je)   The study of the endocrine system.

endogenous (en-doj′ĕ-nus)   Produced from within or inside.

endoscope (en′do-skōp)   An instrument for viewing the internal structure of an organ.

endoscopic (en″do-skop′ik)   Pertaining to a visual examination of the internal structure of an organ with an endoscope.

enteritis (en″ter-i′tis)   Inflammation of the intestine.

enteropathy (en″ter-op′ah-the)   Any disease of the intestine.

environmental (en-vi″ron-men′tal) Pertaining to the environment.

enzymatic (en″zi-mat′ik) Relating to, caused by, or of the nature of an enzyme.

ependymoma (ĕ-pen″dĭ-mo′mah) A tumor arising from the ventricles and spinal cord.

epidermoid (ep″ĭ-der′moid) Resembling the epidermis.

epidural (ep″ĭ-du′ral) Pertaining to an area on, above, or outside the dura mater.

epigastric (ep″ĭ-gas′trik) Pertaining to the upper middle region of the abdomen.

epiphrenic (ep″ĭ-fren′ik) On or above the diaphragm.

epiphyseal plate (ep″ĭ-fiz′e-al plāt) The growth plate; the area between the diaphysis and the epiphysis.

epiphysis (ĕ-pif′ĭ-sis) The secondary center of ossification; proximal and distal ends of a long bone.

epistaxis (ep″ĭ-stak′sis) Nosebleed.

epithelium (ep″ĭ-the′le-um) One of the basic tissues; forms the lining of body spaces, surfaces, and many glands.

eponym (ep′o-nim) A name or phrase formed by a person's name.

equinovarus (e-kwi″no-va′rus) Downward and inward deformity of the foot; clubfoot.

ERCP Endoscopic retrograde cholangiopancreatography.

erect (ĕ-rekt′) The upright position of a patient while standing or seated.

erosion (e-ro′zhun) Eating away; ulceration.

erythrocyte (ĕ-rith′ro-sīt) Red blood cell.

Escherichia coli (esh″ĕ-rik′e-a ko′le) Gram-negative bacteria that are found in the intestine.

esophagitis (ĕ-sof′ah-ji′tis) Inflammation of the esophagus.

esophagogastrectomy (ĕ-sof′ah-go-gas-trek′to-me) Excision of the stomach and esophagus.

esophagogram (ĕ-sof′ah-go-gram) The radiographic visualization of the esophagus with an opaque contrast medium such as barium sulfate.

estrogen (es′tro-jen) A female sex hormone.

etiology (e″te-ol′o-je) The study of disease causes.

evacuation (e-vak″u-a′shun) Removal or emptying, such as from the body.

Ewing's sarcoma (u′ingz sar-ko′mah) A malignant bone tumor.

exacerbation (eg-zas″er-bas′shun) An increase in severity of a disease.

excision (ek-sizh′un) The surgical removal of tissue.

excretion (eks-kre′shun) The process or act of excretion or elimination.

excretory urography (eks′kre-to-re u-rog′rah-fe) Radiographic kidney function test; intravenous pyelography (IVP).

exocrine (ek′so-krin) Secreting externally via a duct.

exogenous (eks-oj′ĕ-nus) Produced from without or outside.

exostosis (ek″sos-to′sis) Accessory bone growth; osteoblastic lesion.

expiration (eks″pĭ-ra′shun) The act of expelling air from the lungs; exhalation.

extension (ek-sten′shun) The straightening or extending of a part.

extrahepatic (eks″trah-hĕ-pat′ik) Situated outside of the liver.

extrinsic (eks-trin′sik) Having external origin.

exudate (eks'u-dāt)   A debris-filled fluid discharge that has escaped from blood vessels as part of the inflammatory response.

F

familial (fah-mil'e-al)   Disease incidence that occurs within a family at a frequency greater than just by chance.

febrile (feb'ril)   Pertaining to fever.

Felty's syndrome (fel'tēz sin'drōm)   A form of rheumatoid arthritis that includes splenomegaly and leukopenia.

femoral anteversion (fem'or-al an"te-ver'zhun)   The inward turning of the leg at the hip.

Ferguson method (fer'gus-on meth'ud)   A method that distinguishes a deforming spinal curve from a compensatory curve.

fiberoptic (fi"ber-op'tik)   Pertaining to a specially coated flexible glass or plastic fiber that has special optical properties.

fibrillation (fi-brĭ-la'shun)   A small uncoordinated involuntary contraction of the heart muscle originating in the right ventricle rather than the sinoatrial node.

fibroid (fi'broid)   Having a fibrous structure.

fibrosarcoma (fi"bro-sar-ko'mah)   A malignant tumor composed of fibrous tissue.

fibrosis (fi-bro'sis)   The least preferred method of healing. The replacement of useful tissue with fibrous tissue; scarring.

filum terminale (fi'lum term-mĭ-nal'e)   The slender thread-like termination of the spinal cord.

fissure (fish'ūr)   A groove or slit-like depression in tissue.

fistula (fis'tu-lah)   An abnormal sinus tract usually connecting two organs.

flatulence (flat'u-lens)   Excessive accumulation of gases in the stomach and intestine, resulting in distension of the abdomen.

flexion (flek'shun)   Bending of a body part.

flocculation (flok"u-la'shun)   The formation of flaky masses or precipitate in solution.

focal (fo'kal)   Localized or focused in a small area.

fontanelle (fon"tah-nel')   A soft spot on an infant's skull.

forensic (fo-ren'zik)   Pertaining to or applied in legal proceedings.

fragmentation (frag"men-ta'shun)   Separation into small segments.

frequency (fre'kwen-se)   The number of occurrences in a period of time.

fungal (fung'gal)   Pertaining to or caused by a fungus.

fungate (fung'gāt)   Grow like a fungus.

fusiform (fu'zĭ-form)   Tapering at both ends; a type of aneurysm.

G

gallium (gal'e-um)   A chemical element, atomic number 31, atomic weight 69.72, symbol Ga.

gangrenous (gang'grĕ-nus)   Pertaining to gangrene.

gastrectomy (gas-trek'to-me)   Partial or complete surgical removal of the stomach.

gastrin (gas'trin)   A hormone that, when ingested, promotes the stimulation of the acid-secreting glands.

gastritis (gas-tri′tus)   Inflammation of the inner lining of the stomach.

gastroduodenostomy (gas″tro-du″o-dĕ-nos′to-me)   Anastomosis of the stomach to the duodenum.

gastroenteritis (gas″tro-en-ter-i′tis)   Inflammation of the lining of the stomach and small intestine.

gastroenterology (gas″tro-en″ter-ol′o-je)   The study of the stomach and intestine and their diseases.

gastroenterostomy (gas″tro-en-ter-os′to-me)   The surgical anastomosis of the stomach and small intestine.

Gastrografin (gas″tro-graf′in)   Trade name of a water-soluble contrast medium.

gastrojejunostomy (gas″tro-jĕ-ju-nos′to-me)   The surgical anastomosis of the stomach to the jejunum.

gastroscope (gas′tro-skŏp)   An instrument that makes possible the observation of the internal lining of the stomach.

genetic (jĕ-net′ik)   Pertaining to hereditary factors.

glial (gli′al)   Pertaining to glia or neuroglia.

glioblastoma (gli″o-blas-to′mah)   Any malignant astrocytoma.

glioma (gli-o′mah)   A tumor composed of neuroglia.

glomerulonephritis (glo-mer″u-lo-nĕ-fri′tis)   Inflammation of the kidney capillaries.

gluteal (gloo′te-al)   Pertaining to the buttocks.

gluten (gloo′ten)   Pertaining to the wheat grain.

gonococcal (gon″o-kok′al)   Referring to the gonococcus organism.

gout (gout)   A hereditary form of arthritis that results from an overproduction of uric acid.

grading (grā′ding)   Determining the severity of a malignant lesion by histological differentiation.

granuloma (gran″u-lo′mah)   A tumor composed of granulation tissue.

granulomatous (gran″-u-lom′ah-tus)   Composed of granulomas.

greenstick fracture (grēn′stik frak′chur)   An incomplete fracture often found in children.

guaiac (gwi′ak)   A reagent used in a stool test for occult fecal blood.

gutta (gut′ah)   A drop.

gynecological (gi″nĕ-ko-loj′i-k′l)   Pertaining to the study of the female genital tract.

H

hamartoma (ham″ar-to′mah)   A benign tumor-like nodule composed of an overgrowth of mature cells and tissues normally present in the affected part, but often with one element predominating.

Harrington rods (har′ing-ton rodz)   Stabilizing metal rods used in scoliosis surgery.

haustra (haws′trah)   Pouches of the colon produced by the teniae coli.

Heberden's nodes (he′ber-denz nōdz)   Small hard nodules found in the distal interphalangeal joints as the result of osteoarthritis.

helix (he′liks)   A coiled structure.

hemangioma (hĕ-man″je-o′mah)   A benign vascular tumor.

hematemesis (hem″ah-tem′ĕ-sis)   The vomiting of blood.

hematochezia (hem″ah-to-ke′ze-ah)   The passage of bright red blood in the stool.

hematocrit (he-mat′o-krit)   The volume percentage of red blood cells in whole blood.

hematogenous (hem″ah-toj′ĕ-nus)   Related to the blood system.

hematological (hem″ah-to-loj′i-k′l)   Pertaining to the morphology of blood.

hematology (hem″ah-tol′o-je)   The study of blood and blood-forming tissues.

hematoma (hem″ah-to′mah)   A blood clot located outside of a blood vessel.

hematuria (hem″ah-tu′re-ah)   Blood in the urine.

hemiparesis (hem″e-par′e-sis)   Muscle weakness or partial paralysis on one side of the body.

hemolytic (he″mo-lit′ik)   Pertaining to red blood cell destruction.

hemorrhage (hem′or-ij)   The escape of blood from a ruptured blood vessel.

hemorrhagic (hem″o-raj′ik)   Pertaining to bleeding or hemorrhage.

hemothorax (he″mo-tho′raks)   A collection of blood in the thoracic cavity.

heparin (hep′ah-rin)   An agent that inhibits blood clotting.

hepatitis (hep″ah-ti′tis)   Inflammation of the liver.

hepatocyte (hep′ah-to-sīt)   Liver cell.

hepatomegaly (hep″ah-to-meg′ah-le)   Liver enlargement.

hepatosplenomegaly (hel″ah-to-sple″no-meg′ah-le)   Enlargement of the liver and spleen.

hereditary (he-red′ĭ-ter-e)   Genetically transmitted from parent to offspring.

hernia (her′ne-ah)   Any protrusion of a part of an organ through an abnormal opening in the structure normally containing it.

herniated (her′ne-āt′ed)   Protruding like a hernia.

hiatal (hi-a′tal)   Pertaining to a cleft, opening, or passageway.

hilum (hi′lum)   A medial depression of an organ where vessels enter and exit the organ.

Hirschsprung's disease (hirsh′sproongz dĭ-zēz′)   Congenital megacolon.

histoplasmosis (his″to-plaz-mo′sis)   A fungal lung disease caused by the inhalation of dust and particulate matter; common among farmers.

histological (his″to-loj-ĭ-k′l)   Pertaining to a microscopic examination of cells.

history (his′to-re)   The written description of patient signs and symptoms.

Hodgkin's disease (hoj′kinz dĭ-zēz′)   A primary neoplastic disease of the lymphatic system.

homeostasis (ho″me-o-sta′sis)   Maintaining stability.

hormone (hor′mōn)   A chemical transmitter produced by cells for a regulatory effect.

hyaline (hi′ah-līn)   Glassy and transparent, as the membranous covering of the alveoli of premature infants.

hydramnios (hi-dram′ne-os)   An overabundance of amniotic fluid.

hydrocarbon (hi″dro-kar′bon)   An organic compound that contains carbon and hydrogen only; a carcinogen.

hydrocephalus (hi-dro-sef′ah-lus)   Accumulation of cerebrospinal fluid in the ventricles of the brain.

hydronephrosis (hi″dro-nĕ-fro′sis)   Distension of the renal pelvis with urine.

hydrostatic (hi-dro-stat′ik)   Pertaining to a liquid in a state of equilibrium or the pressure exerted by a stationary fluid.

hydrothorax (hi-dro-tho′raks)   A collection of serous fluid in the thoracic cavity.

hyperbilirubinemia (hi″per-bil″ĭ-roo″bĭ-ne′me-ah)   An excess of the bile pigment bilirubin in the blood.

hypercalcemia (hi″per-kal-se′me-ah) An excess of calcium in the blood.

hypermobility (hi″per-mo-bil′ĭte) Increased movement.

hypernephroma (hi″per-nĕ-fro′mah) Renal cell carcinoma.

hyperparathyroidism (hi″per-par″ah-thi′roid-izm) Increased activity of the parathyroid glands.

hyperplasia (hi″per-pla′ze-ah) An abnormal increase in cell numbers.

hypertension (hi″per-ten′shun) Persistent high arterial blood pressure.

hypertensive (hi″per-ten′siv) Characterized by or causing increased tension or pressure; a person with high blood pressure.

hypertrophic (hip″per-trof′ik) Pertaining to hypertrophy.

hypertrophy (hi-per′tro-fe) An enlargement in an organ or part due to an increase in cell size; usually pertains to muscle.

hyperuricemia (hi″per-u″rĭ-se′me-ah) An excess of uric acid in the blood.

hypophosphatemia (hi″po-fos″fah-te′me-ah) A deficiency of phosphates in the blood.

hypophysis (hi-pof′ĭ-sis) The pituitary gland.

hypoplasia (hi″po-pla′ze-ah) Incomplete development or underdevelopment of an organ or structure.

hypostatic (hi″po-stat′ik) Referring to poor or stagnant circulation of the organs or tissues.

hypotension (hi″po-ten′shun) Low arterial blood pressure.

hypothalamus (hi″po-thal′ah-mus) The portion of the diencephalon lying beneath the thalamus at the base of the cerebrum.

hypoxemia (hi″pok-se′me-ah) A deficiency of oxygen in the blood.

hypoxia (hi″pok′se-ah) Reduction of oxygen supply to the tissues.

hysterectomy (his″tĕ-rek′to-me) Surgical removal of the uterus.

I

iatrogenic (i-at″ro-jen′ik) Resulting from the activity of a physician.

idiopathic (id″e-o-path′ik) Referring to disease of unknown cause.

immobilization (im-mo″bil-i-za′shun) The prevention of bone and joint movement following injury and treatment.

immunoglobulin (im″u-no-glob′u-lin) A protein with antibody activity, which is essential to fight disease.

immunopathology (im″u-no-pah-thol′o-je) The study of immune reactions associated with disease.

impingement (im-pinj′ment) Encroachment; as in a disk upon the spinal cord.

implantation (im″plan-ta′shun) The grafting of tissue into a specific location.

incarceration (in-kar″ser-a′shun) The unnatural retention or confinement of a part.

incidence (in′sĭ-dens) The number of newly diagnosed cases in a time period, usually a year.

incontinence (in-kon′tĭ-nens) Inability to control excretory functions.

infantile (in′fan-tīl) Pertaining to infancy.

infarct (in′farkt) A localized area of ischemia necrosis.

infarction (in-fark′shun) The death of cells due to anoxia; ischemic necrosis.

inflammation (in″flah-ma′shun) The body's response to injury, which is characterized by the destruction of the affected tissues and the agent itself.

influenza (in″flu-en′zah)   A contagious viral disease commonly referred to as the flu.

inguinal hernia (ing′gwĭ-nal her′ne-ah)   A protrusion of bowel into the groin.

inhalation (in″hah-la′shun)   The drawing of air into the lungs; inspiration.

in situ (in si′tu)   Confined to the site of origin.

intermittent (in″ter-mit′ent)   Occurring at separate intervals.

internist (in-ter′nist)   A physician who specializes in diagnosis and medical treatment.

interstitial (in″ter-stish′al)   Pertaining to the spaces within or between tissues.

intertrochanteric (in″ter-tro″kan-ter′ik)   Referring to an oblique line or crest that runs between the femoral trochanters.

intrathoracic (in″trah-tho-ras′ik)   Within or inside the thorax.

intravenous (in″trah-ve′nus)   Within a vein, as a route of administration.

intubate (in′tu-bāt)   To insert a tube in the airway.

intussusception (in″tus-sus-sep′shun)   Telescoping of the bowel into itself.

invaginate (in-vaj′ĭ-nāt)   To infold one portion of a structure into another.

invasion (in-va′zhun)   The spreading of cancer to an adjacent area.

iodine (i′o-dīn)   An element that in its radioactive form is commonly employed as a contrast aent in diagnostic radiology.

irradiation (ĭ-ra″de-a′shun)   Exposure to radiant energy; x-rays.

ischemia (is-ke′me-ah)   The deficiency of blood to tissue.

isotope (i′so-tōp)   A chemical element having the same atomic number as another but a different atomic weight or mass.

ivory bones (i′vo-re bōnz)   Osteopetrosis.

IVP   Intravenous pyelogram or pyelography.

J

jaundice (jawn′dis)   A yellowish discoloration of the skin or mucous membranes due to hyperbilirubinemia.

juvenile (joo′vĕ-nīl)   Pertaining to youth or childhood, as diseases that occur during that time.

K

keratin (ker′ah-tin)   A hard protein that is the principal constitutent of epidermis.

Kienböck's disease (kēn′beks dĭ-zēz′) Osteochondrosis of the carpal lunate; lunatomalacia.

Köhler's disease (ka′lerz dĭ-zēz)   Osteochondrosis of the tarsal navicular in children.

kyphosis (ki-fo′sis)   An abnormal increased convexity of the kyphotic curve of the dorsal spine; humpback deformity

L

laceration (las″er-a′shun)   A jagged tearing of tissue.

laminated (lam′ĭ-nāt″ed)   Arranged in layers.

laminectomy (lam″ĭ-nek′to-me)   Surgical removal of the lamina.

laparatomy (lap-ah-rot′o-me) An incision through the abdominal wall.

Legg-Calvé-Perthes disease (leg′kal-va′per′thez dĭ-zez′) Osteochondrosis of the femoral head epiphyses.

leiomyoma (li″o-mi-o′mah) A smooth muscle tumor; usually benign.

lesion (le′zhun) A structural change that is abnormal and that is the result of trauma or disease.

lethargy (leth′ar-je) Drowsiness or indifference.

leukemia (loo-ke′me-ah) Cancer of the blood-forming organs.

leukocytosis (loo″ko-si-to′sis) An abnormal increase in the number of circulating white blood cells.

lidocaine (li′do-kān) A drug used as a local anesthetic.

ligament (lig′ah-ment) A band of fibrous tissue connecting bones or cartilages, providing support for joints.

ligation (li-ga′shun) Application of a ligature.

linitis plastica (lĭ-ni′tis plas′ti-ka) A diffuse inflammatory proliferation of the gastric submucosa.

lipase (lip′ās) A fat-splitting enzyme.

lipid (lip′id) Fat.

lipoma (lĭ-po′mah) A benign tumor composed of fatty tissue.

lipping (lip′ing) The development of a bony overgrowth.

Lippman-Cobb method (lip′mun kob meth′ud) A method of measuring the degree of scoliotic angle.

liquefaction (lik″wĕ-fak′shun) Conversion into a fluid; a form of necrosis.

lobectomy (lo-bek′to-me) Surgical removal of a lobe of an organ.

lobular (lob′u-lar) Referring a segment or subunit of a lobe.

loculated (lok′u-la-ted) Confined within, such as an interlobar fissure.

lordotic (lor-dot′ik) Referring to lordosis, a forward curvature, as in the spine.

lucency (loo′sen-se) A clear area in an image produced by the passage of radiant energy through matter.

lumen (loo′men) The cavity within a hollow organ.

lunatomalacia (loo-na″to-mah-la′she-ah) A synonym for osteochondrosis.

lung edge (lung ej) The visible border of the pleura seen on a chest film of a pneumothorax.

lupus erythematosus (loo′pus er″ĭ-them-ah-to′sus) A generalized degeneration of collagen connective tissue.

lymphadenopathy (lim-fad″ĕ-nop′ah-the) The enlargement of lymph nodes due to a disease process.

lymphogranuloma (lim″fo-gran″u-lo′mah) Hodgkin's disease.

lymphoma (lim-fo′mah) A general term for lymphatic cancer.

lymphosarcoma (lim″fo-sar-ko′mah) A general term for lymphatic cancer, excluding Hodgkin's disease.

lysis (li′sis) Destruction or decomposition.

M

magnesium (mag-ne′ze-um) An essential element in nutrition; required for action of many enzymes.

malabsorption (mal″ab-sorp′shun) Impaired intestinal absorption of nutrients.

malaise (mal-āz′) Generalized weakness and lack of energy.

malignancy (mah-lig′nan-se) The ability to metastasize.

malignant (mah-lig′nant) Tending to have morbid consequences; cancerous.

malnutrition (mal″nu-trish′un) Any disorder of nutrition.

mammary dysplasia (mam′er-e dis-pla′se-ah) Fibrocystic disease of the breast.

mammography (mam-og′rah-fe) Radiography of the breast.

manifestations (man″ĭ-fes-ta′shunz) Signs apparent to the senses; results of disease.

manipulation (mah-nip″u-la′shun) Skillful or dextrous treatment by the hands, as in a closed reduction of a bone deformity.

mannitol (man′ĭ-tol) A drug used to control cerebral edema.

marble bones (mar′b′l bōnz) Osteopetrosis.

Marfan's syndrome (Mar-fahnz′ sin′drōm) A generalized, degenerative connective tissue disease.

marrow (mar′o) The soft sponge-like material found in the cavities of bone.

mass (mas) A lump or collection of adhering particles or fibers.

mastectomy (mas-tek′to-me) Surgical removal of the breast.

matrix (ma′triks) The intercellular substance of a tissue.

measles (me′zelz) An acute contagious viral disease also called rubeola.

mediastinum (me″de-as-ti′num) A median septum or partition, as in the chest cavity.

medulla (mĕ-dul′ah) The central or inner portion of an organ.

medulloblastoma (mĕ-dul″o-blas-to′mah) A brain tumor consisting of medulloblasts.

megacolon (meg″ah-ko′lon) A congenital or functional enlargement of the colon.

megaloureter (meg″ah-lo-u-re′ter) Congenital ureteral diltation without obvious cause.

melena (mĕ-le′nah) The evacuation of black tarry stools, indicating gastrointestinal bleeding.

Ménétrier's disease (mān″a-tre-ārz′ dis-zēz′) Giant hypertrophic gastritis with profuse thickening of the gastric mucosa often in the presence of inflammation.

meningioma (mĕ-nin″je-o′mah) A benign tumor of the meninges.

meningitis (men″in-ji′tis) Inflammation of the meninges of the brain and spinal cord.

mesenteric (mes″en-ter′ik) Pertaining to the mesentery.

mesentery (mes′en-ter″e) Membraneous folds of tissue attaching various organs to the abdominal wall.

mesoderm (mes′o-derm) The middle of the three germ layers.

metabolic (met″ah-bol′ik) Pertaining to metabolism.

metaphysis (me-taf′ĭ-sis) The point where the diaphysis and epiphysis meet.

metaplasia (met″ah-pla′ze-ah) A change from one cell type to another.

metastasis (mĕ-tas′tah-sis) The transfer or spread of a cancerous lesion from one place to another.

metastatic (met″ah-stat′ik) Pertaining to metastasis.

metatarsus adductus (met″ah-tar′sus ah-dukt′us) An inward turning or varus deformity of the foot.

metrizamide (mĕ-triz′ah-mīd) A water-soluble contrast medium used in myelography.

migraine (mi'grān)   Severe headaches usually limited to one side of the head.

morbidity (mor-bid'ĭ-te)   The frequency of disability within a population.

morphine (mor'fēn)   An opium derivitive that may be used as an analgesic or respiratory depressant.

mucous (mu'kus)   Pertaining to a mucus discharge.

mucoviscidosis (mu"ko-vis"ĭ-do'sis)   A condition characterized by the accumulation of thick mucus in the body passageways.

mucus (mu'kus)   A sticky fluid secreted by mucous membranes.

multiple myeloma (mul'tĭ-p'l mi"ĕ-lo'mah)   A malignancy involving the plasma cells of bone marrow.

mycobacteria (mi"ko-bak-te're-ah)   Microorganisms resembling the bacillus that causes tuberculosis.

mycosis (mi-ko'sis)   Any disease caused by a fungus.

myelocele (mi'ĕ-lo-sēl)   A protrusion or herniation of the spinal meninges.

myelography (mi"ĕ-log'rah-fe)   Radiological examination of the spinal canal.

myeloma (mi"ĕ-lo'mah)   A tumor of the plasma cells of bone marrow.

myelomeningocele (mi"ĕ-lo-mĕ-ning'go-sēl)   Herniation of the meninges and spinal cord.

myocardial (mi"o-kar'de-al)   Pertaining to the myocardium or heart muscle.

N

narcotic (nar-kot'ik)   A drug that produces insensibility or stupor.

nausea (naw'se-ah)   A feeling of the need to regurgitate or vomit.

necrosis (nĕ-kro'sis)   The morphological changes indicative of cell death caused by enzymatic degradation.

neoplasia (ne"o-pla'ze-ah)   The formation of a neoplasma.

neoplasm (ne'o-plazm)   Any new and abnormal growth.

nephrectomy (nĕ-frek'to-me)   Surgical removal of a kidney.

nephritis (nĕ-fri'tis)   Inflammation of the kidney.

nephrocalcinosis (nef"ro-kal"sĭ-no'sis)   The deposition of calciuum phosphate in the renal tubules, resulting in renal insufficiency.

nephrolithiasis (nef"ro-lĭ-thi'ah-sis)   A condition marked by the presence of renal calculi.

nephrolithotomy (nef"ro-lĭ-thot'o-me)   A surgical incision of the kidney for removal of calculi.

nephrolithotripsy (nef"ro-lith'o-trip"se)   The use of ultrasonic waves to break up kidney stone into smaller pieces and facilitate passage.

nephron (nef'ron)   The structural and functional unit of the kidney.

nephroscope (nef'ro-skōp)   An instrument inserted through an incision to observe the internal aspects of the renal pelvis.

nephrostomy (nĕ-fros'to-me)   Creation of a permanent opening into the renal pelvis.

nephrotomography (nef"ro-to-mog'rah-fe)   Body section radiography of the kidney.

neurosis (nu-ro'sis)   An emotional disorder chiefly characterized by anxiety.

nodular (nod'u-lar)   Like a node or mass.

nosocomial (nos"o-ko'me-al)   Pertaining to a disease acquired while in a hospital.

O

obliteration (ob-lit″er-a′shun) Complete removal, whether by disease, degeneration, surgery, radiation, etc.

obstruction (ob-struk′shun) Blockage; occlusion.

occlusion (ŏ-kloo′zhun) Blockage or obstruction, as of a tube-like passageway.

occult (ŏ-kult′) Hidden or not apparent.

ocular (ok′u-lar) Pertaining to the eye.

olecranon (o-lek′rah-non) The most proximal part of the ulna; the posterior tip of the elbow.

oligodendroglia (ol″ĭ-go-den-drog′le-ah) The nonneural cells of ectodermal origin.

oligodendroglioma (ol″ĭ-go-den″dro-gli-o′mah) A neoplasm composed of oligodendroglia.

organic (or-gan′ik) Pertaining to an organ; consisting of an organized structure.

orthopedic (or″tho-pe′dik) Referring to the correction of deformities of the skeletal system.

Ortolani's sign (or-tah-lah′nēz sīn) A characteristic clicking sound heard in the presence of congenital hip dysplasia.

Osgood-Schlatter disease (oz′good-shlat′er dĭ-zēz′) Osteochondritis of the tibial tubercle.

osseous (os′e-us) Of the nature or quality of bone; bony.

osteitis deformans (os″te-i′tis de-for′manz) Paget's disease of bone.

osteoblast (os′te-o-blast″) An immature bone cell.

osteoblastic (os″te-o-blas′tik) Pertaining to the formation of new bone.

osteochondroma (os″te-o-kon-dro′mah) A benign tumor consisting of bone and cartilage.

osteochondrosis (os″te-o-kon-dro′sis) A disease of the growth ossification centers in children.

osteoclastoma (os″te-o-klas-to′mah) Giant cell tumor of bone.

osteocyte (os′te-o-sīt″) A mature bone cell.

osteogenic (os″te-o-jen′ik) Originating from bone; bone forming.

osteogenesis imperfecta (os″te-o-jen′ĕ-sis) A brittle bone disease resulting in fractures with the least bit of trauma.

osteoid (os′te-oid) The soft, organic part of the bony matrix.

osteolytic (os″te-o-lit′ik) Relating to osteolysis, dissolution of bone.

osteoma (os″te-o′mah) A benign bone tumor.

osteomalacia (os″te-o-mah-la′she-ah) A condition marked by the softening of bone.

osteomyelitis (os″te-o-mi″ĕ-l′tis) An infection of bone.

osteopetrosis (os″te-o-pe-tro′sis) A hereditary disorder resulting in abnormally dense bone.

osteophytic (os″te-o-fĭ′tik) Pertaining to a bony overgrowth.

osteoporosis (os″te-o-po-ro′sis) The decreased mineralization of bone; porous bone.

osteosarcoma (os″te-o-sar-ko′mah) A malignant bone tumor.

osteotomy (os″te-ot′o-me) The surgical cutting of bone.

ovarian (o-va′re-an) Pertaining to the ovary.

ovoid (o′void) Egg-shaped.

P

Paget's disease (paj'ets dĭ-zēz') Osteitis deformans; a disease of the elderly.

palliative (pal'e-a"tiv) A treatment used to control the effects of a disease rather than cure it, such as for relief of cancer.

pancreatitis (pan"kre-a-ti'tis) Inflammation of the pancreas.

panlobar (pan-lo'bar) Pertaining to all of the lung lobe.

pannus (pan'us) An inflammatory exudate present within a joint capsule as a result of rheumatoid arthritis.

Pantopaque (pan-to-pāk) An oil-based contrast medium used in myelography.

paralysis (pah-ral'ĭ-sis) A loss or impairment of motor function of a body part.

paranasal (par"ah-na'zal) Located near the nose.

paranoia (par"ah-noi'ah) A mental disorder characterized by delusions of persecution.

paraparesis (par"ah-par'ĕ-sis) Partial paralysis of the lower extremities.

paraplegia (par"ah-ple'je-ah) Paralysis of the lower extremities and possibly the pelvis.

parasite (par'ah-sīt) A plant or animal that lives on or within another living organism.

paravertebral (par"ah-ver'tĕ-bral) Beside or near the vertebral column.

parenchyma (pah-reng'kĭ-mah) The functioning unit of any organ.

parenteral (pah-ren'ter-al) Not through the alimentary canal but rather by injection through some other route.

pathology (pah-thol'o-je) The study of disease.

pathogenesis (path"o-jen'ĕ-sis) The sequence of events that leads to the development of disease.

pathophysiology (path"o-fiz"e-ol'o-je) The physiology of abnormal function.

pauciarticular (paw"se-ar-tik"u-lar) A form of juvenile rheumatoid arthritis that affects both male and female children and adolescents.

pectus excavatum (pek'tus eks-ka-va'tum) A congenital funnel-shaped depression of the chest wall.

pediatrician (pe"de-ah-trish'un) A physician specializing in the care of infants and children.

peptic (pep'tik) Pertaining to pepsin and other proteolyic enzymes involved in digestion.

percutaneous (per"ku-ta'ne-us) Usually pertaining to an injection through the skin.

perforation (per-fo-ra'shun) A hole or break in a wall or membrane.

perfusion (per-fu'zhun) The passage of fluid through a vessel membrane.

periodontal (per"e-o-don'tal) Pertaining to the gums or the area surrounding the teeth.

periosteum (per"e-os'te-um) The specialized tissue covering the bones.

peristalsis (per"ĭ-stal'sis) The wavy contractions of circular and longitudinal muscle of the alimentary tract.

peritonitis (per"ĭ-to-ni'tis) Inflammation of the peritoneum.

pernicious (per-nish'us) Pertaining to a form of anemia that is related to the body's inability to absorb vitamin B_{12}.

pertussis (per-tus'is) Whooping cough.

petechia (pe-te'ke-ah) Pinpoint purplish intradermal or subcutaneous skin hemorrhage.

phagocytosis (fag″o-si-to′sis)   The engulfing of microorganisms and other foreign matter by phagocytes.

phenacetin (fĕ-nas′ĕ-tin)   An analgesic and antipyretic.

phlebolith (fleb′o-lith)   A venous calculus.

phosphate (fos′fāt)   Any salt or ester of phosphoric acid.

phrenoesophageal (fren″o-ĕ-sof′ah-je′al)   Pertaining to the esophageal hiatus, which is located in the diaphragm.

physical therapy (fiz′e-kal ther′ah-pe)   The medical specialty that uses physical agents and methods of treatment for restoring function lost in muscle, bone, nerve, and joint disorders.

pigeon breast (pij′en brest)   A prominence of the breast bone.

pigeon toe (pij′en to)   Metatarsus adductus.

plaque (plak)   Any patch or flat area, such at the fatty deposits on the arterial intima in association with atherosclerosis.

platybasia (plat″e-ba′se-ah)   A flat cranial base with a small foramen magnum.

pneumococcus (nu″mo-kok′us)   Airborne bacteria of the species *Diplococcus pneumoniae*.

pneumoconiosis (nu″mo-ko″ne-o′sis)   A condition characterized by the accumulation of dust and particulate matter in the lungs.

pneumonia (nu-mo′ne-ah)   A bacterial or viral infection of the lungs.

pneumothorax (nu″mo-tho′raks)   Air in the thoracic cavity.

podagra (po-dag′rah)   A gout-like pain in the great toe.

polyarticular (pol″e-ar-tik′u-lar)   Affecting many joints.

polycystic (pol″e-sis′tik)   Containing multiple cysts, a condition common in the kidneys.

poliomyelitis (po″le-o-mi″ĕ-li′tis)   An acute viral disease that attacks the central nervous system.

polycythemia (pol″e-si-the′me-ah)   An increase in the total red cell mass in the blood.

portal (por′tal)   Pertaining to the liver.

postmenopausal (pōst″men-o-paw′zal)   After menopause.

potassium (po-tas′e-um)   A mineral that in combination with others forms alkaline salts that are important in body processes and play an important role in acid-base balance in the body.

prednisone (pred′nĭ-sōn)   An antiinflammatory agent; a glucocorticoid.

prevalence (prev′ah-lens)   The total number of cases of a disease at any one place and time.

procedure (pro-se′jur)   A series of steps by which a desired result is accomplished.

proctology (prok-tol′o-je)   The study of the rectum and anus and their diseases.

prognathism (prog′na-thizm)   Marked prominence of the mandible.

prognosis (prog-no′sis)   The predicted outcome of a disease.

proliferation (pro-lif-ĕ-ra′shun)   The reproduction or multiplication of similar forms.

prosthesis (pros-the′sis)   An artificial substitute for a missing body part.

proteinuria (pro″te-in-u′re-ah)   The increase of serum proteins in urine.

prothrombin time (pro-throm′bin tīm)   A blood test that measures the activity of clotting factors.

proximal (prok′sĭ-mal)   Nearest to the point of reference.

pruritus (proo-ri′tus)   Itching.

pseudo- (soo′do)   A prefix meaning false.

pseudotumor (soo″do-tu′mor)   Phantom tumor.

psittacosis (sit-ah-ko′sis)   A disease transmitted by parrots; parrot fever.

psychosis (si-ko′sis)   A major mental disorder characterized by derangement of personality and a loss of contact with reality.

psychosomatic (si″ko-so-mat′ik)   Pertaining to symptoms of illnesses involving interrelations of mind and body.

pulsion (pul′shun)   Pushing outward; a type of diverticulum.

purine (pu′rin)   A heterocylic compound found in the DNA and RNA.

purulent (pu′-roo-lent)   Pertaining to a pus-like discharge.

pus (pus)   A purulent discharge.

pyelography (pi″ĕp-log′rah-fe)   Radiographic demonstration of the renal pelvis.

pyelonephritis (pi″ĕ-lo-nĕ-fri′tis)   Infection of the kidney and renal pelvis.

pyloromyotomy (pi-lo″ro-mi-ot′o-me)   A surgical incision made into the pylorus.

pyogenic (pi″o-jen′ik)   Producing pus.

pyothorax (pi″o-tho′raks)   A collection of pus in the thoracic cavity.

pyramid (pēr-ah-mid)   A pointed or cone-shaped structure or part.

Q

quadriceps (kwod′rĭ-seps)   A group of four muscles of the thigh.

R

RA latex fixation (la′-tĕks fik-sa′-shŭn)   A blood test used to determine the presence of the rheumatoid factor and rheumatoid arthritis.

radioisotope (ra″de-o-i′so-tōp)   A radioactive form of an element.

radiolucent (ra-de-o-lu′sent)   Permitting the passage of x-rays, as through anatomical structures.

radionuclide (ra″de-o-nu′klīd)   A radioactive pharmaceutical; isotope.

radiopacity (ra″de-o-pas′ĭ-te)   The property of being radiopaque.

radiopaque (ra″de-o-pāk′)   Not permitting the passage of radiant energy such as x-rays.

radiopharmaceutical (ra″de-o-fahr″mah-su′tĭ-kal)   A radioactive isotope prepared by a pharmacist for later injection of a patient having an examination in the department of nuclear medicine.

radioresistance (ra″de-o-re-zis′tans)   The lack of response of tissue to radiation.

radiosensitivity (ra″de-o-sen″sĭ-tiv′ĭ-te)   The response of tissue to radiation.

radium (ra′-de-um)   A highly radioactive element found in uranium.

Rathke's pouch (rahth′kĕz powch)   A diverticulum from the embryonic buccal cavity, from which the anterior pituitary is developed.

recessive (re-ses′iv)   In genetics, incapable of expression unless the allele is carried by both parents.

recumbent (re-kum′bent)   Lying down.

Reed-Sternberg cell (rēd-stern′berg sel)   A type of cell found in persons with Hodgkin's disease.

reflux (re′fluks)   Backward or return flow.

regeneration (re-jen"er-a'shun) The preferred method of body repair, in which the original function of the cell is restored.

regurgitation (re-gur"jĭ-ta'shun) A backward or reverse flow, as of undigested food.

Reiter's syndrome (ri'terz sin'drōm) A disease of males, characterized by diarrhea, urethritis, conjunctivitis, and polyarthritis.

remission (re-mish'un) The regression of disease; a period of time in which diminution of symptoms occurs.

renal cell carcinoma (re'nal sel kar"sĭ-no'mah) Hypernephroma; adenocarcinoma.

repair (re-pār') The replacement and restoration of the cell or tissue and its function.

resection (re-sek'shun) The surgical removal of a large specimen, primarily for treatment.

resorption (re-sorp'shun) The lysis and assimilation of a substance.

restoration (res"to-ra'shun) To return to normal position and function.

retension (re-ten'shun) The process of holding back or keeping in a position.

retrograde (ret'ro-grād) Going backward, against the flow.

retrolental fibroplasia (re"tro-len'tal fi"bro-pla'se-ah) A condition of premature infants characterized by the presence of opaque tissue behind the lens, leading to retinal detachment and blindness, the result of an excessive concentration of oxygen.

retroperitoneal (re"tro-per"ĭ-to-ne'al) Behind the peritoneum.

rheumatoid arthritis (roo'mah-toid ar-thri'tis) A chronic systemic disease with inflammatory changes of joints.

rheumatoid factor (roo'mah-toid fak'tor) The factor that when present is indicative of rheumatoid arthritis.

rhinitis (ri-ni'tis) Inflammation of the mucous membrane of the nose, resulting in discharge from the nose.

rickets (rik'ets) A condition caused by a deficiency of vitamin D.

rupture (rup'chur) Forcible tearing of tissue, as a herniation.

S

saccular (sak'u-lar) Shaped like a sac.

sacroiliitis (sa"kro-il"e-i'tis) Inflammation of the sacroiliac joint.

saliva (sah-li'vah) Fluid containing ptyalin that is secreted by salivary glands.

salmonella (sal"mo-nel'ah) Any organism belonging to the genus *Salmonella*.

sanguineous (sang-gwin'e-us) Bloody.

sarcoma (sar-ko'mah) A malignant tumor of connective tissue origin.

scar (skahr) The formation of fibrous tissue following healing of certain tissues.

scarlet fever (skar'let fe'ver) A contagious disease caused by beta-hemolytic streptococci.

Schatzki's ring (shat'skēz ring) A narrow constriction of the distal esophagus with a characteristic radiographic appearance.

Scheuermann's disease (shoi'er-manz dĭ-zez') Osteochondrosis of the vertebral epiphyses in children.

schizophrenia (skiz"o-fre'ne-ah) A general term covering a wide range of mental disorders characterized by mental deterioration and involving several characteristic disturbances of multiple inappropriate mental processes.

Schmorl's nodes (shmorlz nōdz)   A common bone defect of a vertebral body into which the nucleus pulposus herniates.

scirrhous (skir'us)   Pertaining to the nature of a hard cancer.

sclera (skle'rah)   The rough outer coat of the eyeball.

sclerosis (skle-ro'sis)   An induration or hardening of tissue.

scoliosis (sko"le-o'sis)   A lateral curvature of the spine.

scurvy (skur've)   A disease due to a deficiency of vitamin C.

sedimentation rate (sed"ĭ-men-ta'shun rāt)   A blood test measuring the settling out of sediment from centrifuged blood in 1 hour.

senile (se'nīl)   Pertaining to old age.

septic (sep'tik)   Produced by the presence of microorganisms in tissue.

septicemia (sep"tĭ-se'me-ah)   Blood poisoning.

sequestrum (se-kwes'trum)   A dead piece of tissue that becomes separated from adjacent living tissue.

serosa (se-ro'sah)   The outermost lining of the alimentary tract.

serotype (se'ro-tīp)   The type of microorganism present with disease.

serous (se'rus)   Resembling or producing serum.

serpiginous (ser-pij'ĭ-nus)   Having a wavy border.

serum (se'rum)   The clear straw-colored liquid part of a plasma that contains no cells or hemoglobin.

SGOT   Serum glutamic-oxaloacetic transaminase; a blood test used to detect the level of liver damage.

SGPT   Serum glutamic-pyruvic transaminase; a blood test used to detect the level of liver damage.

shigella (shĭ-gel'ah)   Any organism belonging to the genus of *Shigella*.

shunt (shunt)   A bypass or redirection.

sibling (sib'ling)   Any two or more offspring of the same parents.

sigmoidoscope (sig-moi'do-skōp)   An endoscope used for evaluation of the sigmoid colon.

sign (sīn)   An observable manifestation.

silica (sil'ĭ-kah)   Particulate dust common in sand and glass.

silicosis (sil"ĭ-ko'sis)   A condition of the lungs caused by the inhalation of silica.

sinusoid (si'nŭ-soid)   A form of specialized capillary in the reticuloendothelium.

sling (sling)   A supporting or immobilizing bandage.

sodium (so'de-um)   An element that is a major part of blood plasma and intercellular fluid.

solitary (sol'ĭ-ter"e)   Single or alone.

sonography (so-nog'rah-fe)   Ultrasonography; a diagnostic imaging technique using sound waves.

spasm (spazm)   An involuntary contraction of muscle.

spica cast (spi'kah kast)   A casting of the pelvis and lower extremities.

spina bifida (spi'nah bif'ĭ-dah)   A failure of the lamina to unite posteriorly.

splenoportography (sple"no-por-tog'rah-fe)   A radiographic procedure involving an injection of a contrast agent into the splenic pulp, affording visualization of the portal venous system.

splint (splint)   A flexible or rigid appliance that immobilizes a body part.

spondylitis (spon"dĭ-li'tis)   Inflammation of the vertebrae.

spondylolisthesis (spon″dĭ-lo-lis′the-sis)   The forward movement of one vertebra upon another.

spondylolysis (spon″dĭ-lol′ĭ-sis)   The dissolution of a vertebra.

spondylosis (spon″dĭ-lo′sis)   Ankylosis of a vertebral joint consistent with degenerative changes.

spontaneous (spon-ta′ne-us)   Voluntary; without external influence.

spontaneous pneumothorax (spon-ta′ne-us nu″mo-tho′raks)   The appearnce of air in the thorax that occurs for no apparent reason.

sprue bowel (sproo bow′el)   A chronic form of the malabsorption syndrome or celiac disease.

sputum (spu′tum)   Expectorate from the lungs.

squamous (skwa′mus)   Scaly; flat and saucer-like.

Staphylococcus (staf″ĭ-lo-kok′us)   A genus of gram-negative bacteria.

stasis (sta′sis)   The stoppage of flow, as in blood, urine, air, etc.

steatorrhea (ste″ah-to-re′ah)   Fat-laden stool, which is often due to celiac disease.

stellate (stel′āt)   Star-like.

stenosis (stĕ-no′sis)   The narrowing of a lumen.

steroid (ste′roid)   A type of medication used to promote body repair.

Still's disease (stilz dĭ-zēz′)   Juvenile rheumatoid arthritis.

stratification (strat″ĭ-fi-ka′shun)   An arrangement in layers, as in gallstones.

Streptococcus (strĕp-tō-kŏk′us)   A genus of gram-negative bacteria.

stricture (strik′chur)   An abnormal narrowing of a duct or tube-like passageway.

stroke (strōk)   A sudden and usually severe attack due to a rupture or blockage of a blood vessel in the brain, resulting in loss of consciousness, paralysis, and other symptoms; cerebrovascular accident.

stunted (stunt′ed)   Shortened; retarded, as in growth.

stupor (stu′por)   Partial or near unconsciousness.

subcutaneous (sub″ku-ta′ne-us)   Below or underneath the skin.

subdural (sub-du′ral)   Referring to an area just below the dura mater.

subluxation (sub″luk-sa-shun)   A partial dislocation.

subpleural (sub-ploor′al)   Located below or underneath the pleura.

suicide (soo′ĭ-sīd)   The taking of one's own life.

supine (soo-pīn′)   Lying on the back.

suppurative (sup′u-ra″tiv)   Pyogenic; the formation of pus.

surfactant (sur-fak′tant)   A chemical detergent that serves to decrease surface tension of the lung.

sweat (swet)   Perspiration.

sweat test (swet test)   A diagnostic test for cystic fibrosis that when positive shows increased concentration of sodium chloride ion in perspiration.

symptom (simp′tum)   Any abnormality that is perceived by the patient.

synovitis (sin″o-vi′tis)   Inflammation of a synovial membrane.

syphilis (sif′ĭ-lis)   A contagious venereal disease.

systole (sis′to-le)   The working phase or contraction period of the heart.

T

tachycardia (tak″e-kar′de-ah) Excessively rapid heartbeat.

talipes (tal′ĭ-pēz) Congenital clubfoot.

talus (ta′lus) The highest tarsal bone of the ankle.

tendinitis (ten″dĭ-ni′tis) Inflammation of a tendon.

tendon (ten′dun) Fibrous tissue that connects muscle to bone.

tension (ten′shun) The act of stretching or making taut.

tentorium (ten-to′re-um) An anatomical part resembling a tent or covering.

terminal (ter′mĭ-nal) Pertaining to an end.

test (test) An examination, as of a specimen removed from a patient.

therapy (ther′ah-pe) The treatment of disease.

thoracentesis (tho″rah-sen-te′sis) The tapping or removal of fluid from the chest cavity by needle puncture.

thrombi (throm′be) Blood clots contained within a blood vessel.

thrombosis (throm-bo′sis) The formation of clotted blood in a blood vessel, particularly a vein.

thrombus (throm′bus) A blood clot or mass of clotted blood.

tibial torsion (tib′e-al tor′shun) A twisting of the tibia.

TNM system A method for staging of cancer; T = tumor, N = node, M = metastasis.

tomography (to-mog′rah-fe) Body section radiography.

tophi (to′fi) Urate deposits occurring in gout.

toxicity (tok-sis′ĭ-te) The quality of being poisonous.

toxin (tok′-sin) A poison.

trabecula (tra-bek′u-lah) The supporting fiber of connective tissue.

traction (trak′shun) The exertion of a pulling force that is applied to a fractured bone or dislocation.

transcolemic Metastatic spread via body spaces or cavities.

transformation (trans″for-ma′shun) A change of form or structure.

transhepatic (trans″hĕ-pat′ik) Through or across the liver, as an injection.

transient (tran′se-ent) Temporary.

transitional (trans-ish″ĭ-nal) Pertaining to a change taking place; usually in cells.

trauma (traw-mah) An injury due to an external force.

Trendelenburg's position (tren-del′en-bergz po-zish′un) The supine position with the head lower than the feet; 45-degree inclination.

Trendelenburg's sign (tren-del′en-bergz sīn) A maneuver for diagnosing congenital hip dysplasia.

treponema (trep″o-ne′mah) A parasitic spirochete causing venereal disease.

trident (tri′dent) Three-pronged.

triglyceride (tri-glis′er-īd) A combination of fatty acids and glycerol; a lipid.

trumpeting (trum′pet-ing) A widening of the long bone metaphyses.

trypsin (trip′sin) A proteolytic enzyme found in the intestine.

T-tube cholangiogram (te′tūb ko-lan′je-o-gram″) A postoperative radiological examination of the bile ducts.

tuberculosis (too-ber″ku-lo′sis) An infectious, inflammatory disease, usually of the lungs.

tumor (too'mor)   An abnormal enlargement of tissue; neoplasm.

TUR   Transurethral resection for prostatic hypertrophy.

U

ulcer (ul'ser)   A depressed lesion on the surface of an organ or tissue.

ulceration (ul"sĕ-ra'shun)   The formation or development of an ulcer.

umbilicus (um-bil'ĭ-kus)   The navel; the site of attachment of the umbilical cord.

undifferentiated (un-dif"er-en'she-a-ted)   Not differentiated; primitive.

unicameral (u"nĭ-kam'er-al)   Having only one cavity or compartment.

unilateral (u"nĭ-lat'er-al)   Appearing only on one side.

unstable (un-sta'b'l)   Not steady; irregular.

urate (u'rāt)   A salt of uric acid.

urea (u-re'ah)   The chief nitrogenous waste in the urine; the end product of protein metabolism.

uremia (u-re'me-ah)   The final stage of renal shutdown when the levels of urea and creatinine are very high.

ureterocele (u-re'ter-o-sēl)   The ballooning of the lower end of the ureter into the urinary bladder.

urethrography (u"rĕ-throg'rah-fe)   Radiographic examination of the urethra.

uric acid (u'rik as'id)   The end product of purine metabolism.

uricosuric (u"rĭ-ko-su'rik)   Pertaining to an agent that promotes the elimination of uric acid.

urinalysis (u"rĭ-nal'ĭ-sis)   Physical, chemical, or microscopic analysis of urine.

urography (u-rog'rah-fe)   Radiographic examination of the urinary tract; kidney function test.

V

vagotomy (va-got'o-me)   Surgical incision of the vagus nerve; minimizes the parasympathetic response, thus reducing the action of the acid-secreting glands.

Valsalva's maneuver (val-sal'vahz mah-noo'ver)   Forcible expiration against a closed glottis.

varicella (var"ĭ-sel'ah)   Chicken pox.

varices (vār'ĭ-sez)   Varicose veins.

vasopressin (vas"o-pres'in)   A hormone that promotes vasoconstriction and elevates blood pressure; antidiuretic hormone.

venography (ve-nog'rah-fe)   A phlebogram; an x-ray examination of the venous system.

ventilation (ven"tĭ-la'shun)   The process in which the air in the lungs is exchanged with the air of the atmosphere.

ventricle (ven'trĭ-k'l)   A fluid-containing space, as of the brain.

villus (vil'lus)   A small vascular process or protrusion that projects upward from a surface membrane.

viral (vi'ral)   Pertaining to a virus.

vitamin D (vi'tah-min de')   The vitamin responsible for bone hardness.

volvulus (vol'vu-lus)   The twisting of a part upon itself, as in the bowel.

W

walk pattern (wok′ pat″ern)   A duck waddle or late sign of congenital hip dysplasia.

Weil's disease (vīlz dĭ-zēz′)   Leptospiral jaundice.

well differentiated (wel dif″er-en′she-āt-ed)   Not similar.

wheeze (hwēz)   Breathing with a rasp or whistling sound.

wormian bone (wer′me-an bōn)   Sutural bone.

X

xenon (ze′non)   Radioactive element used in nuclear medicine for ventilation lung scans.

Z

Zenker's diverticulum (zeng′kerz di″ver-tik′u-lum)   A type of esophageal diverticulum.

Self-Assessment Quiz Answer Key

Chapter One

1.	a	11.	a	21.	a	31.	c	41.	a	50.	a
2.	c	12.	b	22.	d	32.	b	42.	b	51.	b
3.	b	13.	b	23.	b	33.	d	43.	b	52.	a
4.	b	14.	b	24.	b	34.	a	44.	b	53.	c
5.	c	15.	b	25.	a	35.	a	45.	e	54.	d
6.	d	16.	c	26.	c	36.	a	46.	b	55.	c
7.	b	17.	d	27.	d	37.	a	47.	a	56.	e
8.	a	18.	d	28.	b	38.	a	48.	d	57.	b
9.	d	19.	b	29.	a	39.	b	49.	d	58.	d
10.	b	20.	a	30.	a	40.	a				

Chapter Two

1.	d	8.	a	14.	c	20.	a	26.	b	32.	c
2.	c	9.	b	15.	c	21.	c	27.	a	33.	b
3.	a	10.	a	16.	c	22.	e	28.	d	34.	a
4.	a	11.	a	17.	d	23.	a	29.	e	35.	a
5.	c	12.	b	18.	a	24.	b	30.	a	36.	e
6.	d	13.	d	19.	d	25.	d	31.	b	37.	b
7.	a										

Chapter Three

1.	b	8.	a	15.	b	22.	a	28.	c	34.	c
2.	c	9.	a	16.	a	23.	a	29.	d	35.	b
3.	e	10.	b	17.	b	24.	b	30.	a	36.	a
4.	a	11.	c	18.	b	25.	a	31.	b	37.	a
5.	c	12.	b	19.	c	26.	c	32.	c	38.	c
6.	a	13.	c	20.	a	27.	c	33.	d	39.	a
7.	b	14.	b	21.	c						

Chapter Four

1.	a	5.	d	9.	c	13.	c	17.	e
2.	c	6.	b	10.	c	14.	e	18.	a
3.	c	7.	e	11.	a	15.	b	19.	b
4.	a	8.	c	12.	a	16.	b	20.	d

Chapter Five

1.	c	6.	a	11.	c	16.	d	21.	c
2.	a	7.	a	12.	c	17.	b	22.	d
3.	d	8.	c	13.	a	18.	a	23.	b
4.	b	9.	c	14.	a	19.	c	24.	d
5.	b	10.	a	15.	c	20.	a	25.	c

Chapter Six

1.	c	8.	a	15.	c	22.	b	29.	a	36.	c
2.	a	9.	a	16.	d	23.	d	30.	b	37.	d
3.	c	10.	d	17.	b	24.	a	31.	c	38.	d
4.	b	11.	c	18.	c	25.	c	32.	e	39.	b
5.	d	12.	e	19.	a	26.	e	33.	a	40.	e
6.	c	13.	e	20.	a	27.	b	34.	b	41.	a
7.	c	14.	a	21.	a	28.	c	35.	d	42.	e

Chapter Seven

1.	b	6.	c	11.	c	16.	c	21.	a
2.	a	7.	d	12.	e	17.	a	22.	c
3.	a	8.	a	13.	c	18.	b	23.	d
4.	c	9.	b	14.	e	19.	a	24.	a
5.	c	10.	d	15.	a	20.	a		

Chapter Eight

1.	d	17.	d	32.	a	48.	d	64.	c	80.	a
2.	c	18.	b	33.	a	49.	a	65.	a	81.	b
3.	b	19.	a	34.	c	50.	a	66.	c	82.	c
4.	d	20.	a	35.	a	51.	d	67.	b	83.	e
5.	a	21.	a	36.	a	52.	d	68.	d	84.	d
6.	e	22.	d	37.	a	53.	d	69.	a	85.	a
7.	e	23.	c	38.	d	54.	d	70.	a	86.	b
8.	b	24.	b	39.	c	55.	b	71.	a	87.	e
9.	c	25.	a	40.	c	56.	a	72.	c	88.	a
10.	b	26.	c	41.	a	57.	b	73.	a	89.	c
11.	e	27.	a	42.	a	58.	a	74.	a	90.	c
12.	a	28.	c	43.	e	59.	a	75.	a	91.	d
13.	b	29.	a	44.	d	60.	b	76.	c		
14.	a	30.	b	45.	a	61.	b	77.	b		
15.	d	31.	d	46.	a	62.	a	78.	a		
16.	a			47.	d	63.	c	79.	e		

Bibliography

American Cancer Society: A Cancer Source Book For Nurses. New York, American Cancer Society, 1981.

American Cancer Society: Cancer Facts and Figures—1987. New York, American Cancer Society, 1987.

Anderson, WH, and Scotti, FM: A Synopsis of Pathology. 10th ed. St Louis, CV Mosby, 1980.

April, EW: Anatomy. New York, John Wiley & Sons, 1984.

Armstrong, P, and Wastie, ML: X-ray Diagnosis. Oxford, Blackwell Scientific Publications, 1981.

Ballinger, PW: Merrill's Atlas of Roentgenographic Positions and Radiologic Procedures. 6th ed. St. Louis, CV Mosby, 1986.

Bergleiter, R, Birzle, H, and Kuner, EH: Radiology of Trauma. Philadelphia, WB Saunders, 1978.

Bernstein, H: Outlines of Pathology. St Louis, CV Mosby, 1986.

Bevis, EM, and Bower, LF: Fundamentals of Nursing Practice Concepts, Roles and Functions. St Louis, CV Mosby, 1979.

Boyd, W, and Sheldon, H: Introduction to the Study of Disease. 8th ed. Philadelphia, Lea & Febiger, 1980.

Cawson, RA, Marcus, PB, and McCracken, AW: Pathologic Mechanisms and Human Disease. St Louis, CV Mosby, 1982.

Chabner, DE: The Language of Medicine. 3rd ed. Philadelphia, WB Saunders, 1985.

De Santos, LA: The Radiology of Bone Tumors. New York, American Cancer Society, 1980.

Early, PJ, and Sodee, DB: Textbook of Nuclear Medicine. St Louis, CV Mosby, 1985.

Ellis, FH, Jr: Cancer of the Esophagus. New York, American Cancer Society, 1983.

Etter, L: Glossary of Words and Phrases Used in Radiology, Nuclear Medicine and Ultrasound. 2nd ed. Springfield, Ill, Charles C Thomas, 1970.

Fisher, JK, and Germann, DR: Practical Radiologic Diagnosis. Reston, Va, Reston Publishing, 1981.

Grech, P: Casualty Radiography, A Practical Guide for Radiological Diagnosis. London, Chapman & Hall, 1981.

Griffiths, H: Basic Bone Radiology. New York: Appleton-Century-Crofts, 1981.

Hamilton, HK, and Rose, MB: Professional Guide to Diseases. Springhouse, Pa, Intermed Communications. 1982.

Hart, MN, and Kent, TH: Introduction to Human Disease. 2nd ed. East Norwalk, Conn, Appleton-Century-Crofts, 1986.

Jablonski, S: Illustrated Dictionary of Eponymic Syndromes and Diseases and Their Syndromes. Philadelphia, WB Saunders, 1969.

Jett, JR, Cortese, DA, and Fontana, R: Lung Cancer: Current Concepts and Prospects. New York, American Cancer Society, 1983.

Keane, CB, and Miller, BF: Encyclopedia and Dictionary of Medicine, Nursing, and Allied Health. 3rd ed. Philadelphia, WB Saunders, 1983.

Kee, JL, and Tang, HL: Laboratory Diagnostic Tests with Nursing Implications. East Norwalk, Conn, Appleton-Century-Crofts, 1983.

Kissane, JM (ed.): Anderson's Pathology. 2nd ed. St Louis, CV Mosby, 1985.

Livolsi, VA, Merino, MJ, and Neuman, RD: Pathology. New York, John Wiley & Sons, 1984.

Marlowe, JL: Surgical Radiography. Baltimore, University Park Press, 1983.

Mertens, TR, and Winchester, AM: Human Genetics. 4th ed. Columbus, Ohio, Charles E. Merrill, 1983.

Meschan, I: Radiographic Positioning and Related Anatomy. 2nd ed. Philadelphia, WB Saunders, 1978.

Meschan, I, and Ott, DJ: Introduction to Diagnostic Imaging. Philadelphia, WB Saunders, 1984.

Monk, CJ: Orthopedics for Undergraduates. 2nd ed. New York, Oxford University Press, 1981.

Morrill, C, and Torres, LS: Basic Medical Techniques and Patient Care for Radiologic Technologists. 2nd ed. Philadelphia, JB Lippincott, 1983.

Mowschenson, PM: Aids to Undergraduate Surgery. New York, Churchill Livingstone, 1983.

Mulvihill, ML: Human Diseases. 2nd ed. East Norwalk, Conn, Appleton & Lange, 1987.

National Center for Health Statistics: Annual Summary of Births, Marriages, Divorces, and Deaths, United States for 1985. Monthly Vital Statistics Report, Vol. 34, No. 13. DHHS Pub. No. (PHS) 86-1120. Public Health Service, Hyattsville, Md. September 19, 1986.

National Center for Health Statistics: Births, Marriages, Divorces, and Deaths for 1986. Monthly Vital Statistics Report, Vol. 35, No. 12. DHHS Pub. No. (PHS) 87-1120. Public Health Service, Hyattsville, Md. April 2, 1987.

Newton, TH, and Potts, DG: Radiology of the Skull and Brain. Vols. 1 and 2. The Skull. St. Louis, CV Mosby, 1985.

Pagana, KD, and Pagana, TJ: Diagnostic Testing and Nursing Implications: A Case Study Approach. St Louis, CV Mosby, 1982.

Parker, MD: Introduction to Radiography. Philadelphia, JB Lippincott, 1985.

Pearce, DJ: Understanding Chest Radiographs. St Louis, CV Mosby, 1984.

Purtillo, D: A Survey of Human Diseases. Menlo Park, Calif, Addison-Wesley, 1978.

Rosai, J: The Pathology of Tumors. 2nd ed. New York, American Cancer Society, 1979.

Rubin, P (ed.): Cancer of the Gastrointestinal Tract. 2nd ed. New York, American Cancer Society, 1974.

Rubin, P (ed.): Clinical Oncology. 6th ed. New York, American Cancer Society, 1983.

Snopek, A: Fundamentals of Radiographic Special Procedures. 2nd ed. Philadelphia, WB Saunders, 1985.

Sutton, D: Radiology and Imaging for Medical Students. 4th ed. Edinburgh, Churchill Livingstone, 1982.

Taussig, MJ: Processes in Pathology. Oxford, Blackwell Scientific Publications, 1979.

Index

Note: Page numbers in *italics* indicate illustrations; those followed by t indicate tables.